Emotions as Regulation between the Self and the Universe

Dr. Jean Marc Eyssalet
with collaboration
Tania Agursky
Sarah Meron

To our friends Deena, Ruthi and Ilana who have left us

Special thanks to:
Vered Vexler-Moran for the graphics design
Zhou Jinghong for the cover calligraphy
Irena Kleyman for the illustrations

Introduction

Basic assumptions and paradigms of ancient Chinese thought differ from those found in Western philosophy. To understand the Chinese way of thinking we need to avoid patterns familiar from Western philosophy.

The basic assumption of ancient Chinese thought is that the reality of the self and the world as perceived by man is not fixed, but changes continuously and endlessly.[1]

The process of constant change in the Universe, independent of any causal or circumstantial influence, is described by the laws of YIN-YANG 陰陽 (represented by the TAI JI 太極 symbol) and the laws of Five Modalities (movements, phases, elements, WU XING 五行), established during the ZHOU dynasty (1121-256 BC). This way of thought was systematized by ZOU YAN 鄒衍 (305 – 240 BC) during the Warring States period, by DONG ZHONG SHU 董仲舒 (179-104 BC) and by other scholars during the HAN (206 BC to 220 AD) and SUI (581-618) dynasties.

Chinese thought is rooted in the written language, which is based not on sounds but on visual representation. Traditional Chinese characters (ideograms, sinograms, HAN ZI 漢字) have multiple meanings, one source of complication for translation; another is the combination of characters in Chinese texts. The different ways in which a Chinese character, or combination of characters, may be translated are complementary, not contradictory. In addition, the Chinese language has changed since the time of the writing and organizing of medical thought in the classical medical text, NEI JING 內經.

According to the ancient Chinese, the Universe is based on the Trinity of Powers: Heaven, Earth and Man. Heaven represents oneness,

---

1 sub-mutational according to L. Vandermeersch

unity, impersonal consciousness, without 'substantial forms'[2] or shapes. Heaven rules Earth, which represents multiple separate and changing 'substantial forms' (matter, substances and shapes). The flow of constantly changing communication between Heaven and Earth is called energy (QI 氣). The Chinese approach does not see Man as the centre of the Universe, but as an integral part of the Universe, connecting Heaven and Earth. QI 氣 of Heaven flows through Man.

All movements (changes, QI 氣) in Heaven, Earth and Man can be described according to the laws of YIN-YANG 陰陽 and the laws of Five Modalities/Elements (WU XING 五行).

Man, through his Heart-Consciousness (XIN 心), is a witness during his lifetime to everything that happens and changes in the Universe in time and space. Heart-Consciousness (XIN 心) is the great mystery of life from the moment of conception until the moment of death. ZHUANG ZI, Chapter 4, calls Man's Heart 'Authentic (original, true) Heart (CHANG XIN 帝心)'. LU ZI, in *The Secret of the Golden Flower*, calls it the *Heavenly Heart* (TIAN XIN 天心) and writes:

...but the conscious spirit dwells below in the heart. This lower fleshly heart has the shape of a large peach: it is covered by the wings of the lungs, supported by the liver, and served by the bowels. This heart is dependent on the outside world. If a man does not eat for one day even, it feels extremely uncomfortable. If it hears something terrifying it throbs; if it hears something enraging it stops; if it is faced with death it becomes sad; if it sees something beautiful it is dazzled.[3]

Heart-Consciousness (XIN 心) is linked to Individual Spirit (SHEN 神), which represents Heaven in Man and embraces his Earth aspect - body ('substantial forms'). SHEN 神 is a 'subtle process (JI 機)' organizing

---

2 A theory of **substantial forms** asserts that forms (or ideas) organize matter and make it intelligible. Substantial forms are the source of properties, order, unity, identity, and information about objects. The idea of substantial forms dominates ancient Greek philosophy and medieval philosophy. See Wikipedia

3 R. Wilhelm; Translated from German by C. F. Baynes

the flow of QI 氣, which directs the formation and maintenance of the body. SHEN 神 can be seen as the composer, conductor and orchestra of the unique oeuvre of Man. Each person is a unique piece of music, with a unique perspective on the world. SHEN 神 is the source of man's spontaneous creativity, which enables spiritual transformation. SHEN 神 and Heart (XIN 心) express the continuity of the unique Consciousness of a person, from conception to death. However, throughout our lives SHEN 神 is also awareness of the moment.

SHEN 神 embraces the other four BEN SHEN 本神 (Roots of SHEN): HUN 魂, YI 意, PO 魄 and ZHI 志. Each BEN SHEN 本神 leads a stage in the development of the individual, from the moment of conception till death.

The human body results from a proper functioning of the five ZANG 臟 (organs-functions): Heart, Liver, Spleen, Lung and Kidney. Each ZANG 臟 is connected with one of the five BEN SHEN 本神. SHEN 神 is connected with Heart; HUN 魂 with Liver, YI 意 with Spleen, PO 魄 with Lung and ZHI 志 with Kidney.

Emotions and their central role in life in ancient Chinese thought
This book presents differing but complementary views on the nature of emotions/passions.

Emotions are born from innumerable changing interactions:
- between Heart-Consciousness and destiny (heredity),
- between QI 氣 and 'substantial forms' (body),
- between BEN SHEN 本神 and 'substantial forms' - the body created by the five ZANG 臟 and connected with the mother's body and PO 魄,
- between the masculine and feminine aspects of a person,
- between a man and a woman,
- between personal history, family history and interaction with society (cultural influences, virtues and moral values),
- between man and his environment (climate, weather, air), lifestyle, food and beverages.

Each ZANG 臟 is related to its own emotion, but at the same time all emotions are related to Heart (XIN 心). Emotions are expressed through their impact on Heart and through 'Center of Chest' (TAN ZHONG 膻中), which is responsible for the creation, storage and distribution of QI 氣, Blood and body liquids. Intense or long-lasting emotions interfere with body functions and provoke disease.

A similar point of view is expressed by neurobiologist A. Damasio:
I see the essence of emotion as the collection of changes in body state that are induced in myriad organs by nerve cell terminals, under the control of a dedicated brain system, which is responding to the content of thoughts relative to a particular entity or event.[4]

According to ancient Chinese thought, normal human life is based on the five emotions:
1. Anger (NU 怒)
2. Joy (XI 喜)
3. Sorrow (BEI 悲)
4. Fear (KONG 恐)
5. Thought (SI 思)

The description of the influence of emotions in this book is based on the following chapters of NEI JING 內經, attributed to the legendary Yellow Emperor:
- NEI JING LING SHU, Chapter 8, *Roots of Spirit* (BEN SHEN 本神) (describing the basic aspects of Man's life and also the harmful effects of emotions)
- NEI JING SU WEN, Chapter 39, *Discourse on Origin of Pain* (describing the harmful effects of emotions)
- NEI JING LING SHU, Chapter 22, *Quiet and Agitated Mental Disorders* (DIAN KUANG BING 癲狂病) (describing extreme emotional states)

LING SHU, Chapter 8 (BEN SHEN 本神), opens with the statement addressed by the Yellow Emperor to his teacher QI BO: *The first law*

---

[4] Damasio, A. R. *Descartes' Error: Emotion, Reason, and the Human Brain*, p. 139

in the art of acupuncture is the necessity of rooting in SHEN (BEN YU SHEN 本于神). It is this that is the key to treatment in Chinese medicine: communication Heart to Heart, SHEN 神 to SHEN 神, between therapist and patient on both conscious and subconscious levels. This chapter of LING SHU describes the development of body and mind, and questions whether life is a person's individual responsibility or is part of his destiny (decreed by Heaven). The text refers to the body, but the emphasis is on existence, personal growth and development, wisdom.

It also explains 13 entities of Chinese thought:
1. DE 德, virtue, the mandate of life
2. QI 氣, energy, all types of movement and change
3. SHENG 生, life
4. JING 精, fundamental vitality
5. SHEN 神, Individual Spirit, Consciousness
6. HUN 魂, Wood Modality aspect of SHEN, related to father and birth
7. PO 魄, Metal Modality aspect of SHEN, related to mother, body and fetal life
8. XIN 心, Heart-Consciousness
9. YI 意, Soil Modality aspect of SHEN, intent, ideas
10. ZHI 志, Water Modality aspect of SHEN, will, determination
11. SI 思, thought, thinking process
12. LU 慮, contemplation
13. ZHI 智, intelligence, wisdom

LING SHU, Chapter 8, continues with a description of damage caused by intense or long-lasting emotions to BEN SHEN 本神, to body functions and to man's behavior. The emotions described in LING SHU, Chapter 8 are:
1. Apprehension, distress, obsessive thinking, worry (CHU TI SI LU 怵惕思慮), which cause fear and dread (KONG JU 惶恐)
2. Sorrow and grief (BEI AI 悲哀)
3. Joy and pleasure (XI LE 喜樂)
4. Melancholy and sadness (CHOU YOU 愁憂)
5. Overflowing anger (SHENG NU 盛怒)
6. Fear and dread (KONG JU 惶恐)

SU WEN, Chapter 39, explores the immediate pathologic effects on body functions of the six emotions/passions and of the three energies of external origin:
1. Anger (NU 怒)
2. Joy (XI 喜)
3. Sorrow (BEI 悲)
4. Fear (KONG 恐)
5. Cold (HAN 寒)
6. Heat (JIONG 炅)
7. Panic (JING 驚)
8. Exhaustion (LAO 勞)
9. Thought / excessive thinking (SI 思)

LING SHU, Chapter 22, presents a dense, complex description of mental disorders: DIAN 癲 - quiet mental disorders (depression) and KUANG 狂 - agitated mental disorders (mania).

Treatment of emotional imbalance in Chinese Medicine
According to Chinese medicine, methods of treatment for acute or chronic emotional disorders are: acupuncture, moxibustion, herbal medicine, food therapy, attentive body movements (DAO YIN 導引, QI GONG 氣功, TAI JI QUAN 太極拳) and attentive breath exercises.

Treatments described in this book for problems stemming from emotions are based on selecting acupuncture points according to:
- the traditional function of acupuncture points, especially of the five 'antique' points (WU SHU 五輸) and LUO 絡, YUAN 元, MU 募, SHU 俞, XI 郄, and the regulation of Connecting Channels (LUO 絡) and Divergent (BIE 別) Channels
- influence specific to a symptom or sign, even if there is no clear explanation of the influence
- regulation of the flow in Six Layers (LIU JING 六經)
- regulation of Eight Extraordinary Meridians
- recommendations for treating syndromes (ZHENG 證) according to traditional Chinese medicine

It is possible to describe the pathologic changes in body functions caused by emotional imbalance as a syndrome (ZHENG 證) of traditional Chinese medicine, and treat points prescribed for this syndrome. Sometimes a state of emotional imbalance may be described by several syndromes - for example, depression may be described as *Constrained QI Syndrome* (YU ZHENG 鬱證) or as *Liver QI Congested and Knotted* (GAN QI YU JIE 肝氣鬱結) or as *Heart and Spleen Dual Deficiency* (XIN PI LIANG XU 心脾兩虛).

The concept of syndrome (ZHENG 證) appeared relatively late in the history of Chinese medicine, during the MING Dynasty and the beginning of the QIN Dynasty (17th century). During this period many schools of Chinese medicine therapy existed and there was a need for standardization. Symptoms and signs were classified as syndromes (ZHENG 證) in order to describe a disorder and adopt herbal treatments and acupuncture points for each syndrome. At this time, under the influence of *Compendium of Materia Medica* BEN CAO GANG MU by LI SHI ZHEN, herbal treatments were considered to be of great importance. The questioning of a patient for the purpose of determining the syndrome was aimed at 'matter' (organ function, Blood, body liquids, heat, cold), while subtle aspects of the personality were left aside.

Although traditional Chinese medicine syndromes have their limits in the overall observation of a patient, they have their place in contributing to the treatment of emotional imbalance.[5]

---

5   Flows B. and Lake J., *Chinese Medical Psychiatry* Sionneau P. *Troubles Psychiques en Medicine Chinoise*

1

Five Modalities (WU XING 五行) on the Three Levels of the Universe (Heaven, Earth and Man)

The Universe is based on the Trinity of Powers (SAN CAI 三才): Heaven, Earth and Man (TIAN DI REN 天地人).[1] Man is standing with his hands spread up to Heaven and his feet planted on the ground, representing the link between Heaven and Earth. Man is not the center of the Universe. Man's existence is due to the dynamic crossroads of opposing and complementary influences:
- the subtle influences of QI 氣 flow, and
- the coarse influences of 'substantial forms' (XING 形).

Man is the witness to, and the result of, all these influences.

The flow of QI 氣 and the changes in 'substantial forms' in the Universe (Heaven, Earth and Man) may be interpreted by the laws of:
- YIN-YANG 陰陽,
- WU XING 五行, Five Modalities (Wood, Fire, Soil,[2] Metal, Water),
- LIU JING 六經, Six Layers of QI flow,
- BA GUA 八卦, Eight Trigrams[3].

YIN-YANG 陰陽, which do not exist in reality, are represented by the symbol called Supreme Ultimate, Great Summit (TAI JI 太極). The TAI JI 太極 symbol describes the Unity; in it, the color of YIN is black and the color of YANG is red. Traditionally the TAI JI symbol is displayed in the vertical direction (Figure 1): red color – YANG 陽, on the left; black color – YIN 陰, on the right (the observer being in the middle).

To understand YIN-YANG 陰陽, imagine a Chinese painter who paints the TAI JI symbol, symbol of the Universe. Before representing the symbol, the painter meditates. Then he chooses a plank of wood and two colors: black and red. First, the artist draws a circle and fills it

---

1 Legge J.
2 In Five Modalities TU 土 is translated as Soil (not as Earth) to avoid confusion with the Trinity of Powers Heaven-Man-Earth 地
3 YI JING, the Book of Changes, includes 64 hexagrams composed of 8 trigrams

with black color, (which will become the color specific to YIN 陰) symbolizing basis, emptiness, void, darkness. Then he takes the red color and paints the red dot at the bottom of the circle (Winter Solstice, midnight) which marks the beginning of all cycles (change of direction, beginning of growth and increased light):
- The beginning of the specified movement,
- Midnight on the Chinese clock,
- Winter Solstice, the shortest day in the calendar according to the sun,
- North in ancient Chinese maps.) In ancient Chinese maps, South was shown at the top, North at the bottom).

Figure 1. On the TAI JI 太極 **symbol space and time are described by** YIN-YANG 陰陽

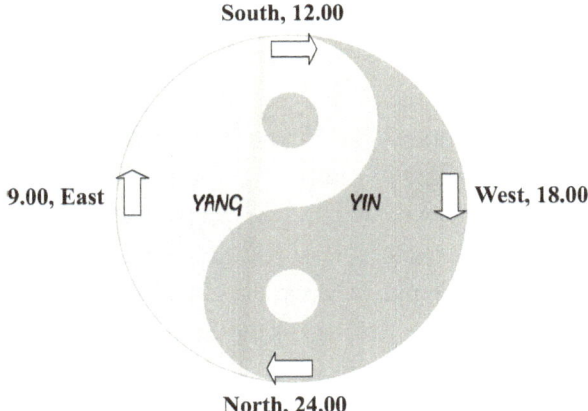

The artist continues to paint red color (the color of YANG 陽) over black on the left side of the circle, in the shape of a tadpole - tail down and head up. This makes two tadpoles: red tadpole head up, and black tadpole head down. The artist leaves the 'black eye' in the center of the head of the red tadpole, and draws the 'red eye' in the center of the head of the black tadpole.

YIN-YANG 陰陽 are the dynamic condition of the expression of the perception of objects and movement in time and space. Time and space interlock in the TAI JI symbol: at the bottom - midnight and North, at the top - noon and South. The process of painting, first all black, then red for YANG, emphasizes that YIN 陰 and YANG 陽 are not equal: YIN 陰, the black background below YANG 陽, allows and supports the manifestation of YANG.

The 'red eye' in the center of YIN symbolizes the birth of YANG out of YIN. The 'black eye' in YANG shows that YIN appears when YANG declines.

A. Man, through his Heart-Consciousness (XIN 心) and Spirit (SHEN 神), is the witness to all that happens in the Universe

In Chinese thought the mind and body are not opposed. There is no existence of any part of a person, including his feelings and emotions, separate from his body. All the subtle influences that determine the individual, including feelings, emotions and desires, are recorded in his body.

Man is the witness, through his Heart-Consciousness (XIN 心) to all the functions and changes of 'substantial forms' (body structures and patterns of consciousness) which take place between Heaven and Earth. Heart-Consciousness (XIN 心) is the uninterrupted meeting of all the influences that connect Man to the Universe in time and space, from conception to death. Heart-Consciousness is also the crossroad between the inborn and the acquired.

Body structure and function are based on organized movement which, like sound, rhythm and harmony in a musical work, determines the dynamic balance of a person living in a body connected to the environment. Therefore all expressions of QI 氣 (for example, cold and heat, sweet and salty flavors, fear and joy) are movements that speed up or slow down the associated body functions.

In Man, Heart (XIN 心) is closely linked with Individual Spirit (SHEN 神) and the two are often used as synonyms in Chinese texts. Heart (XIN 心) usually refers to Consciousness, while SHEN 神 represents a centered observer of oneself and of the Universe.

LING SHU, Chapter 8, which describes the Chinese perception of body and mind, begins: *The first law in the art of acupuncture is the necessity of rooting in SHEN (BEN YU SHEN 本于神).*[4]

Figure 2. The character SHEN 神 'Individual Spirit' in ancient seal and classical script

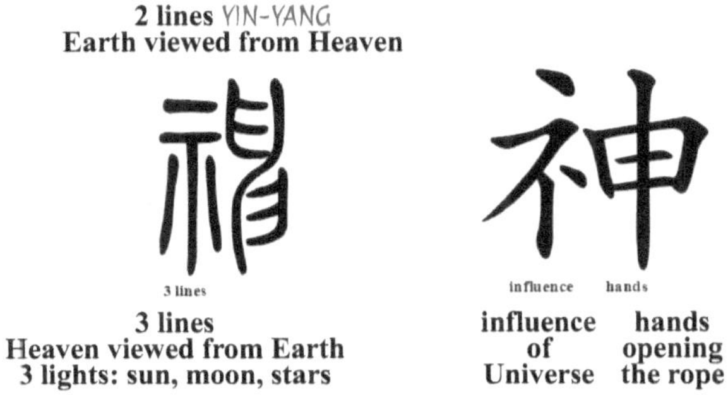

2 lines YIN-YANG
Earth viewed from Heaven

3 lines
Heaven viewed from Earth
3 lights: sun, moon, stars

influence
of
Universe

hands
opening
the rope

SHEN 神 is the expression and identification of needs and desires, directing the mechanisms which organize personality, morality and self-identity. The character SHEN 神 (Figure 2) shows the radical 礻/示 'the celestial influence in the Universe';[5] the two top lines 二 are a symbol of YIN-YANG, the three lines below 小 represent the three celestial luminaries: sun, moon and stars-planets. The phonetic 申 shows hands opening a tied rope - a symbol of expansion, extension, communication between Man and the Universe. SHEN 神 is translated as Spirit of Life, Personal or Individual Spirit, mind, Consciousness, and sometimes Holy Spirit or gods. However, the meaning of the character SHEN 神 is not fully compatible with any of these terms. SHEN 神 is not something to be believed in or worshiped.

The notion of SHEN includes various aspects:
- The origin of SHEN 神 is in the meeting between Source QI (YUAN QI 原氣/元氣) which transfers the mother's Source JING 精 (egg cell) and Source QI which transfers the father's Source JING 精

---

4 See page 89
5 Wieger, Lesson 3

(sperm). SHEN 神 is active continuously during the entire life of an individual, from conception to death.

- SHEN 神 is the spiritual - the most subtle aspect of Consciousness, but also the designer of everything that characterizes the human body. Therefore SHEN 神 embraces both material and non-material aspects of life: JING 精, QI 氣, mind and 'substantial forms' (Blood, body liquids, physical body structure).
- SHEN 神 is the Individual Spirit that unites all levels of Consciousness and may be considered the axis of Consciousness, self-image and the image of the world that each person develops.
- SHEN 神 is the individual organized Consciousness of the Universe receiving stimuli from Heaven and Earth at every moment. SHEN 神 is the creative power of Man, in whom Heaven and Earth are linked, the axis at the intersection between the personal and the universal. At every moment we encounter the Universe (through our body and through the filters of personal (emotional) and family history, cultural background, people we meet, traumas, age. SHEN 神 at every moment expresses a dialogue between the Universe (denoted by the red color at South on the TAI JI symbol) and the unique (the 'black eye' in the middle of the red tadpole on the TAI JI symbol). SHEN 神 is a meeting of heredity (individual genes) and the environment (air and food) (Figure 3).

Figure 3. SHEN 神 **is a meeting between heredity (individual genes) and environment (air and food)**

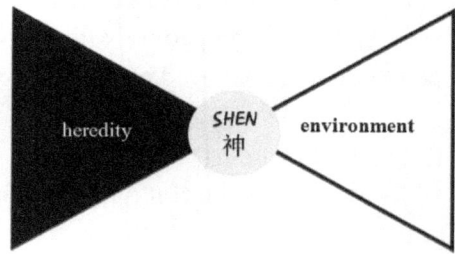

- SHEN 神 through Heart-Consciousness (XIN 心) is a meeting place between the instant Consciousness of 'the moment - now', and the continuous Consciousness of time and 'substantial forms' in space:

Figure 4. The vertical plane: Heaven and Earth link through SHEN 神/Heart (XIN 心) providing an awareness of the moment

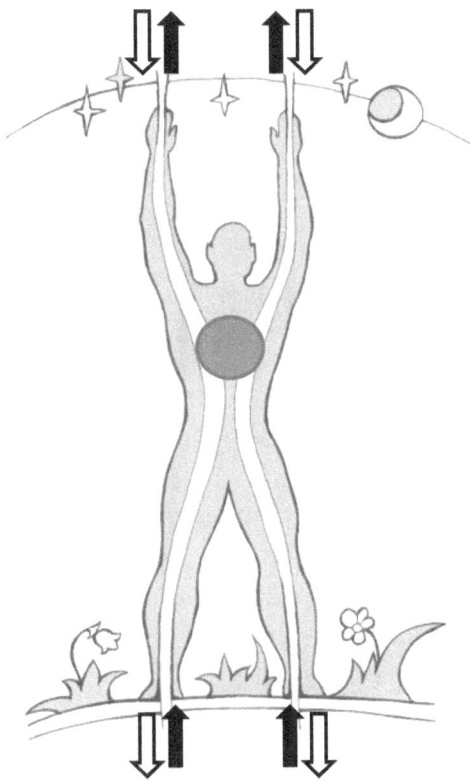

- Consciousness of here and now (the vertical plane: Heaven-Man-Earth) links Heaven and Earth and represents the awareness of the moment. The interaction between Heaven and Earth passes through Heart of Man in both directions, opening to listening to the moment (Figure 4). This Consciousness is influenced by heredity (genome).
- The continuity of Consciousness (the horizontal cyclical plane), is constant awareness of changes taking place in the person and in 'substantial forms' around him during interactions in space and time (expressed by four seasons and four regions) (Figure 5). Therefore, Consciousness on the horizontal plane is continuously affected by the environment.

Figure 5. The horizontal plane: time and space (represented on the TAI JI symbol by four seasons and four regions)

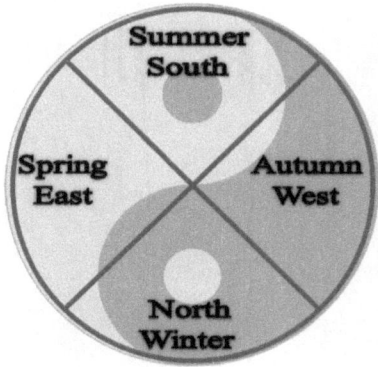

B. Five Modalities (WU XING 五行) as the music of the Universe

Five Modalities (movements, phases, elements) (WU XING 五行) (Wood, Fire, Soil, Metal and Water) symbolize the five types of QI 氣 movement in the Universe (Heaven-Man-Earth) – the five vibrations (a metaphor for pentatonic music) that change rhythm of the Universe (Figure 6).

Figure 6. Five Modalities represented on the TAI JI symbol. In the figure to the left, Soil is located on the periphery between Fire and Metal, in the figure to the right Soil at the center of the circle

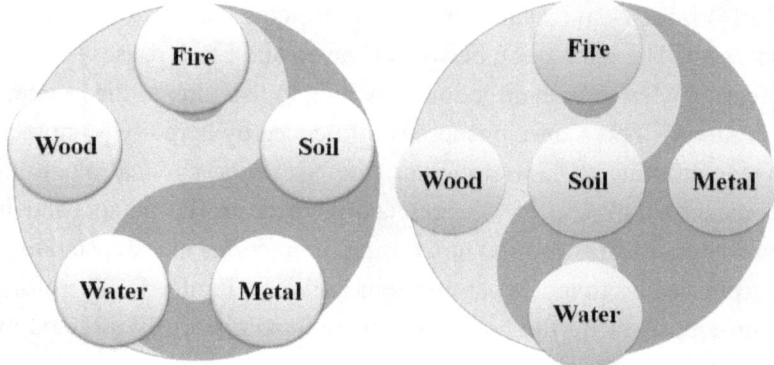

Five Modalities as expressed on Three Levels - Heaven, Earth and Man are:
- At the non-material level of Heaven, Five Modalities denote the five planets, the five QI 氣 which influence Earth (wind, heat, dampness, dryness and cold) and seasons.
- At the level of Earth, representing density and 'substantial forms', Five Modalities denote the five regions of space, five colors, five sounds, five tastes and five odors. Earth produces vegetables, seeds, animals and fruits according to the five types of QI.
- At the level of Man, Five Modalities are five aspects of SHEN 神, five ZANG 臟 (Liver, Heart, Spleen, Lung, Kidney) which form the organs of transit (FU 腑: Gallbladder, Small intestine, Stomach, Large intestine, Bladder), five body tissues, five types of body liquids, five senses and sense organs and their orifices, and five emotions. Each Modality is perceived by color and form, sound, taste, touch and smell through the five sense organs of Man. Each Modality dominates a specific period in life.

Wood Modality (MU 木)

Wood Modality symbolizes the ascending movement of Earth to Heaven, the growth of YANG, the passage from the density of matter-'substantial forms' to the non-material, from stability to movement. Trees and plants denote Wood Modality. Wood Modality is characterized by instability, upward movement exteriorization and change. Wood Modality symbolizes the rising of clouds and the flowing of blood upwards to the head in man.

Wood at the level of Heaven
Wind (FENG 風) (SU WEN, Chapter 5) - is the heavenly QI that creates Wood Modality. The planet Jupiter denotes Wood Modality.
Season: spring, the onset of outward QI movement, procreation.

Wood at the level of Earth
Direction of QI movement: eruption in all directions, especially outward and upward along the vertical axis.

Manifestation: 1. changing direction; 2. branching; 3. creation, reproduction and development; 4. centrifugal spiral.
Nature: warm
Messages transmitted through the five senses:
Color: green-blue, turquoise - colors of life (vegetation, water, sky)
Sound: JUE 角 - sound close to Mi in solfège
Smell: fermentation, sour (yeast dough, fermentation of fruit)
Taste: sour
Touch: rigid, like a tree
Climate: windy
Region / direction: East

Wood at the level of Man
Liver (GAN 肝) represents Wood Modality in the human body.
Periods of Wood domination in life are: birth, childhood, adolescence, and other periods of crisis and change. The exteriorization of Wood is expressed in a drive to communicate with the environment through language, empathy, humanity, and when unbalanced is expressed in anger and antagonism.

Fire Modality (HUO 火)
Fire Modality symbolizes the sublime YANG development and the beginning of YIN. Fire Modality is a symbol of light, brightness, and the Spirit of man.

Fire at the level of Heaven
Heat is the heavenly QI that creates Fire Modality (SU WEN, Chapter 5). Fire Modality is characterized by light, sun, heat and radiance. The planet Mars represents Fire Modality.
Season: summer, symbolizing the flow of QI on the surface, growth and radiance.

Fire at the level of Earth
Direction of QI movement: balanced flow on the surface, internal-external communications.

Manifestation: 1. fire, flame; 2. light and light sources in the sky (lightning, stars, moon, sun); 3. star-shaped flowers (chrysanthemum); 4. dry leaves presenting a web of fibers (plant communications network); 5. all ways of communication;
Nature: hot
Messages transmitted through the five senses:
Color: red
Sound: ZHI 徵 – close to Sol in solfège
Smell: burnt
Taste: bitter
Touch: fiber, fabrics made of coarse fibers such as cotton or jute cloth
Climate: hot
Region / direction: South

Fire at the level of Man
Heart (XIN 心) represents Fire and is regarded as the Emperor of the body. The light of Consciousness, 'blooming', maturity and flexibility of Fire Modality are the basis for all kinds of intra-body and internal-external communications (feelings, emotions, thermoregulation, circulation, blood flow, love, speech) and joy.

Metal Modality (JIN 金)

Metal Modality symbolizes descent from Heaven to Earth, the passage from the non-material to the density of 'substantial forms', from movement to stability. Metal Modality represents rain falling from Heaven to Earth.

Metal at the level of Heaven
Dryness is the heavenly QI that creates Metal Modality (SU WEN, Chapter 5). Metal Modality is characterized by cooling, purification, separation, dissolution, destruction. The planet Venus represents Metal Modality.
Season: autumn, which symbolizes QI of purification, judgment and harvest.

Metal at the level of Earth
Direction of QI movement: inward – gathering inside, covering, protecting from the outside, downward movement.
Manifestation: 1. areas of tension and borders, cell membranes, skin, bark, soap bubbles; 2. crystals; 3. cracks in non-elastic material.
Nature: cool
Messages transmitted through the five senses:
Color: white
Sound: SHANG 商 - close to Re in solfege
Smell: metallic (blood, onions, garlic)
Taste: pungent
Touch: crisp
Climate: dry
Region / direction: West

Metal at the level of Man
Lung (FEI 肺) represents Metal and bodily borders (the skin surface and alveoli). Metal dominates fetal life and pregnancy. The interiorization, separation, boundaries and purification characteristic of Metal are expressed in life by judgment and justice or, when unbalanced, by sadness and depression.

Water Modality (SHUI 水)

Water Modality symbolizes YIN dominance, exhaustion of YANG, but also YANG emergence inside YIN and growth of YANG. Water also symbolizes 'sources', support and root of life.

Water at the level of Heaven
Cold is heavenly QI that creates Water Modality (SU WEN, Chapter 5). Water Modality is characterized by liquidity, flow (overcoming obstacles) and also by hardening, distribution and storage. The planet Mercury represents Water Modality.
Season: winter, symbolizing storage and retreat.

Water at the level of Earth

Direction of QI movement: slowing down and stopping, retreat (rest) and storage, the source of all directions. Water cannot be eliminated - it moves from place to place, changing to vapor or ice, or being absorbed into the soil.

Manifestation: 1. water flow; 2. movement of the snake; 3. hollow rigid structures like bones or bamboo; 4. transfer of heredity; 5. freezing, hibernation.

Nature: cold

Messages transmitted through the five senses:

Color: black (color of standing water) and all dark colors

Sound: YU 羽 - close to La in solfège

Smell: rot (fungi, mold cheeses - Camembert), salty (seawater)

Taste: salty

Touch: liquid

Climate: cold

Region / direction: North

Water at the level of Man

Kidney (SHEN 腎) represents Water in the human body: storage, transfer of heredity, toughness (bones) and flow of fluids, and is expressed through the will to live, determination, intelligence, wisdom or, when unbalanced, through fear.

Soil Modality (TU 土)

Soil Modality represents the steady center, from which the changes of YIN-YANG are observed, and traces and influences are recorded and stored.

Soil at the level of Heaven

Humidity is heavenly QI that creates Soil Modality (SU WEN, Chapter 5). Soil Modality is characterized by filling forms and margins, consolidation, stability, relaxation and balance. The planet Saturn represents Soil Modality.

Season: The year has four seasons, but there are Five Modalities. The Soil Modality season is the transition between summer and autumn known as 'Indian Summer', which smoothes the transition from YANG - summer to YIN – autumn. The last 18 days of each season (corresponding to the end of January, the end of May, the end of July and the end of October), which assist the transition from season to season, also represent QI of Soil.

Soil at the level of Earth
Direction of QI movement: stabilizing opposing forces
Manifestation: 1. increase of volume (fat tissue); 2. casting forms (clay pots); 3. filling cracks and spaces; 4. slowing down, release; 5. centripetal spiral movement;
Nature: balanced, neutral
Messages transmitted through the five senses:
Color: yellow-brown (soil range from off-white to near-black)
Sound: GONG 宫 - close to Fa in solfège
Smell: perfume (all pleasant scents, for example, the smell of a rose)
Taste: sweet
Touch: full and flexible
Climate: humid
Region: Center

Soil at the level of Man
Spleen (and pancreas) (PI 脾), Soil Modality, located in the center of the body, balances and stabilizes the body. The stability of Soil is expressed in loyalty, sincerity, thinking and, when unbalanced, by obsessive thinking and worry.

Laws of change of Five Modalities (WU XING 五行)

Chinese thought links all phenomena in nature. This perception was expressed first by the laws of YIN-YANG. Interconnections between the Five Modalities are based on two natural laws, expressing the balance:
• Law of Generation (nurture, creation) - SHENG 生
• Law of Control (repression, overcoming) - KE 赳

To express these laws graphically, Soil Modality is moved from the center of the TAI JI symbol to the circumference between Fire and Metal (Figure 6) and thus it eases the transition between YANG (Fire) retreating and YIN (Metal). Chinese thought uses the laws of change of Five Modalities to explain natural phenomena, and Chinese medicine uses these laws to describe imbalance in a person and to establish treatment.

Law of Generation (SHENG 生) **of Five Modalities**
The Law of Generation SHENG is also known as the Law of Mother and Son, which means that every Modality generates and nourishes the next Modality in a clockwise direction (Figure 7).

Figure 7. Law of Generation (SHENG 生) **of Five Modalities**
Wood generates Fire; Fire generates Soil; Soil generates Metal; Metal generates Water; Water generates Wood.

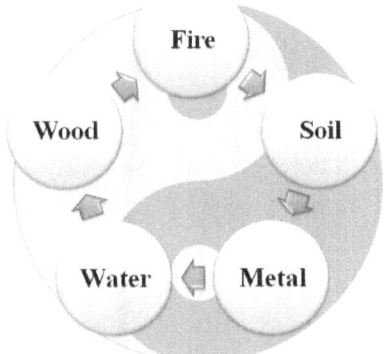

Law of Control (KE 克) **of Five Modalities**
The law of Control KE of Five Modalities, which describes the impact of each Modality on the second Modality in a clockwise direction, is also known as the Law of 'grandfather-grandson' (the first Modality in a clockwise direction is the son, therefore the second is the grandson) (Figure 8).

Figure 8. Law of Control (KE 尅) **of Five Modalities**
Wood controls Soil; Fire controls Metal; Soil controls Water; Metal controls Wood; Water controls Fire.

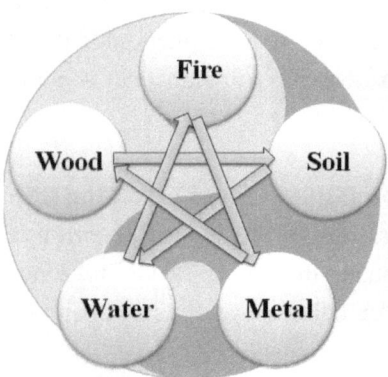

Each of the Five Modalities affects the other four Modalities, according to two natural laws (generation and control). Each Modality has four different connections that create the range of mutual influences, allowing balance. For example, in the case of Wood Modality (Figure 9): Wood is generated by Water; Wood generates Fire; Wood Controls Soil; Wood is controlled by Metal.

Figure 9. Relationship between Wood Modality and other Modalities
Wood is generated by Water; Wood generates Fire; Wood Controls Soil; Wood is controlled by Metal.

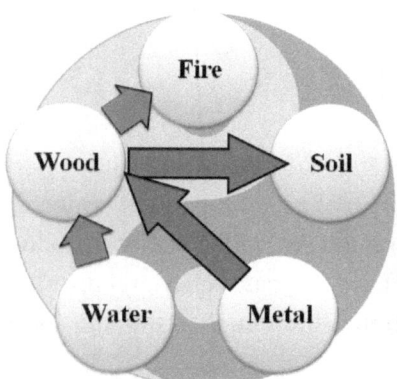

Harmful Relationships between Five Modalities: Reversed Generation and Reversed Control Laws

Harmful relationships between Five Modalities are those opposing the natural flow of QI between Heaven and Earth. When something is terribly wrong there is a danger of a rebellion against stable family tradition. In Reverse Generation (Abuse) (CHENG 乘) the son harms, abuses his mother, and in Reverse Control (Insult) (WU 侮) the grandson insults his grandfather.

The Reversed Law of Generation of Five Modalities - Abusive Relationship (CHENG 乘)

According to the Reversed Law of Generation of Five Modalities, each Modality harms the previous Modality in a counterclockwise direction (Figure 10).

Figure 10. Abusive relationship, reversed generation (CHENG 乘) **of Five Modalities**

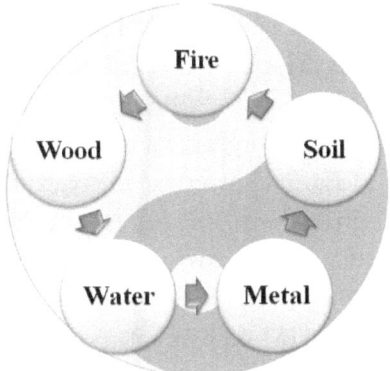

Reversed Law of Control of Five Modalities – 'Insult' relationship (WU 侮)

According to the Reversed Law of Control–Insult (WU 侮) of Five Modalities, each Modality insults the second Modality counterclockwise; the grandson insults his grandfather (Figure 11).

Figure 11. Insult relationship, reversed control (WU 侮) **of Five Modalities**

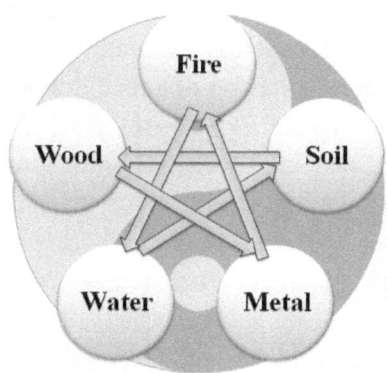

C. Man on Three Levels (Heaven, Earth and Man) expressed by Five Modalities (WU XING 五行)

The Universe is based on the Trinity of Powers (SAN CAI 三才): Heaven, Earth and Man. Man himself is expressed on these Three Levels: Heaven, Earth and Man (Figure 12).

- Man is expressed on the subtle level of Heaven (Upper Level) as five aspects/Roots of SHEN 神 (BEN SHEN 本神): SHEN 神, HUN 魂, YI 意, PO 魄, ZHI 志; these organize a man's life (body and mind).
- Man at the level of Earth (Lower Level) is expressed by means of the 'substantial forms' - five ZANG 臟 (Heart, Liver, Spleen, Lung and Kidney), which build body tissues with the help of QI 氣, Blood, the five flavors and body liquids
- Man at the level of Man (Middle Level) links the subtle influence of Heaven with 'substantial forms' of Earth through the expression of the five emotions/passions/desires.

Emotions result from the communication between BEN SHEN 本神 and ZANG 臟. Repetitive, long-lasting or excessive emotions/desires result from an imbalance between BEN SHEN 本神 and ZANG 臟. For example, repetitive anger is indicative of an imbalance between HUN 魂 and Liver. Pathologies caused by emotions can be treated by acupuncture according to syndromes as described in Chinese medicine.

Figure 12. Man on Three Levels (Heaven-Man-Earth) expressed by Five Modalities. Emotions communicate between (BEN SHEN 本神) **and** ZANG 臟

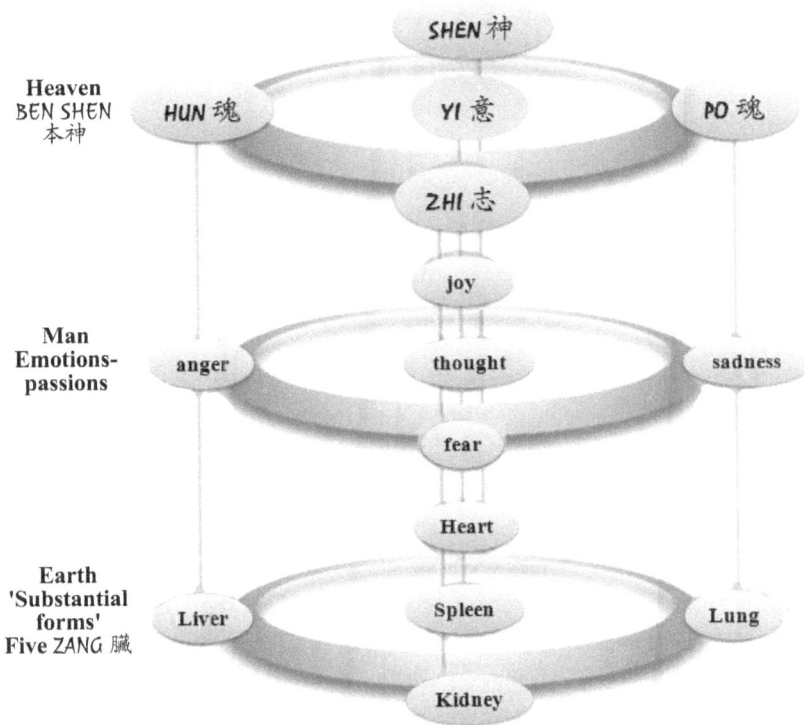

Five Modalities express Three Levels of Man (Heaven, Man, Earth)
Upper Level (Heaven): five aspects of SHEN
(BEN SHEN 本神)

The character BEN 本 is a radical translated as 'root, origin, source, basis'.[6] Each BEN SHEN 本神 is attributed to one of the Five Modalities, and is related to a ZANG 臟. SHEN 神 is connected to Heart-Fire-South. HUN 魂 dwells in Liver-Wood-East, YI 意 in Spleen-Soil-Center, PO 魄 in Lung-Metal-West, ZHI 志 in Kidney-Water-North (Figure 13).

---

6 Wieger, Lesson 1; http://zhongwen.com/d/165/x187.htm

Figure 13. BEN SHEN 本神 - **five aspects of** SHEN 神 - **represented on the** TAI JI **symbol**

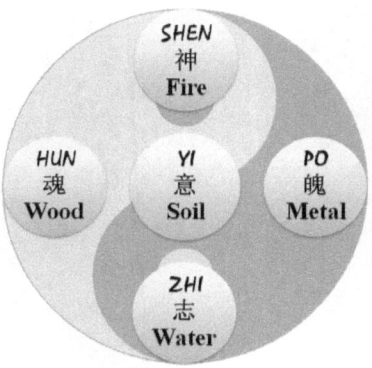

Fire Modality - South on the TAI JI symbol - SHEN 神[7]

Fire Modality is at the South of the TAI JI symbol. Fire Modality represents YANG – red color, which dominates the upper part of the TAI JI symbol, though YIN is always present in the background and is represented by the 'black eye' in the middle of the red color. South is also the symbol of conception, the creation of SHEN through the interaction of JING 精 of father and JING 精 of mother. The 'black eye' – YIN in the center of YANG – is the symbol of the 'substantial forms', female egg cell that produces the body after meeting with the sperm cell. SHEN is eruption of life, and is present until the last breath. In ancient China, the South symbolized a pregnant empress - bearing the future emperor.

Fire in Man is SHEN 神 inseparable from Heart (XIN 心). SHEN 神 is the most subtle aspect of Consciousness and is also the designer of everything that characterizes the human body ('substantial forms'). SHEN combines material and non-material aspects: fundamental vitality (JING 精), energy (QI 氣), mind and body (Blood, organs, tissues) and also includes the four other BEN SHEN 本神, which describe the expression of SHEN in space and time throughout a person's life.

---

[7] see page 12 and Figure 2 for the character SHEN 神

Metal Modality - West on the TAI JI symbol - PO 魄

West, the location of sunset, represents a balance between YANG and YIN. On the West YANG declines and YIN emerges, so Metal Modality symbolizes YIN, the beginning of YIN dominance. Metal Modality in man is Lung. PO 魄 represents the 'Metal' aspect of BEN SHEN 本神 which dwells in Lung.

Figure 14. The character PO 魄 - Metal Modality aspect of BEN SHEN 本神, 'the purified influence of earth' in ancient seal and classical script

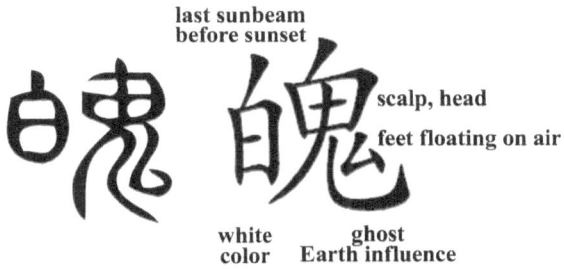

The character PO 魄 (Figure 14)[8] includes the phonetic 白 'the last ray of sun before sunset'; it symbolizes purity and is translated as 'white color'. The radical GUI 鬼 shows 'a skull or head with feet floating on air beneath',[9] and is translated as 'ghost'. GUI 鬼 are 'the centripetal influence of earth'. PO 魄 conveys 'the purified influence of earth', and is sometimes translated as *'vegetative soul' or 'anima'*.[10]

PO 魄 represents the characteristics of Metal Modality:
- Inertia, separation, dissolution, introversion, deep sleep and death;
- Building and maintenance of the physical body;
- White color of the body, which represents the density of 'substantial forms': the nervous system, bones, milk and sperm;

---

8 http://zhongwen.com/d/190/x122.htm
9 Wieger, Lesson 40
10 *The Secret of the Golden Flower*, Wilhelm R.; Translated from German by Baynes, see page 73

- Aggressiveness, predation (activity of the hypothalamus – a part of the limbic system - paleomammalian complex);
- The feminine aspect (YIN 陰) of BEN SHEN 本神, responsible for the relationship with the mother, starting with the development of the fetus in the womb. PO 魄 in the adult continues to represent the relationship to the mother, descent, convergence, assembling.

PO 魄 and fetal development

Each BEN SHEN 本神 is active in the human body from conception to death. PO 魄 (the feminine aspect of BEN SHEN 本神) is especially active during the first phase of human life, assuring the dialog with the mother's body and SHEN, while directing other BEN SHEN during fetal development.

Fetal development proceeds on the Three Levels: Heaven-Universe, Earth-body and Man-emotions.

- On the subtle level of Heaven-Universe:
  PO 魄 allows the reception of LING 靈, 'spiritual accomplishment', 'an affirmation of the generation of the body'. The radical 雨 'rain' in the character LING 靈 is a metaphor for QI 氣 of Heaven and Earth which passes through the mother's body and enables fetal growth, like 'rain falling from Heaven to Earth' providing 'water' for growth.[11] In China, rain is used as a metaphor for sexuality.
  Metal generates Water: PO 魄 assists the reception and storage of Source (inborn) JING 精 in Kidney, Eight Extraordinary Meridians and Organs of Extraordinary Longevity (QI HENG ZHI FU 奇恒之腑) to assure a sufficient flow of QI and body growth and maintenance for the duration of life.

- On the level of Earth-'substantial forms'- body:
  PO 魄 governs the generation of the body during fetal development according to the original, inherited plan, assured by the mother's blood transferred through the placenta to the fetus.

---

11 Wieger, Lesson 72

The paradox of PO 魄 on the 'substantial forms' - body level is that:
- on one hand, PO 魄 assures an opening to Heaven by 'non-action' - allowing human existence and body rehabilitation through deep sleep.
- on the other hand, PO 魄 activates 'the purified centripetal influences of earth', necessary for the generation and maintenance of organs. These centripetal influences are transferred through the mother's blood to the fetus, often bringing harmful or alien memories. 'Ghosts of the past', issues that have not been completed or properly resolved, and guilt are transferred to the fetus through egocentric hostile forces - GUI 鬼. GUI 鬼, the radical in the character PO 魄, is translated as 'ghost' and represents the centripetal influence of earth.

- On the level of Man-emotions:
PO 魄 assures a complete attachment during pregnancy, followed by a natural separation - birth. PO 魄 symbolizes maternal protection, rehabilitation and the feminine aspect of nature. Many emotional disorders can be related to an imbalance of PO 魄.

Wood Modality - East on the TAI JI symbol - HUN 魂

East, the location of sunrise, like West, the location of sunset, represents balance between YIN and YANG. However, on the East YANG emerges and YIN declines, so Wood Modality symbolizes the beginning of YANG dominance.

Wood Modality in man is Liver. HUN 魂 represents the Wood aspect of BEN SHEN which inhabits Liver. The character HUN 魂 (Figure 15) includes the phonetic 云 'word', 'speech',[12] 'cloud' or 'vapor'.[13] GUI 鬼, translated as 'ghost' and representing 'the influence of earth', is the radical in both HUN 魂 and PO 魄.[14] HUN is the 'talking, earthly' aspect of SHEN 神 and is sometimes translated as *'spiritual soul'*.[15]

---

12 http://zhongwen.com/d/187/x238.htm
13 Wieger, Lesson 93
14 Wieger, Lesson 40
15 *The Secret of the Golden Flower*, Wilhelm R.; see page 73

Figure 15. The character HUN 魂 **- Wood Modality aspect of** BEN SHEN 本神**, 'talking' influence of earth in ancient seal and classical script**

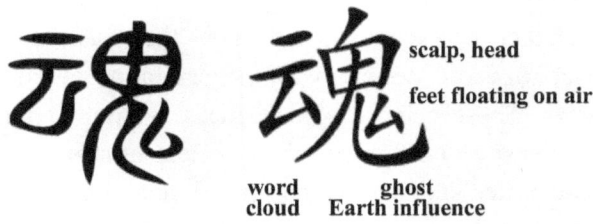

Unlike PO, HUN 魂 is not identified with the human body, but allows communication between the body and environment through breathing and speech. HUN - YANG - Wood represents rising, an activation of SHEN 神. HUN is the dragon of SHEN 神, connecting and unifying all movement of QI 氣. HUN is perspective, passion, creativity, imagination, body movement, self-esteem and the rectitude of Man between Heaven and Earth.

HUN 魂 expresses itself in human life through:
- Birth, which is a passage from a fluid environment to air.
- Cutting of the umbilical cord - separating mother and child, and activating the functions of the nine orifices of the five senses - communication with the environment.
- The first cry, the first breath which opens the lungs and provides separation of the small blood circulation from the large blood circulation. The first cry is the ancestor of communication with society by means of speech. Speech, communication, transmission of personal experience, is the basis for learning laws and acquiring knowledge of the body and the exterior world, providing exchange of opinions, personal expression and self-evaluation, which allow the rectitude of Man between Heaven and Earth.
- Any change of mind and body during lifetime, before and after birth, moving, acting.
- Sight (eyes are connected with Liver), dreaming (seeing with closed eyes).

- Waking from sleep.
- Connection with the father, representing the language and laws of society.
- Impulse, heroism, generosity, associated with masculinity.
- Personal name (in ancient China the father named his children).
- Relationships and communication with the exterior world.

Water Modality - North on the TAI JI symbol - ZHI 志

Water Modality represents the North, midnight at the bottom of the TAI JI symbol, opposed to Fire Modality on the South. YANG-red dominates the top left of the TAI JI symbol and YIN-black dominates the bottom and right. But there is the 'red eye' in the center of YIN which symbolizes the root of YANG (Kidney YANG and ZHI 志). ZHI 志 represents the Water aspect of BEN SHEN and dwells in Kidney.

ZHI 志 is the will or passion to live, the ability to realize life (self realization) and determination. ZHI 志 is the gathering of inheritance, Source JING 精 which assures existence, and allows the strength, judgment and ability to realize the unique potential of the individual.

Figure 16. The character ZHI 志 **- Water Modality aspect of** BEN SHEN 本神 **in ancient seal and classical script**

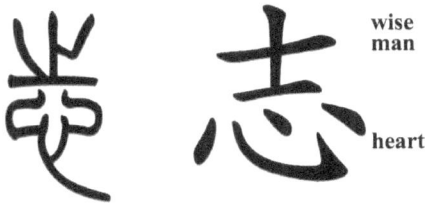

The character ZHI 志 (Figure 16) shows the radical 心 'heart' below the phonetic 士 symbolizing 'a wise man' (one who knows).[16] ZHI 志 is the heart of what is happening now,[17] the truth of Heart, translated as 'the capacity of realization', 'will' or 'determination' and also as 'desires or passions which characterize emotional life'.

---

16 Ryjik, 60
17 Wieger, lesson 79

ZHI 志 anchors SHEN 神 in reality. According to HUAI NAN ZI:
When ZHI 志 finds its place, SHEN 神 has its anchor.[18]

SU WEN, Chapter 2, recommends rules for the use of ZHI 志 to adapt to each season of the year to ensure a long and healthy life.

Soil Modality - the Center of the TAI JI symbol - YI 意

Soil Modality is the Center of the TAI JI symbol, the confluence of North-South and East-West. Soil Modality represents a permanent record of influences, changes and cycles of the four other Modalities.

YI 意 represents the Soil aspect of BEN SHEN and dwells in Spleen. The character YI 意 (Figure 17) shows the radical 心 'heart' below the phonetic 音 'sound', comprising 立 'a man standing on his two feet' and 曰 'singing with open mouth' (with the tongue inside).[19]

Figure 17. The character YI 意 - Soil Modality aspect of BEN SHEN 本神 in ancient seal and classical script

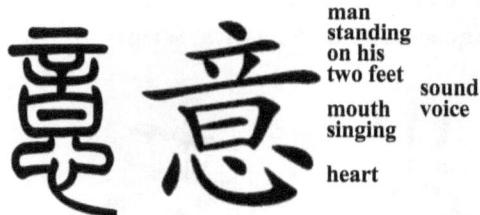

YI 意, the sound of the music of Heart-Consciousness, is translated as 'intentionality', 'intent' or 'ideas'. YI 意 records all reminiscences and traces of Consciousness and creates ideas and intent. SHEN 神 identifies flavors, and acquires JING 精 and body liquids from food as directed by Spleen-YI 意, providing formation, growth and maintenance of the coarse forms of the physical body and the subtle forms of language, ideas, ways of thinking and intuition.

---

18 See page 123, Chapter 4
19 Wieger, Lesson 73

Interaction between BEN SHEN 本神 **during life**

SHEN 神, HUN 魂 and PO 魄 together direct man's development and functions from the beginning of life. SHEN directs the organization of life from conception. PO 魄 directs fetal development and the relationship with the mother. HUN 魂 directs birth and the relationship with the father, and is connected to the first and last names. YI 意 directs the process of registration: memories, images and intents. ZHI 志 directs the union of body and soul: vitality, determination, adaptability.

In Figure 18, the interaction between BEN SHEN 本神 on the TAI JI symbol is represented as a mushroom. SHEN 神, HUN 魂 and PO 魄, active from the initial stages of fetal development, form the cap of the mushroom while YI 意 and ZHI 志, the supporting stem, become more active after birth.

Figure 18. Interaction between BEN SHEN 本神 **presented on the** TAI JI **symbol as a mushroom in which** SHEN 神, HUN 魂 **and** PO 魄 **are the cap, while** YI 意 **and** ZHI 志 **are the stem**

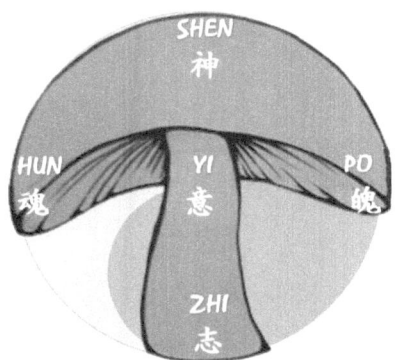

Five Modalities express Three Levels of Man (Heaven, Man, Earth)
Lower Level (Earth): the five ZANG 臟

Earth level, the lowest level in Figure 12, presents the five ZANG 臟, centers of body formation, the builders of 'substantial forms' (body tissues) with the help of QI 氣, Blood, body liquids and five flavors.

ZANG differ from the organs called liver, heart, spleen, lung and kidney in Western medicine.[20] Five ZANG express Five Modalities in Man (Figure 19):
- Liver represents Wood Modality
- Heart represents Fire Modality
- Spleen represents Soil Modality
- Lung represents Metal Modality
- Kidney represents Water Modality

Figure 19. Five ZANG 臟 presented on the TAI JI symbol

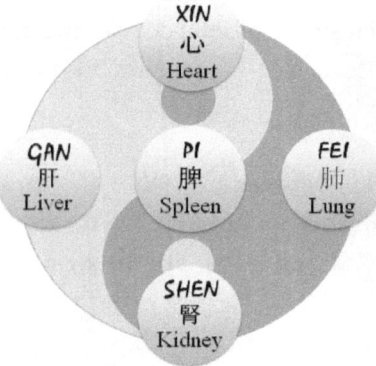

Man's life is expressed through his body formed by ZANG 臟, which in themselves are non-personal and similar in every person. However, ZANG function according to heredity, personal history and difficulties, and therefore each person's body is different and unique.

The character ZANG 臟 shows the radical 月 'flesh', and the phonetic 藏 'conceal', 'hide', 'hoard', 'storage'.[21] The character 藏 contains 艹/艸 'vegetation', 丬 'wall', 弋 'spear', and 臣 'a minister', 'an important person bowing'.[22] The character ZANG 臟 conveys the meaning 'a body structure well protected (by vegetation, wall and spear) storing a treasure, important function'.

---

20 Eyssalet, *Les Cinq Chemins du Clair et de l'Obscur*
21 http://zhongwen.com/d/197/x166.htm
22 http://zhongwen.com/d/194/x195.htm

What do ZANG 臟 store?

- Each of the five ZANG 'stores' Source (inborn) and acquired (postnatal) JING 精,[23] necessary to maintain life. Spleen, Lung and Liver supply acquired JING (which maintains and operates Source JING) obtained from food, beverages and air. Kidney is responsible for the storage of Source JING in man. Heart-Consciousness activates Source JING and, with the help of JING QI 精氣 (QI which transfers Source and acquired JING), ensures the functions and maintenance of 'substantial forms' (body) and mind, thus sustaining life.

- Each of the five ZANG 'stores' one of the five BEN SHEN 本神 (Figure 13). SHEN 神 is connected to Heart. HUN 魂 dwells in Liver, YI 意 in Spleen, PO 魄 in Lung, ZHI 志 in Kidney. Each BEN SHEN 本神, through its ZANG, forms the body and personality of the individual according to the original design (genome) and provides all modifications of the body-mind (change of lifestyle decisions), and relates to a specific period of a person's life history in time and space. SU WEN, Chapter 23, makes clear the connection between ZANG and BEN SHEN 本神:

五 WU	心 XIN	肺 FEI	肝 GAN	脾 PI	腎 SHEN
臟 ZANG	藏 CANG	藏 CANG	藏 CANG	藏 CANG	藏 CANG
所 SUO	神 SHEN	魄 PO	魂 HUN	意 YI	志 ZHI
藏 CANG					

Five ZANG 臟 store.
Heart stores SHEN 神.
Lung stores PO 魄.
Liver stores HUN 魂.
Spleen stores YI 意, intent.
Kidney stores ZHI 志, determination, will.

---

23 See page 101 for the character JING 精

Each ZANG 臟 includes its specific:
- Function of transit (hollow) organ (FU 腑) (Gallbladder, Small intestine, Stomach, Large intestine, Bladder),
- Body tissue (muscle, blood vessels, fat, skin, bones),
- External expression ('flowering') (nails, face, lips, body hair, hair),
- Body liquid (tears, sweat, saliva active in digestion, nasal liquids, saliva active in mouth lubrication),
- Orifice (eyes, tongue, mouth, nose, ears, anus and urethra),
- Sense organ (vision, touch, taste, smell, hearing),
- Meridians (JING MAI 經脈) (each ZANG and FU has its own meridian, which nourishes it and provides communication with other organs).

Each ZANG 臟 is identified by its specific:
- Emotion
- Flavor (acid, bitter, sweet, pungent, salty)
- Smell
- Voice
- Complexion
- Radial pulse
- Dreams

Fire Modality - South on the TAI JI symbol – Heart (XIN 心)

Fire Modality in the human body is represented by ZANG - Heart (XIN 心). Heart is the ruling prince of the body, but SHEN 神 (linked to Heart) is man's true governor. The character XIN 心 describes 'Heart with blood vessels crossing it'. 心 is the only character depicting ZANG organs that does not include the radical 月 'flesh', because Heart is beyond flesh. XIN 心 is also translated as 'awareness', 'mind' or 'Consciousness'.[24]

Fire Modality (XING HUO 火行) in the Universe and in man has two aspects:
- Fire as a source of light - ruling prince, prince-Fire (JUN HUO 君火);
- Fire as a source of heat - minister-Fire (XIANG HUO 相火).

---

24 http://zhongwen.com/d/164/x223.htm

Prince-Fire, symbolizing light and radiance, is represented by ZANG-Heart and its transit organ (FU 腑) Small Intestine (XIAO CHANG 小腸).

Minister-Fire is represented by ZANG-Master of Heart (Viceroy of Heart, XIN ZHU 心主), also called 'Envelope of Heart Communication' or 'Communication System of Heart'[25] (XIN BAO LUO 心包絡), and by its transit organ (FU 腑) SAN JIAO 三焦 (Triple-Warmer, Triple Heater). Master of Heart and SAN JIAO are not associated with any body structure in man but are a function of body organization and regulation (function without 'substantial form').

Heart, like SHEN 神, can be considered in two interrelated ways:
1. Heart-Prince, in charge of the four other ZANG (Liver, Spleen, Lung, Kidney), similarly to SHEN 神, which is in charge of the four other BEN SHEN 本神.
2. Heart representing Fire Modality and governed by the laws of the Five Modalities.

Heart–Prince forms the blood vessels, and governs the flow of Blood in the blood vessels (MAI 脈) and the flow of QI in the meridians (JING MAI 經脈), including acupuncture points (XUE 穴) located on the meridian pathways. Meridians (JING MAI 經脈) 'irrigate' the body, assuring the functioning of the vascular and nervous systems. Activation of XUE 穴 through acupuncture, moxibition, massage or essential oils allows therapeutic regulation of BEN SHEN 本神 and of ZANG-FU (all body functions): cardiovascular/circulatory, digestive/excretory, endocrine, integumentary/exocrine, lymphatic/immune, muscular/skeletal, nervous (central and peripheral, including feelings and emotions), renal/urinary, reproductive and respiratory systems.

Heart–Prince is radiance expressed as internal-external communications, and is therefore responsible for all subtle aspects of the senses which transmit messages from the exterior perceived by the sensory organs. Each ZANG function includes sense perception

---

25 Usually translated as pericardium

(Spleen is responsible for taste, Liver - sight, Kidney - hearing, Lung - smell), but Heart - the ruler - oversees them all and therefore rules perception. Clear vision and brightness of eyes, and the perception of refined tastes and smells, are overseen by Heart. The sense of touch – connected to the entire body - is governed by Heart. Kidney governs hearing, but Heart governs the ability to listen.

Heart-SHEN 神 rules Consciousness, including emotional life, and is the first ZANG to be affected by intensive or prolonged emotions. Heart also regulates the rhythm of sleeping and waking, therefore Heart disorders cause insomnia or nightmares.

Heart governs the flow of body liquids and thermoregulation (by sweat) with the help of SAN JIAO 三焦. Sweat following a flood of emotions is a sign of QI deficiency; cold sweat is a sign of YANG deficiency; a small quantity of sweat accompanied by thirst, excitability, palpitations or increased heart rate is a sign of Blood deficiency (anemia).

'Flowering' of Heart is face. Change of complexion reflects the condition of Heart. SHEN and Heart conditions can also be observed in the eyes.

The tongue is the 'orifice' of Heart - 'Heart bud'. The diagnosis of imbalance between Fire and Water in the body is made through observing changes in the body and coating of the tongue. A pale tongue is a sign of cold; a red tongue is a sign of heat; and a violet tongue - congestion of blood and QI.

The Heart pulse, one of the six radial pulses, is felt on the fold of the left wrist (CUN). Heart pulses are:
- flooded - HONG 洪;
- at regular intervals, similar to pearls on a string rolling one after another;
- floating FU 浮;
- slightly dispersed SAN 散.

Metal Modality - West on the TAI JI symbol – Lung (FEI 肺)

Metal Modality in the human body is represented by Lung (FEI 肺). Lung is the Prime Minister of the human body. PO 魄, which stores and organizes QI and 'substantial forms' in fetus, is BEN SHEN 本神 stored in Lung. Lung controls breathing, moves QI downwards, cools and purifies QI, organizes the flow of Nourishing QI (RONG/YING 營/榮) in the meridians. The daily cycle of Nourishing QI flow in the meridians starts from Lung Meridian. Radial pulses are felt on Lung Meridian. Lung connects the body surface (skin and body hair - the body tissue of the Lung) with internal organs and tissues of the body. The character FEI 肺 shows the radical 月 'flesh', and the phonetic 市 'market' or 'plants intertwined', [26] and conveys the meaning that Lung is 'flesh in which exchange takes place'.

Metal-Lung nourishes Water-Kidney-ZHI (Generation law): Lung moves body liquids downwards to Kidney and cools the fire of Heart and Liver.

Lung and its transit organ (FU 腑) Large Intestine (DA CHANG 大腸), represent the purification and cleansing characteristics of Metal Modality. Large Intestine purifies the body by removing waste and 'judges' which food residues and liquids to reabsorb and which to discharge.
The nose - the orifice of Lung - directs the sense of smell. Lung forms skin – the body boundaries.

Sadness, sense of failure, separation and alienation are caused by Lung QI deficiency or Lung injury by Fire. These emotions are accompanied by a feeling of pressure or tightening in the chest, shortness of breath, cold sweat, fatigue at any effort, weak voice and pale complexion, thin and pale tongue.

---

26 http://zhongwen.com/d/170/x205.htm, Eyssalet, *Les Cinq Chemins du Clair et de l'Obscur*

The Lung pulse, one of the six radial pulses, is felt on the fold of the right wrist (CUN), Lung pulses are:
- floating, FU 浮;
- short, DUAN 短;
- without resistance as if touching fur, MAO 毛.

Wood Modality - East of the TAI JI symbol - Liver (GAN 肝)

Wood Modality in man is Liver (GAN 肝). Liver is the General of the Army in the human body. HUN 魂, associated with childbirth, is BEN SHEN 本神 stored in Liver. Wood-Liver represents a link between Water and Fire on the ascending phase of the TAI JI symbol. Wood-Liver is generated by Water-Kidney and generates Fire-Heart. Liver, nourished by Source QI stored by Kidney, assures the vital impulse of Heart (SHEN 神).

The character GAN 肝 shows the radical 月 'flesh' and the phonetic 干 'pestle', which conveys the meaning 'crushing', 'resistance', 'injury', 'a clashing of swords'.[27] Liver is the Army General, the 'fighting' flesh. According to SU WEN, Chapter 8, Liver is responsible for planning and contemplation, consideration of the situation, strategy (MU LU 謀慮).

Liver is in charge of the strategy of 'smooth' QI flow in Man. In Lower JIAO, Liver (together with Kidney) produces Defensive QI (WEI QI 衛氣), responsible for the thermoregulation (sweat), immune, nervous, tendino-muscular and reproductive systems. WEI QI 衛氣, through HUN 魂, is related to waking, sleeping and dreaming. Liver governs eyes (orifice and eyesight). There is a Daoist saying that eyes reflect Spirit - HUN 魂.

Liver is in charge of the strategy of the movement and storage of Blood. Liver moves the Blood to the location where it is needed and together with Spleen governs the menstrual cycle. Liver is in charge of the function of the external genitalia and sexuality in woman and man (erection) since Liver Meridian passes through the genitals.

---

27 Wieger, Lesson 102

Liver absorbs JING 精 from food and with the help of Spleen transfers it to the whole body, especially to the eyes, nervous system, tendons and muscles.

Liver is closely connected with its transit organ (FU 腑) Gallbladder (DAN 膽), which represents the YANG aspect of Liver. Gallbladder governs decisions.

Gallbladder is one of the six Organs of Extraordinary Longevity (QI HENG ZHI FU 奇恒之腑), and therefore stores JING 精, administrated by Kidney.

Gallbladder is *Rectitude of the Center* (ZHONG ZHENG 中正) (SU WEN, Chapter 8). *Rectitude of the Center* in Man is the balanced flow of QI from Earth to Heaven (from Kidney-Water to Heart-Fire, passing through Liver-Gallbladder), and also the regulation of *clear* above the diaphragm and *turbid* below.[28]

Liver imbalance is expressed as *Liver QI congestion* (preventing the smooth flow of QI and Blood) or an excess of *Liver QI/YANG* injuring Heart, Lung and Spleen and causing the ascent of blood to the face, resulting in headache, redness of eyes, shouting and anger.

The Liver pulse, one of the six radial pulses, is felt on the middle position (GUAN) on the left wrist. Liver pulses are:
- Sinking, CHEN 沉;
- Long, CHANG 長;
- Wiry, XUAN 弦.

Water Modality - North on the TAI JI symbol - Kidney (SHEN 腎)
Water Modality in Man is Kidney (SHEN 腎). Water – fluid, vapor and solid (ice) - symbolizes both fluidity and rigidity in nature. Kidney

---

28 *Clear* (QING 清) are substances ready to use and QI which above the diaphragm. *Turbid* (ZHOU 濁) are raw substances need to be processed in order to be absorbed and QI below the diaphragm.

structures the body through bones - the skeleton. Bones also protect the interior: ribs protect the chest, the skull protects the brain. Kidney also nourishes the bone marrow. The character SHEN 腎 shows the radical 月 'flesh' and the phonetic 臤[29] 'strength', which consists of the radical 臣 'minister (an important person bowing)' and 又 'a strong fist'.[30] SHEN 腎 conveys the meaning that Kidney is strong flesh (body) with an important mission.

As Water irrigates and stabilizes all forms of life, so Kidney anchors, saturates and stabilizes the whole body. Kidney governs the storage of inborn, Source JING 精 by Source QI (YUAN QI 原氣/元氣), originating from the lineages of the mother and the father and from the mother during pregnancy. After birth, Source JING 精 is complemented by acquired JING 精 absorbed from food and air. ZHI 志, 'determination', 'will', is BEN SHEN 本神 stored in Kidney.

Kidneys are the only ZANG organ divided into two (in ancient China Lungs were considered to be one undivided organ). The left Kidney is considered YIN and the right Kidney - YANG. The left side of the body is YANG but left Kidney is YIN, like the 'black eye' emerging in the red part of the TAI JI symbol. The right side of the body is YIN, but right Kidney is YANG, like the 'red eye' emerging in the black part of the TAI JI symbol (Figure 20).

Kidney YIN, the left Kidney, is responsible for the YIN aspect of Kidney function;
- Regulation of body liquids: cooling and moistening the body;
- Storage of Source JING 精 by Source QI (YUAN QI 原氣/元氣),

Kidney YANG (also known as MING MEN 命門 - Gate of Destiny), the right Kidney, is responsible for the YANG-Kidney-Fire aspect of function:

---

29 http://zhongwen.com/d/181/x199.htm
30 http://zhongwen.com/d/166/x218.htm, Wieger, Lesson 82

- Distribution of JING 精 through the three fundamental Extraordinary Meridians: DU MAI 督脈, REN MAI 任脈 and CHONG MAI 衝脈, providing the basis for the growth and development of body and brain;
- Formation of the genital organs, sperm and the uterus, providing transmission of heredity: the passage of Source QI (YUAN QI 原氣 / 元氣) transferring Source JING 精 to the next generation; Liver is responsible for sexual desire and the functioning of the external genitalia;
- Production of Defensive QI (WEI QI 衛氣) together with Liver in Lower JIAO.[31] Kidney YANG (root of SAN JIAO) is related through WEI QI 衛氣 to physical activity (movement, coordination) and to thermoregulation.

Figure 20. Kidney YIN and Kidney YANG presented on the TAI JI symbol

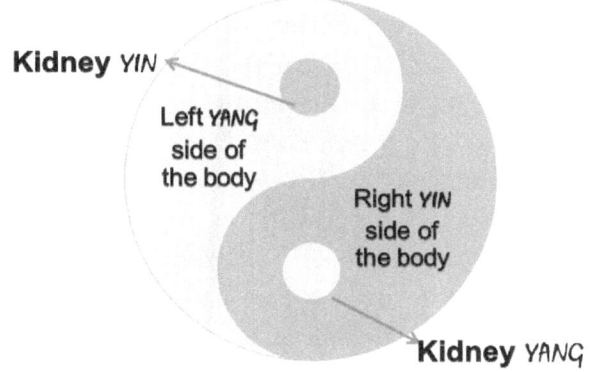

According to Chinese medicine, the function of Urinary Bladder (PANG GUANG 膀胱), transit organ (FU 腑) of Kidney, includes all filtration, re-absorption and secretion in the nephron. Bladder is described as *the capital city of the body*[32]. Bladder Meridian is the longest in the body (67 points), flowing from the inner eye cantus to the little toe. There are points on Bladder Meridian which affect BEN SHEN 本神 and the YANG aspect of ZANG-FU function (SHU).

---

31 See page 42
32 SU WEN, Chapter 8

Insufficiency of Kidney is expressed as fatigue accompanied by cold sweating, cold, noise sensitivity, pain in knees and lower back, urinary disorders, dark complexion, gray tongue coating.

The Kidney pulses, two of the six radial pulses, are felt on the distal position (CHI) of both wrists. The pulse of the left hand (the left side of the body is YANG) shows the state of Kidney YIN (body water and JING 精 reservoirs); the pulse of the right hand (the right side of the body is YIN) shows the state of Kidney YANG (MING MEN 命門). Kidney pulses are:
- Sinking, CHEN 沉;
- Sometimes slippery, HUA 滑;
- Full, SHI 實;
- Like a stone felt in a stream, SHI 石

Soil Modality - Center on the TAI JI symbol – Spleen (PI 脾)
Soil Modality in man is Spleen (PI 脾), responsible for regular functioning in daily life. It is compared to a servant or receptionist of the other four organs (Liver, Heart, Lung and Kidney). Spleen and Stomach are a couple, ZANG-FU, in the center of the body (Middle JIAO), connected to the process of absorption of JING 精, liquids, five flavors, and Nourishing QI (RONG/YING 營/榮) from food and beverages. YI 意, intent, ideation, the storage of all experiences in life, is BEN SHEN 本神 stored in Spleen.

The character PI 脾 shows the radical 月 'flesh' and the phonetic 卑 'a pitcher for use on weekdays' (in ancient China a special vessel was used on holidays).[33] PI 脾 conveys the meaning 'flesh for regular use', and is translated as 'Spleen' or as 'spleen-pancreas' to express the digestive function.[34]

---

33 Eyssalet, *Les Cinq Chemins du Clair et de l'Obscur*
34 The spleen produces white blood cells and red blood cells and disposes of damaged or dead cells. The spleen also produces antibodies and is part of the immune system. The pancreas is of great importance in digestion. Pancreatic juices contain enzymes that help digest proteins, carbohydrates and fats. The hormones secreted by the pancreas are responsible for regulating blood glucose levels.

Spleen raises *clear* liquids and Nourishing QI (RONG/YING 營/榮) to Upper JIAO (Heart and Lung). In Upper JIAO, Nourishing QI becomes part of ZONG QI 宗氣 (QI of the rhythm of breath and Blood flow), or starts flowing in meridians (JING LUO MAI), or is transformed into Blood, and thus nourishes the body and Consciousness.

Spleen and YI 意 also link conscious and subconscious patterns of:
• Memories and traces of memories,
• Feelings,
• Emotions, passions,
• Body language and facial expression,
• Images, including body image,
• Words to build thoughts,
• The states of consciousness,
• Thoughts,
• Intent,
• Ideas.

Any excess of Liver fire or Heart fire originating from emotions/passions is expressed in the body, which is nourished by Spleen and Stomach. In acupuncture, points on Stomach Meridian are often used to cleanse and regulate the fire of passions.

Spleen dysfunction causes indigestion with abdominal bloating, loose stools, edema with reduced quantities of urine, hiccups, heartburn, heaviness of the body, difficulty in body movement, and also compulsive behavior, sadness, recurrent thoughts and nightmares, swollen wet tongue with teeth marks and white coating, yellowish complexion, puffy face.

The Spleen pulse, one of the six radial pulses, is felt on the middle position (GUAN) of the right wrist. The Spleen pulse is slow, retarding (HUAN 緩), similar to the strut of a hen (slow walking, easy steps). HUAN 緩 has a sense of 'thickness' and when felt in other radial pulses is called 'Stomach QI pulse'.

Five Modalities express Three Levels of Man
(Heaven, Man, Earth)
Middle Level (Man): five emotions (WU ZHI 五志)

The Middle Level of Man (Figure 12) is represented by five emotions (desires, passions).[35] The level of Man-emotions connects the level of Earth-ZANG (Heart, Liver, Spleen, Lung and Kidney), with the level of Heaven-BEN SHEN 本神, the organization of human existence.

Five Emotions (WU ZHI 五志) are (Figure 21):
1. Anger (NU 怒)
2. Joy (XI 喜)
3. Sorrow (BEI 悲)
4. Fear (KONG 恐)
5. Thought (SI 思)

Figure 21. Five emotions (WU ZHI 五志) **presented on the TAI JI symbol**

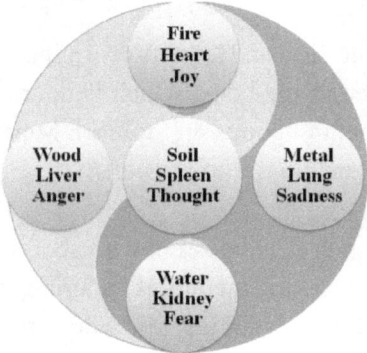

Emotions are born from innumerable changing interactions:
- between Heart-Consciousness and destiny (heredity),
- between QI and 'substantial forms' (body),
- between BEN SHEN 本神 and 'substantial forms' (body created by the five ZANG 臟 and connected with the mother's body and PO 魄),

---

35 Passion (from the Greek verb πασχω meaning to suffer) is a very strong feeling about a person or thing. Passion is an intense emotion, a compelling enthusiasm or desire for something, according to Wikipedia

- between the masculine and feminine aspects of man,
- between a man and a woman,
- between personal history, family history and interaction with society (cultural influences, virtues and moral values),
- between man and his environment (climate, weather, air), lifestyle, food and beverages.

In man and animals, regulation of emotions is related to the diaphragm, which separates *clear* ZONG QI 宗氣 (QI of the rhythm of breath and Blood flow)[36] from *turbid* QI originating from food and ancestors (genome).

Chinese texts use five emotions (WU ZHI 五志) and seven emotions/passions (QI QING 七情) to describe mental life. The number five in traditional Chinese thought expresses the proper functioning of Five Modalities in man. The number seven (seven passions, seven flavors) is used to highlight the deviation from normal functioning which may cause disease. The seven passions differ in different Chinese texts, but usually they are the same five emotions with the addition of sorrow (grief) (BEI 悲), panic (fright) (JING 驚), or dread (JU 懼).

Figure 22. The character QING 情 'emotion, passion, color of Consciousness' in ancient seal and classical script

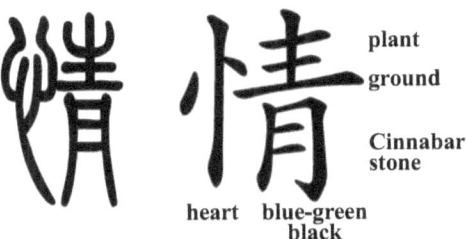

Is there a significant difference between the five emotions (WU ZHI 五志) and the seven passions (QI QING 七情)? The characters QING 情 and ZHI 志 project different messages.

---

36 Usually referred to as Ancestral QI, but this name may cause confusion since ZONG QI 宗氣 is not connected directly to heredity

The character QING 情 shows the radical 心/忄 'heart' in its horizontal version and the phonetic 青 'nature's color: blue-green, deep blue, black' (Figure 22).[37] QING 情 describes a natural tendency or 'natural color of Heart-Consciousness': love, emotion, passion, truth, taste, sexual attraction.

ZHI 志 (Figure 16), 'the truth of Heart', is translated as 'emotion/passion'; it is also 'BEN SHEN 本神 which dwells in Kidney'- 'determination', 'ability to realize', 'willpower', 'desire to live', 'a passion for life'.[38] Passion/emotion (ZHI 志) emphasizes will and decisions made consciously or subconsciously by the mind and body.

The dual meaning of ZHI 志 allows a connection between the Upper Level-Heaven-BEN SHEN 本神, and the Middle Level-Man-emotions (Figure 12). ZHI 志 'anchors' BEN SHEN 本神 and expresses determination and the ability to realize life through the rhythm of life expressed by each emotion-passion. Emotions/passions (ZHI 志) are not only used in a negative sense; they are messages from the subconscious, and contribute to all aspects of human functioning.

Fire Modality - South on the TAI JI symbol
joy (XI 喜) and pleasure (LE 樂)

Joy and pleasure (XI LE 喜樂) are emotions of Heart. Joy emerges from the opening and awareness of Heart, responsible for the free flow of the network of meridians and blood vessels and for interaction with the environment.

The character XI 喜 shows 壴 'a hand beating a drum' above 口 'an open mouth' (Figure 23). XI 喜 is joy expressed spontaneously by singing to the rhythm of the drum.[39] Rhythm and music symbolize happy Heart. Music also provides a metaphor for SHEN 神 - composer, conductor and orchestra of the totality of the person. XI 喜 is happiness in the

---

37 http://zhongwen.com/d/177/x161.htm, Wieger, Lesson 115
38 See page 33
39 Wieger, Lesson 165

here and now, spontaneous, expressing free communication between Heaven and Earth, the joy of life. Natural and spontaneous laughter expresses genuine happiness and joy.

The character LE 樂 shows 白 'a large drum' and 玄玄 'two bells' on 木 'a wooden platform', and is translated as 'elation', 'joy', 'pleasure' and 'delight' (Figure 23).[40] LE 樂 describes a communal celebration accompanied by music, elation and shared happiness and pleasure. The character 樂 pronounced as YUÈ, is translated as 'music accompanying worship and confirming harmony between Heaven and Earth'. XI 喜 is spontaneous personal joy, LE 樂 is joy of openness and social relaxation. LE 樂 creates joy and XI 喜 expresses joy.

Figure 23. The characters XI 喜 'joy' and LE 樂 'pleasure' in ancient seal and classical script

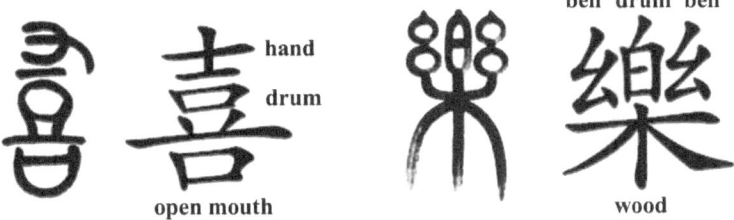

Center of Chest (TAN ZHONG 膻中) is *the official functioning as minister and envoy. Joy and happiness* (XI LE 喜樂) *originate in it* (SU WEN, Chapter 8).[41] XI 喜 and LE 樂 emerge from Center of Chest (which corresponds to Master of Heart), responsible for communication and the rhythm of QI flow. Joy and pleasure provide the rhythm of harmonized QI flow expressed as a feeling of expansion, connection and happiness of the body. Exaggerated or prolonged joy and pleasure weaken QI flow and cause fatigue. It should be remembered that Heart is responsible for mental life and all emotions and passions. All intense emotions injure Heart.

---

40 Wieger, Lesson 88
41 Translation of Unschuld P. U. and Tessenow H.

Metal Modality - West on the TAI JI symbol
sorrow (BEI 悲), sadness (YOU 憂),
grief (AI 哀), melancholy (CHOU 愁)

The characters BEI 悲, YOU 憂, AI 哀, CHOU 愁 describe different aspects of sadness, sorrow, grief, depression and melancholy, all expressing Metal Modality, which regulates introverted movement, descent, cooling, justice. All kinds of sadness express separation and brutality characteristic of a deficiency of Metal Modality. Excess of Metal Modality is expressed by deep depression with a tendency to suicide.

Figure 24. The characters BEI 悲 **'sorrow',** YOU 憂 **'sadness',** AI 哀 **'grief',** CHOU 愁 **'melancholy' in ancient seal and classical script**

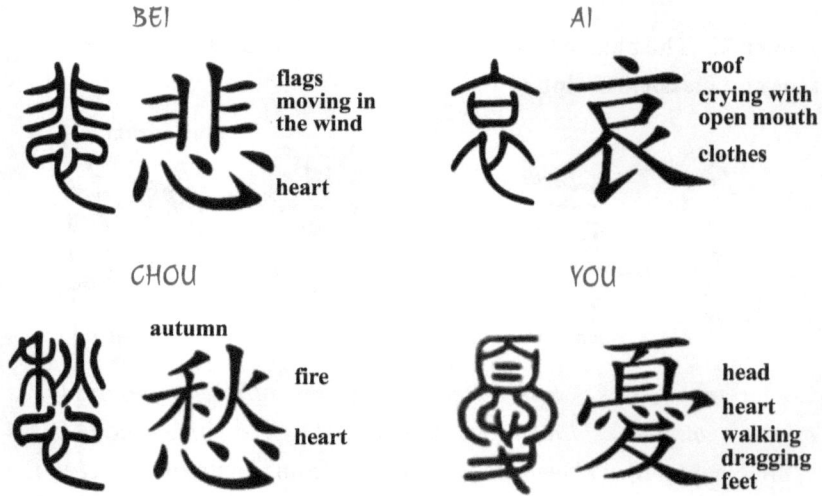

The character YOU 憂 shows 夂 'a man walking slowly, dragging his feet' with his 心 'heart' and 百 'head' separated and troubled (Figure 24).[42] The character YOU 憂 describes sadness accompanied by worry, a sense of oppression, blockage, heavy and dark thoughts, internal and external stress, suffering. YOU 憂 is translated as 'sadness', 'sadness accompanied by worry', 'sorrow', 'concern', 'anxiety', describing a situation in which a man, as if in exile, does not find his right place.

---

42 Wieger, Lesson 160

The character BEI 悲 shows the radical 心 'heart' below the phonetic 非 'flags moving in the wind' symbolizing 'no, negation, denial' (Figure 24).[43] BEI 悲 is the negation of Heart, denial of inner self creating a painful reality, and is translated as 'sorrow', 'sadness', 'grief'. BEI 悲 describes a loss of feeling or relationship, lack of self-value or radical separation.

The character AI 哀 'grief', 'sorrow', 'pity' – shows 宀 'under the roof' (in the house), 口 'a man crying with open mouth' and 衣 'tearing his clothes' - a symbol of mourning in Chinese culture (Figure 24).[44] BEI AI 悲哀 often appear together in Chinese texts to describe grief.

The character CHOU 愁 shows the radical 心 'heart', and the phonetic 秋 'autumn' (火 'fire' drying 禾 'ripening grain' or 'grain receiving color of fire') (Figure 24).[45] 'Autumn in the Heart' symbolizes Metal Modality and describes a slow process of losing the joy of life, loss of self, sadness, melancholy. CHOU 愁 is reminiscent of leaves falling in autumn, describing nostalgia and regrets.

Wood Modality - East on the TAI JI symbol – anger (NU 怒)
Anger (NU 怒) is the emotion expressing the failure of Liver to regulate the smooth flow of QI. The virtue attributed to Liver is REN 仁 'benevolence', 'humanity', 'kindness' - the opposite of anger. The character REN 仁 shows 亻 'a man standing' and 二 'the number 2'.[46] REN 仁 conveys the meaning 'the ability to consider others', 'good communication with the other'.

The character NU 怒 shows the radical 心 'heart' below 奴 'slave': (又 'a hand grasping' 女 'a woman-slave kneeling' - the image of a person without rights) (Figure 25).[47] NU 怒 means 'anger', 'slavery of heart', 'slavery of mind', 'violence against the feminine aspect of a person'.

---

43 http://zhongwen.com/d/180/x100.htm
44 Wieger, Lesson 1
45 http://zhongwen.com/d/183/x84.htm
46 Wieger, Lesson 2
47 Wieger, Lesson 67

Explosive or suppressed anger causes upward movement of QI and Blood and injures the anchoring of the body to the ground.

Figure 25. The character NU 怒 **'anger' in ancient seal and classical script**

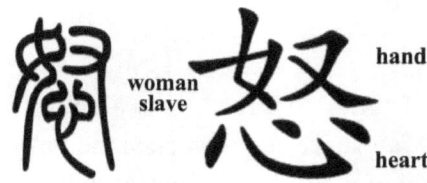

Lack of regulation of Liver is related to all kinds of misunderstandings in family life, work, public relations and politics: feelings of exploitation, dissatisfaction, revolt, betrayal and aggression. Liver and Gallbladder suffer both from the outbreak of anger and from suppressed anger.

Water Modality - North on the TAI JI **symbol**
fear (KONG 恐**) and dread (**JU 懼**)**

Fear (KONG 恐) and dread (JU 懼) are emotions that damage Kidney. The character KONG 恐 shows the radical 心 'heart', and the phonetic 巩 (凡 'a hand' which 工 'is working') translated as 'to hold' (Figure 26).[48] KONG 恐, 'a hand holding the heart' describes the 'active and hot' fear leading to flight, which interferes with the function of Heart and causes fibrillation, palpitation and rapid or irregular heartbeat.

Figure 26. The characters KONG 恐 **'fear' and** JU 懼 **'dread' in ancient seal and classical script**

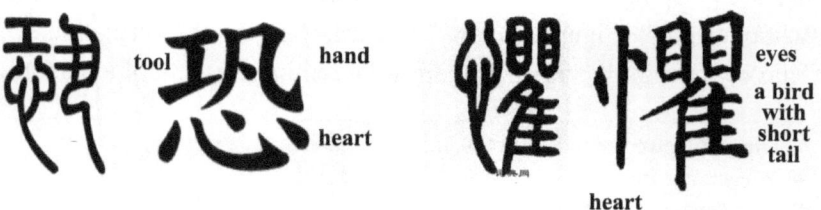

48 Wieger, Lessons 38, 11

The character JU 懼 shows the radical 心 'heart' in its vertical version 忄; the phonetic 瞿 presents 目目 'two eyes' above 隹 'a bird with a short tail' - a bird looking to both sides (an owl) (Figure 26).[49] JU 懼 describes 'passive and cold' paralyzing fear, dread or terror, occurring when at night a person sees the eyes of an owl and his heart freezes in the face of the unexpected, the unknown.

Fear (KONG 恐) and dread (JU 懼) weaken JING 精 storage in Kidney-ZHI 志, and therefore the ability to anchor the body. Fear and dread injure the pelvis, the perineum, the lower back and the legs. In fear and dread, Kidney YANG (MING MEN 命門) does not control the lower orifices (anus and urethra) and JING 精 is lost through feces and urine.

Fear provokes Kidney deficiency, Kidney-Water does not control Fire-Heart, and empty Heart YANG rises. Heart and Kidney Meridians belong to the SHAO YIN layer of the QI flow. The 'knot' point of SHAO YIN is CV23 (point 23 on the Extraordinary Meridian REN MAI 任脈), located close to the thyroid. Hypothyroidism may be related to fear.

Soil Modality - Center of the TAI JI symbol
thought, worry (SI 思)

Soil Modality stabilizes the other four Modalities. Spleen-Soil stabilizes and nourishes all ZANG (Heart, Liver, Lung and Kidney), keeping all parts of the body together through the absorption of QI, JING 精, flavors and liquids from food and beverages entering Stomach. YI 意 (BEN SHEN 本神 stored in Spleen) registers sensations, images, words, intents and thoughts, and creates new ideas and thoughts.

Thinking is the emotion of Spleen. In Chinese medicine, thinking is considered to be an emotion, or to be precise: the relationship between the mind and emotions which may become dust covering other emotions.

---

49 http://zhongwen.com/d/196/x223.htm, Wieger, Lesson 158

Thinking assures balance and links all the other emotions. Any disruption of Spleen function causes over thinking, excessive, obsessive thinking and worry.

Figure 27. The character SI 思 'thought, worry' in ancient seal and classical script

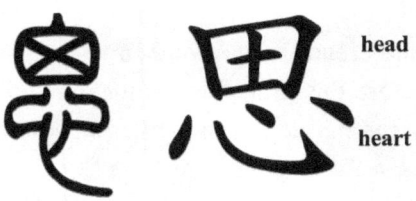

The character SI 思 shows the radical 心 'heart' below the phonetic 田 'head' (Figure 27),[50] 'the pressing of head on Heart-Consciousness', translated as 'thought', but also as 'worry', 'excessive and obsessive thinking'.

In SU WEN and LING SHU, when SI 思 causes disease it is translated as obsessive thinking. Obsessive thinking obstructs the activity of the brain, and blocks the absorption of food in Stomach and the intestines. Recurrent thoughts interfere with nourishment of Lung by Spleen (Law of Generation) and are expressed by melancholy and sorrow (CHOU YOU 愁憂) or anxiety and depression.

Summary

Man is re-balanced at every moment, on the Three Levels of the Universe (Heaven-Man-Earth) expressed by Five Modalities: Five *Roots of* SHEN (BEN SHEN 本神), five emotions and five ZANG 臟 (Figure 12). Disease is the result of an imbalance between the Three Levels of the Universe, but usually manifests in one ZANG 臟. Intense emotions/passions signify communication problems between Man and the Universe.

---

50 Wieger, Lesson 40

2

SHEN 神, ethics and emotions

In ancient China, emotions/passions were considered to be signs of error, causes or consequences of immoral, non-ethical behavior or faults at the spiritual level. The following Chinese texts discuss emotions in relation to the Universe (Heaven and Earth), consciousness, mental life and ethics:

a. ZHUANG ZI, 莊子, Chapter 15, late Warring States period (476–221 BC);
b. HUAI NAN ZI, 淮南子,[51] Chapters 7 and 1, HAN Dynasty (206 BC–220 AD);
c. WU XING DA YI, 五行大義, Chapter 18, attributed to SHAO YU of the School of Five Elements/Modalities (WU XING 五行), SUI Dynasty (581-618 BC).

A. Emotions according to ZHUANG ZI 莊子, Chapter 15

悲	BEI	sorrow	喜	XI	joy	好	HAO	love
樂	LE	pleasure	怒	NU	anger	惡	WU	hate
者	ZHE	(are)	者	ZHE	(are)	者	ZHE	(are)
德	DE		道	DAO		心	XIN	heart
之	ZHI	of	之	ZHI	of	之	ZHI	of
邪	XIE	damage	過	GUO	overflow	失	SHI	loss

Sorrow and pleasure (BEI LE 悲樂) *are pernicious* (XIE 邪) (energies) *of* DE 德 (the individual link with DAO 道).
Joy and anger (XI NU 喜怒) (cause) *an overflow* (GUO 過) *of* DAO 道.
Love and hate (HAO WU 好惡) *are loss of Heart-Consciousness* (XIN 心).

---

51 *The Masters/Philosophers of Huainan*, Chinese philosophical classic

ZHUANG ZI, Chapter 15, describes types of damage caused by three pairs of emotions:
- Sorrow and pleasure (BEI LE 悲樂)
- Joy and anger (XI NU 喜怒)
- Love and hate (HAO WU 好惡)

These three pairs of emotions harm the three essential aspects of man which assure proper communication with Heaven and Earth:
- DE 德,[52] the efficient functioning of the person, the individual link with DAO 道
- DAO 道, the Ultimate Way, the direction of the dance of the Universe
- XIN 心, Heart-Consciousness

Sorrow and pleasure poison Lung and Heart, which distribute Clear QI in meridians and vessels from Upper JIAO (chest). ZHUANG ZI considers sorrow and pleasure as pernicious (XIE 邪) energies of DE 德 - the dynamic authenticity, the individual connection to DAO 道.

Joy and anger (XI NU 喜怒) injure Heart and Liver, causing YANG to rise and 'overflow' (GUO 過) in Upper JIAO. This overflow injures the harmony of the vertical axis (Heaven-Man-Earth) and contradicts DAO 道, the authentic direction.

Heaven and Earth communicate with each other in Heart of Man. Heart-Consciousness should be empty, without obstructions. Love and hate (HAO WU 好惡), strong positive or negative attachments, cause the loss (SHI 失) of the emptiness of Heart-Consciousness (or of DE 德 in another version of this text).

The character HAO 好, love, shows 女 'a woman' with 子 'a child'.[53] The character WU 惡 shows 亞 'a deformed object' that 心 'Heart-Consciousness' does not accept and is translated as 'hate'.[54]

---

52 See page 52 for etymology of the character DE 德
53 Wieger, Lesson 67
54 http://zhongwen.com/d/180/x99.htm

B. Emotions according to HUAI NAN ZI 淮南子
Chapters 7 and 1

HUAI NAN ZI, The Masters of Huainan, is a Chinese philosophical classic from the HAN dynasty (206 BC – 220 AD).

HUAI NAN ZI, Chapter 7, discusses damage caused by the same three pairs of emotions as appear in ZHUANG ZI:
- Sorrow and pleasure (BEI LE 悲樂)
- Joy and anger (XI NU 喜怒)
- Love and hate (HAO ZENG 好憎) (ZHUANG ZI denotes hate by a different character - WU 惡)

HUAI NAN ZI, Chapter 7, repeats ZHUANG ZI, Chapter 15:

夫	FU	so	而	ER	and			
悲	BEI	sorrow	喜	XI	joy	好	HAO	love
樂	LE	pleasure	怒	NU	anger	憎	ZENG	hate
者	ZHE	are	者	ZHE	are	者	ZHE	are
德	DE		道	DAO		心	XIN	heart
之	ZHI	of	之	ZHI	of	之	ZHI	of
邪	XIE	damage	過	GUO	overflow	暴	BAO	violence
也	YE	period	也	YE	period	也	YE	period

Sorrow and pleasure (BEI LE 悲樂) *are pernicious* (XIE 邪) (energies) *of* DE 德.
Joy and anger (XI NU 喜怒) (cause) *an overflow* (GUO 過) *of* DAO 道.
Love and hate (HAO ZENG 好憎) *are violence* (BAO 暴) *to Heart-Consciousness* (XIN 心).

HUAI NAN ZI, Chapter 1, describes damage caused by eight emotions arranged in four pairs:

- Joy and anger (XI NU 喜怒)
- Sadness (accompanied by worry) and sorrow (YOU BEI 憂悲) (sadness replaces pleasure discussed in texts above)
- Love and hate (HAO ZENG 好憎)
- Attachment and lust (SHI YU 嗜欲) (not discussed in the other texts)

夫 FU	so							
喜 XI	joy	憂 YOU	sadness	好 HAO	love	嗜 SHI	relationship
怒 NU	anger	悲 BEI	sorrow	憎 ZENG	hate	欲 YU	desire
者 ZHE	are	者 ZHE	are	者 ZHE	are	者 ZHE	are
道 DAO		德 DE		心 XIN	heart	性 XING	nature
之 ZHI	of	之 ZHI	of	之 ZHI	of	之 ZHI	of
邪 XIE	damage	失 SHI	loss	過 GUO	overflow	暴 BAO	violence
也 YE	period	也 YE	period	也 YE	period	也 YE	period

Joy and anger (XI NU 喜怒) *are pernicious* (XIE 邪) (energies) *of* DAO 道.
Sadness and sorrow (YOU BEI 憂悲) *are loss of* DE 德.
Love and hate (HAO ZENG 好憎) (cause) *an overflow* (GUO 過) *of Heart-Consciousness* (XIN 心).
Attachment and lust (SHI YU 嗜欲) *are violence* (BAO 暴) *to Intimate Nature* (XING 性).

HUAI NAN ZI, Chapter 1, states in the first sentence that joy and anger are pernicious (XIE 邪) energies of DAO 道, as compared to 'overflow' of DAO 道 in the other texts. Both pernicious energies and overflow separate the individual from the Unity-DAO 道.

In the second sentence, sadness accompanied by worry (YOU 憂) and sorrow are loss (SHI 失) of DE 德. Sadness and sorrow (similarly to sorrow and pleasure discussed in the previous texts) obstruct the flow in Upper JIAO, harm Lung and Heart[55] and disturb communication

---

55 See page 52

with the environment. Therefore sadness and sorrow are pernicious energies, which cause loss of DE 德.

In the third sentence, love and hate overflow (GUO 過) Heart-Consciousness and compromise its emptiness, just as do loss, violence or fatigue in the other texts. Love and hate interfere with the emptiness of Heart-Consciousness, making it impossible for the individual to preserve the smooth flow of QI - to be in a correct place and to see others in their correct place.

The fourth sentence of HUAI NAN ZI, Chapter 1, discusses two emotions not mentioned before: attachment (compulsive relationships) and lust (SHI YU 嗜欲) which do violence (BAO 暴) to Intimate Human Nature, personal qualities (XING 性). The character XING 性 shows the horizontal version of the radical 心/忄 'heart', and the phonetic 生 'life'.[56] XING 性 is the spontaneous consciousness of the moment, a natural personal perspective.

It can be seen that in ancient China the emotions were considered to be a hindrance to the proper existence of Man between Heaven and Earth.

The following table summarizes the three texts discussed above:

emotions	joy, anger 喜怒	sorrow, pleasure 悲樂	sadness, sorrow 憂悲	love, hate 好憎/惡	attachments lust 嗜欲
ZHUANG ZI Chapter 15	overflow of DAO 道	pernicious energies of DE 德		loss of Heart (XIN 心)	
HUAI NAN ZI Chapter 7	overflow of DAO 道	pernicious energies of DE 德		violence to Heart (XIN 心)	
HUAI NAN ZI Chapter 1	pernicious energies of DAO 道		loss of DE 德	overflow of Heart (XIN 心)	violence to XING 性

---

56 Wieger, Lesson 71

C. Intimate Natures (XING 性) and emotions (QING 情) according to Fundamentals of the Five Elements
(WU XING DA YI 五行大義), Chapter 18

Fundamentals of the Five Elements/Modalities (WU XING DA YI 五行大義), attributed to SHAO YU of the School of Five Elements/Modalities (WU XING 五行), SUI Dynasty (581-618 BC), is a collection of knowledge about Heaven and the stars, Earth and its regions, time and human activity.

左 ZUO								
傳 ZHUAN								
子 ZI	child							
產 CHAN	birth							
云 YUN	say							
則 ZE	from	故 GU	so	因 YIN	as for	生 SHENG	life
天 TIAN	heaven	曰 YUE	says	地 DI	earth	萬 WANG	10.000
之 ZHI	of	明 MING	bright	之 ZHI	of	物 WU	creature
明 MING	bright	也 YE	period	性 XING	Nature	因 YIN	so
天 TIAN	heaven			性 XING	Nature	其 QI	their
有 YOU	have			生 SHENG	generate	所 SUO	which
三 SAN	three			也 YE	period	生 SHENG	generate
光 GUAN	light					而 ER	and
						用 YONG	function
						之 ZHI	of

ZU ZHUAN in the Chapter 'Birth' said: Heaven is lit by the three lights, so it is said that it is brightness.
As for the Intimate Nature (XING 性) of Earth, its Intimate Nature is procreation. It generates Myriad Beings. So its function is procreation.

生	SHENG	generate	五	WU	5	
其	QI	its	行	XING	Modality	
六	LIU	6	者	ZHE	are	
氣	QI		為	WEI	called	
用	YONG	function	五	WU	5	
其	QI	its	性	XING	Nature	
五	WU	5	也	YE	period	
行	XING	Modality				

六	LIU	6
氣	QI	
者	ZHE	are
通	TONG	communicate
六	LIU	6
情	QING	emotion
也	YE	period

(Earth) *generates its six types of* QI 氣 *by means of Five Modalities* (WU XING 五行).

Five Modalities (WU XING 五行) *are the five Intimate Natures* (XING 性).

The six types of QI 氣 *communicate with the six emotions* (QING 情).

翼	YI								
奉	FENG					性	XING	Nature	
云	YUN	said				者	ZHE	are	
五	WU	5	六	LIU	6	仁	REN	humanity	
行	XING	modality	律	LU	tubes	義	YI	justice	
在	ZAI	in	在	ZAI	in	禮	LI	rituals	
人	REN	man	人	REN	man	智	ZHI	wisdom	
為	WEI	are	為	WEI	are	信	XIN	loyalty	
性	XING	Nature	情	QING	emotion	也	YE	period	

情	QING	emotion
者	ZHE	are
喜	XI	joy
怒	NU	anger
樂	LE	pleasure
哀	AI	grief
好	HAO	love
惡	WU	hate
也	YE	period

YI FENG *said: Five Modalities* (WU XING 五行) *of Man are his Intimate Natures* (XING 性).

The six Musical Tubes of Man are his emotions (QING 情).

Intimate Natures (XING 性) *of Man are: humanity, justice, observance of ritual, wisdom and loyalty* (REN YI LI ZHI XIN 仁義禮智信).

The emotions of Man are: joy (XI 喜), *anger* (NU 怒), *pleasure* (LE 樂), *grief* (AI 哀), *love* (HAO 好) *and hate* (WU 惡).

WU XING DA YI, Chapter 18, quotes ZU ZHUAN[57] and presents the three luminaries of Heaven (sun, moon and stars) and the procreative ability of Earth. Then WU XING DA YI, Chapter 18, quotes YI FENG 翼奉.

Under the lights of Heaven, Earth has the ability to generate Myriad Beings by means of Five Modalities with the help of the six types of QI: YANG, YIN, wind, rain, shadow and light (as presented at the end of this chapter). The six types of Earth QI in Man – the six types of vibrations (comparable to the sounds produced by the six musical tubes) - are the music of his six e motions (QING 情): joy (XI 喜), anger (NU 怒), pleasure (LE 樂), grief (AI 哀), love (HAO 好) and hate (WU 惡).

At the level of Heaven, Five Modalities in Man are expressed by means of the five virtues, his Intimate Natures (XING 性): humanity, justice, observance of ritual, wisdom and loyalty (REN YI LI ZHI XIN 仁義禮智信).

REN 仁 - 'humanity', 'kindness', 'benevolence' - is an Intimate Nature, a virtue attributed to Wood-Liver. The character REN 仁 shows 亻 'a man standing' and 二 'the number 2'.[58] REN 仁 denotes the ability to consider others, kindness, good interpersonal communication, the opposite of anger.

YI 義 – justice - is an Intimate Nature, a virtue attributed to Metal-Lung. The character YI 義 shows the radical 羊 'sheep' and the phonetic 我 'two crossed spears' or 'a hand holding a spear', symbolizing conflict.[59] YI 義 is a 'just resolution of a conflict, confirmed by eating a sheep'.

LI 禮 - observance of ritual and tradition, a proper action at the right time - is an Intimate Nature, a virtue attributed to Fire-Heart. The character LI 禮 shows the radical 礻 'influence of the Universe',[60] and the phonetic 豊 'a jug containing legumes to worship and honor

---

57 *The Commentary of* ZUO, that is traditionally regarded as a commentary on the ancient Chinese chronicle *Spring and Autumn Annals* (CHUN QIU 春秋).
58 Wieger, Lesson 2
59 Wieger, Lesson 71
60 The radical 礻 is also a component of the character SHEN 神. See page 13

the ancestors'.⁶¹ LI 禮 conveys an image of communication with the Universe through a ceremony or a ritual.

ZHI 智 - wisdom, intelligence, common sense, discrimination between good and evil - is an Intimate Nature, a virtue attributed to Water-Kidney. The character ZHI 智 shows the radical 日 'a mouth speaking', and the phonetic 知 'knowledge' composed of 矢 'an arrow that hits the target' and 口 another, open 'mouth'.⁶² ZHI 智 conveys the image of a sage saying precise words that hit the target like a short arrow.

XIN 信 - loyalty, trust, honesty, confidence - is an Intimate Nature, a virtue attributed to Soil-Spleen. The character XIN 信 shows 亻 'a man standing' and 言 'word', and conveys the image of a person who stands by his word, someone who can be trusted.⁶³

WU XING DA YI, Chapter 18, continues:

五	WU	5	六	LIU	6
性	XING	Nature	情	QING	emotion
處	CHU	located	處	CHU	located
內	NEI	interior	外	WAI	exterior
御	YU	direct	御	YU	direct
陽	YANG		陰	YIN	
喻	YU	example	喻	YU	example
收	SHOU	gather	收	SHOU	gather
五	WU	5	六	LIU	6
藏	ZANG	organ	體	TI	body tissues

The five Intimate Natures (XING 性) are located inside (the body) and direct YANG, and so they gather the five ZANG.

The six emotions (QING 情) are located outside (the body) and direct YIN, and so they gather the six body tissues.

---

61 Wieger, Lesson 97
62 Wieger, Lesson 131, http://zhongwen.com/d/180/x188.htm
63 Wieger, Lesson 25

故	GU	so					
情	QING	emotion	性	XING	Nature	性 XING	Nature
勝	SHENG	triumph	自	ZI	my	情 QING	emotion
性	XING	Nature	內	NEI	interior	之 ZHI	of
則	ZE	direct	出	CHU	emerge	交 JIAO	intersect
亂	LUAN	disorder	情	QING	emotion	閒 JIAN	interval
性	XING	Nature	從	CONG	from	不 BU	not
勝	SHENG	triumph	外	WAI	exterior	容 RONG	contain
情	QING	emotion	來	LAI	come	系 XI	silk thread
則	ZE	so					
治	ZHI	order					

So, when emotions (QING 情) dominate Intimate Natures (XING 性), there is disorder; when Intimate Natures dominate emotions, there is order.

Intimate Natures (XING 性) emerge from the interior; emotions (QING 情) come from the exterior.

The interval at the intersection between Intimate Natures (XING 性) and emotions (QING 情) does not contain than a silk thread.

Life consists of constant confrontations between Intimate Natures and emotions. Intimate Natures emerge from the interior of the body and direct YANG, bringing wisdom and inner peace. Emotions emerge from the exterior and direct YIN, bringing disorder.

Intimate Natures are associated with ZANG 臟, while emotions are associated with body tissues which communicate with the environment by means of the sense organs.

Intimate Natures and emotions cannot be separated. Could Intimate Natures exist without emotions, or emotions without Intimate Natures?

WU XING DA YI, Chapter 18, quotes an early Chinese dictionary from the HAN Dynasty (SHUO WEN JIE ZI 說文解字):[64]

---

64 Explaining Graphs and Analyzing Characters, 2nd-century

說	SHUO	dictionary	情	QING	emotion	性	XING	Nature
文	WEN		人	REN	man	人	REN	man
曰	YUE	said	之	ZHI	comma	之	ZHI	comma
			陰	YIN		陽	YANG	
			氣	QI		氣	QI	
			有	YOU	have	善	SHAN	good
			欲	YU	desire	者	ZHE	of
			嗜	SHI	attachment	也	YE	period
			也	YE	period			

SHUO WEN *said: emotions* (QING 情) *are the YIN QI of man; they create desires and unhealthy relationships (attachments).*
Intimate Natures (XING 性) *are the YANG QI of man; they are good.*

						故	GU	so
性	XING	Nature	情	QING	emotion	性	XING	Nature
者	ZHE	of	者	ZHE	of	為	WEI	are
人	REN	man	陰	YIN		本	BEN	root
之	ZHI	of	之	ZHI	from	情	QING	emotion
質	ZHI	rich	數	SHU	multitude	為	WEI	are
所	SUO	which	內	NEI	interior	末	MO	branch
稟	BING	gift	傳	CHUAN	transmit			
受	SHOU	receive	著	ZHU	affect			
產	CHAN	birth	流	LIU	flow			
			通	TONG	communicate			
			於	YU	with			
			五	WU	5			
			藏	ZANG	organs			

Intimate Natures (XING 性) *are the precious material in man, the inborn gift which he receives at birth.*
Emotions (QING 情) *are a multitude of YIN. In the interior* (of the body), *they transmit, spread, influence and communicate with five ZANG.*
So Intimate Natures (XING 性) *are the roots, and emotions* (QING 情) *are the branches.*

WU XING DA YI then quotes *Contract to Rescue SHEN (YUAN SHEN QI 援神契)'* from *Classic of Filial Piety (XIAO JING 孝經)*.[65]

Intimate Natures are associated with ZANG; emotions are associated with body tissues but also communicate with five ZANG (Five Modalities):[66]
- Joy (XI 喜) communicates with Heart
- Anger (NU 怒) communicates with Liver
- Grief (AI 哀) communicates with Lung
- Pleasure (LE 樂) (usually associated with Heart) is apparently associated here with Spleen
- Love (HAO 好) and Hate (WU 惡) are apparently associated here with Kidney

性	XING	Nature	情	QING	emotion	動	DONG	movement
主	ZHU	direct	則	ZE	are	靜	JING	serenity
安	AN	peace	主	ZHU	direct	相	XIANG	together
靜	JING	serenity	動	DONG	movement	交	JIAO	intersect
恬	TIAN	in a way	觸	CHU	touch	故	GU	so
然	RAN	so	境	JING	occasion	閒	JIAN	interval
守	SHOU	keep	而	ER	and	微	WEI	subtle
常	CHANG	constancy	變	BIAN	change	密	MI	very tight
						也	YE	period

Intimate Natures (XING 性) direct peace and serenity naturally and keep constancy.
Emotions (QING 情) direct instability. They touch the circumstances and there is change.
Instability and serenity intersect, that is why the interval between them is very subtle and tight.

---

65 Confucian classic treatise, probably dates to the 4th century BC
66 See also page 74 at the end of Chapter 2

Intimate Natures are YANG, roots of man, associated with unity, goodness, peace, serenity, constancy. Intimate Natures are explained as templates of morality in Chinese culture. They emerge from the interior – from five ZANG 臟 - and therefore are **inborn** similarly to all other ZANG 臟 functions.

Emotions are YIN, branches; they cause *desires and unhealthy relationships*; they emerge from the exterior and are **acquired after birth**; they represent instability, but also movement and change, and therefore life. Without emotions there is no life: no dilemmas, no different situations, no existential questions and no creativity. Intimate Natures and emotions are intertwined – the interval between them is very subtle and tight.

The paradox is that YANG (related to the exterior) is inside ZANG 臟, while YIN (related to the interior) explores the outside world. YANG, a symbol of unity, is directed by Intimate Natures; YIN, related to Myriad Beings, is directed by emotions and 'substantial forms'.

WU XING DA YI, Chapter 18, presents a simple and apparently naïve view of life, emphasizing the non-separation between living beings. In a healthy person the body organs keep their virtues (Intimate Natures) by functioning together, assisting each other, and thus assuring homeostasis. Intimate Natures express social ethics, joint activities for the purpose of the common good. Examples of virtues (Intimate Natures) in nature are schools of fish, flocks of migrating birds, or mammals functioning together, assisting each other in order to survive. Body cells cooperate with each other throughout life and decide whether to reproduce or to commit suicide, assuring the life of the organism.[67] This cooperation is especially important during the embryonic development in which there is a constant collaboration between cells to assure cell approximation, separation or suicide. According to Chinese thought, the pregnant mother's body enables the collaboration between Heaven and Earth to ensure a new life.

---

67 Ameisen J. C. *La sculpture du vivant*

Intimate Natures of human physiology, including brain function, may be seen as:

- REN 仁 - 'humanity' - a concern for the best for the entire body,
- LI 禮 - 'observance of ritual' - coordination between intentions and actions,
- XIN 信 - 'loyalty to oneself' or 'honesty' - coordination between what I am and what I express to the outside world,
- YI 義 - 'justice' - the ability to balance instantly any unusual phenomenon in the body,
- ZHI 智 - 'wisdom' - the intelligence of the inherited program (genome) and its ability to adapt to the environment.

HUN 魂 and Intimate Natures (XING 性); **PO 魄 and emotions**
WU XING DA YI, Chapter 18, cites HE SHANG GONG 河上公 (Daoist School), 1st century AD:

河	HE		五	WU	5	六	LIU	6
上	SHANG		性	XING	Nature	情	QING	emotion
公	GONG		之	ZHI	of	之	ZHI	of
章	ZHANG	chapter	鬼	GUI	Earth spirit	鬼	GUI	Earth spirit
句	JU	phrase	曰	YUE	called	曰	YUE	called
云	YUN	said	魂	HUN		魄	PO	
			為	WEI	is	為	WEI	is
			雄	XIONG	masculine	雌	CI	feminine

HE SHANG GONG says: *the Earth spirit* (GUI 鬼) *of the five Intimate Natures* (XING 性) *is called* HUN 魂 *and it is masculine.*
The Earth spirit (GUI 鬼) *of the six emotions* (QING 情) *is called* PO 魄 *and it is feminine.*

The characters HUN 魂 and PO 魄 both include the radical GUI 鬼 'the centrifugal influences of Earth - ghosts, demons, forces of nature or the Earth spirits (*Daimon* in Greek mythology)'.[68]

---

68 See page 31

HUN 魂 is the Earth spirit (GUI 鬼) of male nature, which opens towards the environment and transcends identity with the body. HUN 魂 rules birth, laws, speech and breath. HUN 魂 (which dwells in Liver), symbolized by a dragon, is the ascending phase of SHEN 神, East on the TAI JI symbol, representing acceleration and unity of QI. HUN 魂 is concerned with communication with the other and with the environment, through body movements, language, imagination and dreams. HUN 魂, related to the five Intimate Natures which represent YANG, assures the exteriorization and expansion of Consciousness (SHEN 神) and the drive to communicate.

PO 魄 (which dwells in Lung) represents the descending phase of SHEN 神, West in the TAI JI symbol, opposite HUN 魂 – East. PO 魄 is the Earth spirit (GUI 鬼) of feminine nature which rules the 'substantial forms' (body): fetal development, body formation, deep sleep and death. PO 魄 is related to passivity, separation, fragmentation, aggression and predation. PO 魄, (related, as we saw above, to YIN and to Myriad Beings) is directed by emotions and 'substantial forms' which separate man from his true self.

PO 魄 is involved with life 'for oneself' and maintains life: provides food and air, a protected space (house) and a regular time for withdrawal (sleep). PO 魄 assisted by GUI 鬼 (the Earth spirits), builds and maintains 'substantial forms' (body) by means of the substances essential for body formation and maintenance. These substances also bring into the body extraneous identities, attachments and obstructions. Sometimes GUI 鬼 may be hostile and harmful, and they are described in Daoism as Three Corpses (SAN SHI 三尸) or Three Worms (SAN CHONG 三蟲) which reside in three body parts: abdomen, chest and head.

PO 魄, the feminine aspect of SHEN, is transmitted to the embryo by the mother. In the fertilized egg cell, the influence of the father's genome (DNA and RNA) is in the nucleus.

The mother's DNA and RNA, however, are located both in the nucleus of the fertilized egg cell and also outside the nucleus in the cytoplasm (extranuclear genes). The mother's extranuclear genes determine the cell division of the fetus.[69]

HUN 魂 and PO 魄 according to WU XING DA YI, and the 'fragmentary autonomous psychic systems of the unconscious' of C. Jung

Psychoanalyst C. Jung in *The Commentary on The Secret of the Golden Flower* refers to the fragmentary autonomous psychic systems of the unconscious, which may overwhelm the consciousness and determine human relationships and human activity:

> *Moreover, their autonomy can be observed in daily life, in affects that obstinately obtrude themselves against our will and, in spite of the most strenuous efforts to repress them, overwhelm the ego and force it under their control.*[70]

Jung emphasizes the alienating characteristics of the fragmentary autonomous systems:

> *If tendencies towards dissociation were not inherent in the human psyche, fragmentary psychic systems would never have been split off; in other words, neither spirits nor gods would ever have come into existence. That is also the reason why our time has become so utterly godless and profane: we lack all knowledge of the unconscious psyche and pursue the cult of consciousness to the exclusion of all else. Our true religion is a monotheism of consciousness, a possession by it, coupled with a fanatical denial of the existence of fragmentary autonomous systems. But we differ from the Buddhist yoga doctrines in that we even deny that these systems are experienceable. This entails a great psychic danger, because the autonomous systems behave like any other repressed contents: they necessarily induce wrong attitudes since the repressed material reappears in consciousness in a spurious form.*[71]

---

69 Ameisen J. C. La *Sculpture du Vivant*
70 Jung, C. *The Commentary on The Secret of the Golden Flower*, page 49
71 Jung, C. *The Commentary on The Secret of the Golden Flower*, page 50

According to Jung, autonomous fragmented psychic systems of the unconscious create symbols of the unnatural. Daimon (GUI 鬼) provide an example of symbols in mental life. Jung stresses the importance of the transmission of symbols to consciousness, and the importance of parables for the balance between mental life and bodily function.

Dreams allow us to meet the subconscious mind; HUN 魂 is associated with dreaming. Every night during paradoxical dreams HUN organizes the symbols and parables. Without dreaming, an objective awakened state of mind would become a victim of ghosts from the subconscious.

Jung also emphasizes that the daimon is not related to external factors:
We completely forget that the reason mankind believes in the "daimon" has nothing whatever to do with external factors, but is simply due to a naive awareness of the tremendous inner effect of autonomous fragmentary systems.[72]

PO 魄 is a problematic aspect of the Individual Spirit (SHEN 神) because it anchors 'substantial forms' (body). PO 魄, associated with the six emotions, contributes to body formation and maintenance, but PO 魄 is not identified with the body itself. A human body (a personal space) exists by mandate of Heaven and Earth.

The Secret of the Golden Flower, Chapter 2, discusses the relationship between the anima (PO 魄) and the human body:
Ordinary men make their bodies through thoughts (YI 意). The body is not only the 7 ft. tall outer body… In the body is the anima (PO 魄). The anima (PO 魄), having produced consciousness, adheres to it. Consciousness depends for its origin on the anima (PO 魄). The anima (PO 魄) is feminine, the substance of consciousness. As long as this consciousness is not interrupted, it continues to beget from generation to generation, and the changes of form of the anima (PO 魄) and the transformations of substance are unceasing.[73]

---

72 Jung, C. *The Commentary on The Secret of the Golden Flower,* page 51
73 *The Secret of the Golden Flower*, Wilhelm R.;translated from German by Baynes

WU XING DA YI, Chapter 18, continues and connects the six emotions with the six types of Earth QI:

六 LIU 6	好 HAO love	怒 NU anger	哀 AI grief
氣 QI	為 WEI is	為 WEI is	為 WEI is
通 TONG communicate	陽 YANG	風 FENG wind	晦 HUI darkness
六 LIU 6	惡 WU hate	喜 XI joy	樂 LE pleasure
情 QING emotion	為 WEI is	為 WEI is	為 WEI is
者 ZHE comma	陰 YIN	雨 YU rain	明 MING light

The six types of QI communicate with the six emotions (QING 情).
Love (HAO 好) *is YANG; hate* (WU 惡) *is YIN;*
Anger (NU 怒) *is wind; joy* (XI 喜) *is rain;*
Grief (AI 哀) *is shadow; pleasure* (LE 樂) *is light.*

The six emotions are implanted at the inception of body formation and reflect, at conscious and unconscious levels, traces of fetal life, childhood and adolescence. The six emotions are expressed in various ways during one's lifetime. According to WU XING DA YI, Chapter 18:

1. Love (HAO 好) connects, unifies and represents YANG.

2. Hate (WU 惡) separates, opposes and represents YIN.

3. Anger (NU 怒) represents wind - Wood Modality, *Liver QI 'excess'*, causing an exaggerated ascent of QI and blood to the head, resulting in an imbalance of the nervous and visual systems.

4. Joy (XI 喜), related to Heart, represents rain. In Chinese culture, rain is a metaphor for sexuality. Raining is a symbol of communication between Heaven and Earth, providing water for conception and growth.[74] The character denoting wedding is 囍 'double joy'. Sexual relations provide irrigation which spontaneously allows

---

[74] See page 30

the conception of new life. The character LING 靈, 'spiritual accomplishment', 'approval of 'substantial forms' issued by Heaven and transferred to Earth', includes the radical 雨 'rain'.[75]

5. Grief (AI 哀),[76] related to Lung, is suffering that injures Heart and conceals the joy of life, just as clouds blot out the light.

6. Pleasure (LE 樂), considered to be the pleasure of love. is related to Heart and represents light, brightness (MING 明). The character MING 明 is comprised of 日 'sun' and 月 'moon'.[77]

emotion	love 好	hate 惡	joy 喜	anger 怒	grief 哀	pleasure 樂
WU XING DA YI Chapter 18	YANG connection	YIN separation	rain blessing	wind 'excess' of Liver	shadow	light

Wind and rain lead us to our next chapter, to the text of HUAI NAN ZI 淮南子, in which the influence of the environment and weather on the emotions is investigated.

---

75 Wieger, Lesson 72
76 See page 52 for the character AI 哀
77 Wieger, Lesson 42

3

Emotions, QI of the Universe, lifestyle and society

In ancient China, passions/emotions were considered as emerging from the endless interactions between Man and QI of Heaven and Earth (Universe) - the four seasons and the weather (cold, heat, humidity, dryness and wind). The emotions were also considered to be influenced by lifestyle, food and beverages, a man's personal and family history, and society (cultural influences, virtues and moral values), as seen in the following Chinese texts:
- HUAI NAN ZI 淮南子, Chapter 7 [78]
- SU WEN, Chapter 5
- LING SHU, Chapter 4
- SU WEN, Chapter 77
- NAN JING 難經, Chapter 49 [79]

A. Heaven and Man - QI and emotions
HUAI NAN ZI 淮南子, Chapter 7

HUAI NAN ZI, Chapter 7, compares four parallel types of QI flow in Heaven and in Man:

天	TIAN	heaven	人	REN	man	
有	YOU	has	亦	YI	also	
風	FENG	wind	有	YOU	has	
雨	YU	rain	取	QU	take	
寒	HAN	cold	與	YU	give	
暑	SHU	heat	喜	XI	joy	
			怒	NU	anger	

Heaven has wind, rain, cold and heat.
Man also has the ability of taking and giving, joy and anger (XI NU 喜怒).

---

[78] *The Masters/Philosophers of Huainan*, Chinese philosophical classic from the HAN dynasty (206 BC – 220 AD)
[79] HAN dynasty (206 BC – 220 AD)

Heaven and Man have four parallel types of QI flow:
- Wind blowing things away, and Man's ability to take;
- Rain falling from Heaven (a gift of Heaven), and Man's ability to give;
- Cold which obstructs QI flow, and the introverted YIN type of anger (NU 怒), which causes QI congestion;
- Heat which invigorates QI flow, and joy (XI 喜) which 'warms' Heart, facilitates communication with the environment.

B. Heaven and Man – seasons, QI 氣 and emotions
SU WEN, Chapter 5

天	TIAN heaven	以	YI so	人	REN man	故	GU so	
有	YOU has	生	SHENG generate	有	YOU has	喜	XI joy	
四	SI 4	寒	HAN cold	五	WU 5	怒	NU anger	
時	SHI season	暑	SHU heat	藏	ZANG organs	傷	SHANG damage	
五	WU 5	燥	ZAO dryness	化	HUA transform	氣	QI	
行	XING Modality	溼	SHI humidity	五	WU 5	寒	HAN cold	
以	YI so	風	FENG wind	氣	QI	暑	SHU heat	
生	SHENG birth			以	YI so	傷	SHANG damage	
長	ZHANG grow			生	SHENG generate	形	XING body	
收	SHOU collect			喜	XI joy			
藏	CANG store			怒	NU anger			
				悲	BEI sorrow			
				憂	YOU sadness and worry			
				恐	KONG fear			
				恐	KONG fear			

Heaven has four seasons and Five Modalities (WU XING 五行) *and thus* (there is) *birth, growth, collection and storage, and cold, heat, dryness, dampness and wind are generated.*

Man has five ZANG 藏 *which transform the five* QI 氣 *to generate joy, anger, sorrow, sadness* (accompanied by worry) *and fear* (XI NU BEI YOU KONG 喜怒悲憂恐).

Indeed, joy and anger (XI NU 喜怒) *damage* QI 氣. *Cold and heat damage 'substantial forms'*-body (XING 形).

SU WEN, Chapter 5, describes the nine types of QI of Heaven (generated by four seasons and Five Modalities), the five emotions of Man, and the damage they cause. This Chapter, a hymn to creation, teaches numerology and explains the dialogue between Heaven and Man.

The influence of Heaven is described by the number 9 (4 types of QI corresponding to seasons and 5 types of QI corresponding to Modalities): birth, growth, collection, storage, cold, heat, dryness, dampness and wind.

Man functions according to the number 5 (5 Modalities operate through 5 ZANG organs). The 5 ZANG (which build the body) are expressed by the 5 emotions:
- Joy (XI 喜)
- Anger (NU 怒)
- Sorrow (BEI 悲)
- Sadness (accompanied by worry) (YOU 憂)
- Fear (KONG 恐)

QI of Heaven and emotions may damage Man:
- QI generated by Heaven: cold and heat damage the 'substantial forms' (body) by affecting Lung, Kidney and Spleen function.
- QI of Man: the emotions joy (XI 喜) and anger (NU 怒) damage harmonious QI flow. Joy affects Heart and anger affects Liver, causing excess of QI in Upper JIAO – the chest and head.

C. Influence of emotions and cold on man,
LING SHU, Chapter 4

Interior or exterior cold (QI of Water Modality) contracts Lung-Metal (Reversed Generation) and damages its function of lowering. Damage to Lung by exterior cold is caused by cold weather or the consumption of cold food or beverages. Damage to Lung by interior cold is caused by two pairs of long-lasting emotions which slow the QI flow and 'cool' the body:

- Melancholy (CHOU 愁), sadness accompanied by worry (YOU 憂) (damage Heart, Lung and Spleen),
- Fear (KONG 恐) and dread (JU 懼) (damage Heart and Kidney).

LING SHU, Chapter 4, describes the damage caused by the combination of emotions and cold on Lung function:

愁	CHOU	melancholy	形	XING	form	以	YI	
憂	YOU	sadness	寒	HAN	cold	其	QI	therefore
恐	KONG	fear	寒	HAN	cold	兩	LIANG	both
懼	JU	dread	飲	YIN	drink	寒	HAN	cold
則	ZE	this	則	ZE	this	相	XIANG	interact
傷	SHANG	damage	傷	SHANG	damage	感	GAN	influence
心	XIN	heart	肺	FEI	lung	中	ZHONG	center
						外	WAI	exterior
						皆	JIE	all
						傷	SHANG	damage

故	GU	so
氣	QI	
逆	NI	rebel
而	ER	and
上	SHANG	ascend
形	XING	body

Melancholy, sadness (accompanied by worry), *fear and dread* (CHOU YOU KONG JU 愁憂恐懼) *damage Heart-Consciousness* (XIN 心).
Cooling the body and drinking cold beverages damage Lung.
Therefore these two types of cold interact and damage the center and the exterior (of the body).
So rebel QI (QI NI 氣逆, counterflow QI, which flows in a contrary direction) *ascends to the upper body.*

These two types of cold (the four emotions and body cold) combine together and damage QI flow in the body center (Heart-Consciousness) and on the surface (Lung-skin). Lung, the prime minister of the body, does not function properly – cannot enable the descent of QI and body liquids. Lung QI 'rebels' (QI NI 氣逆), flows upwards, against the direction of the normal flow of Lung QI causing respiratory distress. LING SHU, Chapter 4, describes Rebel Lung (QI NI 氣逆) syndrome, expressed as dyspnea (difficulty or shortness of breath) or slow breathing (for example, during an asthma attack).

D. Influence of emotions, life events and interaction with society, SU WEN, Chapter 77

凡	FAN	usually	雖	SUI	although	嘗	CHANG	experience	五	WU	5
未	WEI	not	不	BU	not	富	FU	rich	氣	QI	
診	ZHEN	examine	中	ZHONG	center	後	HOU	after	留	LIU	stagnate
病	BING	disease	邪	XIE	evil	貧	PIN	poor	連	LIAN	cause
者	ZHE	comma	病	BING	disease	名	MING	called	病	BING	disease
必	BI	necessary	從	CONG	towards	曰	YUE	said	有	YOU	have
問	WEN	ask	內	NEI	interior	失	SHI	loss	所	SUO	or
嘗	CHANG	experience	生	SHENG	create	精	JING		并	BING	combine
貴	GUI	high rank	名	MING	called						
後	HOU	after	曰	YUE	said						
賤	JIAN	low rank	脫	TUO	spoil						
			營	YING	nourish						

Usually, before a patient is examined, he should be asked whether he has experienced low rank after high rank (lost social status). *Even if he has not been influenced by external pernicious factors, this* (loss of status) *can cause an internal disease called* TUO YING 脫營 *(spoliation of Nourishing QI).*

If he had been rich and has become poor, it is called SHI JING 失精 (loss of JING). *The five types of QI stagnate and together cause disease.*

凡 FAN usually	暴 BAO sudden	皆 JIE together	厥 JUE its
欲 YU desire	樂 LE pleasure	傷 SHANG damage	氣 QI
診 ZHEN examine	暴 BAO sudden	精 JING	上 SHANG up
病 BING disease	苦 KU suffering	氣 QI	行 XING circulate
者 ZHE of	始 SHI begin	暴 BAO sudden	滿 MAN fill
必 BI have to	樂 LE pleasure	怒 NU anger	脈 MAI vessels
問 WEN ask	後 HOU after	傷 SHANG damage	去 QU leave
飲 YIN drink	苦 KU suffer	陰 YIN	形 XING body
食 SHI food		暴 BAO sudden	
居 JU living		喜 XI joy	
處 CHU place		傷 SHANG damage	
		陽 YANG	

Usually, if you want to examine a patient, you need to ask him about his beverages, food, residence, sudden pleasures and sudden suffering, about pleasures which bring suffering.

All these damage JING QI 精氣 *(*QI *which carries* JING*). Sudden anger (*NU 怒*) damages* YIN*; sudden joy (*XI 樂*) damages* YANG*.*

(Anger causes) the QI *flow to ascend. (Joy causes) overflow in the meridians and blood vessels (*MAI 脈*), and (*SHEN*) leaves the body.*

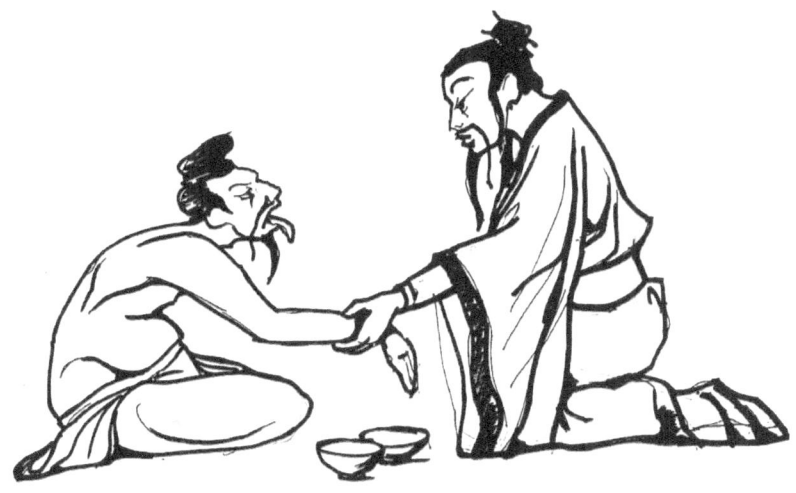

診 ZHEN	examine	故 GU	so	始 SHI	begin	醫 YI	doctor
有 YOU	has	貴 GUI	high rank	富 FU	rich	不 BU	not
三 SAN	3	脫 TUO	take away	後 HOU	after	能 NENG	able
常 CHANG	constant	勢 SHI	lost	貧 PIN	poor	嚴 YAN	rectify
必 BI	necessary	雖 SUI	although	雖 SUI	although	不 BU	not
問 WEN	ask	不 BU	not	不 BU	not	能 NENG	able
貴 GUI	high rank	中 ZHONG	center	傷 SHANG	damage	動 DONG	move
賤 JIAN	low rank	邪 XIE	pernicious	邪 XIE	pernicious	神 SHEN	
封 FENG	investigate	精 JING		皮 PI	skin		
君 JUN	prince	神 SHEN		焦 JIAO	burn		
敗 BAI	injure	內 NEI	interior	筋 JIN	tendon		
傷 SHANG	damage	傷 SHANG	damage	屈 QU	flex		
及 JI	till	身 SHEN	body	痿 WEI	paralysis, muscle flaccidity		
欲 YU	desire	必 BI	necessary	躄 BI	rheumatism		
侯 HOU	push	敗 BAI	damage	為 WEI	make		
王 WANG	king	亡 WANG	destruct	攣 LUAN	contracted		

Examination of the patient includes three constants (the Three Treasures: JING, QI, SHEN). *The patient should be asked about his social status* (high or low), *damage to his dignity, and his ambition to improve social status.*

Loss of high social status, even without the influence of external pernicious factors, damages JING SHEN 精神 (SHEN carrying JING) *in the interior* (of the body), *and leads to unavoidable damage and destruction of the body.*

If the patient had been rich and became poor, even if there was no influence of external pernicious factors, his skin burns, his tendons are flexed; muscular flaccidity (WEI 痿) *and rheumatism* (BI 躄) *cause limb contractions.*

If the physician is unable to rectify (the patient), *he cannot move the patient's* SHEN 神.

離 LI separation	憂 YOU sadness	血 XUE blood	工 GONG work
絕 JUE break up	恐 KONG fear	氣 QI	不 BU not
菀 YU regret	喜 XI joy	離 LI separation	能 NENG capable
結 JIE knot	怒 NU anger	守 SHOU keep	知 ZHI know
	五 WU 5		何 HE what
	藏 ZANG organs		術 SHU are
	空 KONG hollow		之 ZHI its
	虛 XU empty		語 YU manifestation

Separations cause remorse and stagnation.
Sadness (accompanied by worry), *fear, joy and anger* (YOU KONG XI NU 憂恐喜怒) *empty five* ZANG. *Blood and* QI *leave their right place. If the physician does not know all that* (how to question the patient), *what kind of art does he practice?*

SU WEN, Chapter 77, proposes the questioning of the patient with regard to social events in his life and his emotions, and presents the damage caused by emotions and unfavorable events in social life. The causes of disease have not changed much since the time when this chapter was written. The physician must obtain information from the patient about:
- The Three Treasures (SAN BAO 三寶: JING 精, QI 氣, SHEN 神),[80]
- Nutrition, beverages,
- Residence,
- Sudden traumatic events (both happy and those causing suffering),
- Social and economic status, changes in social status, bankruptcy, social ambitions,
- Separations,
- Emotions: sadness accompanied by worry, fear, joy and anger (YOU KONG XI NU 憂恐喜怒).

According to SU WEN, Chapter 77, the types of damage caused by emotions are:

---

80 The Three Treasures are the condition for Man's existence.

- Sudden anger (NU 怒) damages YIN. The ascent of Liver YANG QI exhausts and damages YIN - the lower body (pelvis, lower abdomen).
- Sudden joy (XI 喜) damages YANG - the flow of QI and Blood in vessels. SHEN 神, related to Blood, is injured and leaves the body.
- Sadness (accompanied by worry, YOU 憂), fear (KONG 恐), joy (XI 喜) and anger (NU 怒) exhaust the five ZANG. ZANG do not function properly and Blood and QI are damaged.

E. Influence of emotions and lifestyle on the five ZANG
NAN JING, Chapter 49

憂 YOU	sadness	恚 HUI	rage	飲 YIN	drink	久 JIU	long
愁 CHOU	melancholy	怒 NU	anger	食 SHI	food	坐 ZUO	sit
思 SI	thought	氣 QI		勞 LAO	tired	濕 SHI	humid
慮 LU	worry	逆 NI	rebel	倦 JUAN	exhaust	地 DI	earth
則 ZE	this	上 SHANG	up	則 ZE	this	強 QIANG	
傷 SHANG	damage	而 ER	and	傷 SHANG	damage	力 LI	force
心 XIN	heart	不 BU	not	脾 PI	spleen	入 RU	enter
形 XING	body	下 XIA	down			水 SHUI	water
寒 HAN	cold	則 ZE	this			則 ZE	this
飲 YIN	drink	傷 SHANG	damage			傷 SHANG	damage
冷 LENG	cold	肝 GAN	liver			腎 SHEN	kidneys
則 ZE	this						
傷 SHANG	damage						
肺 FEI	lung						

Sadness (accompanied by worry), *melancholy, excessive thinking and worry* (YOU CHOU SI LU 憂愁思慮) *damage Heart-Consciousness* (XIN 心). *Cold in the body and cold beverages damage Lung.*

Rage and anger (HUI NU 恚怒) *cause the upward flow of rebel QI* (QI NI 氣逆, which flows in an exaggerated fashion in the correct direction) *with no descent, and damage Liver.*

Beverages and food (in exaggeration), *physical fatigue and exhaustion damage Spleen.*

Sitting for a long time on damp ground or forcing oneself to enter (cold) *water damage Kidney.*

NAN JING, Chapter 49, repeats LING SHU, Chapter 4, adding some information and specifying the effects of emotions, weather and lifestyle on the function of the five ZANG.

Heart and Liver are injured by emotions. Damage to Lung, Spleen and Kidney is caused by the weather and by inappropriate behavior.

❖ *Sadness* (accompanied by worry), *melancholy, excessive thinking and worry* (YOU CHOU SI LU 憂愁慮思) *damage Heart-Consciousness* (XIN 心).

LING SHU, Chapter 4, and NAN JING, Chapter 49, both describe damage to Heart-Consciousness caused by two pairs of emotions. The first pair of emotions, sadness and melancholy (YOU CHOU 憂愁) which injure PO 魄 and Heart-Consciousness, is similar in both texts.

The second pair of emotions which damages Heart-Consciousness differs in the two texts:
- Fear and dread (KONG JU 恐懼) damage Kidney-ZHI 志 and destabilize SHEN 神 and Heart-Consciousness (LING SHU, 4);
- Excessive thinking and worry (SI LU 思慮)[81] damage Spleen-YI 意 and destabilize SHEN 神 and Heart-Consciousness (NAN JING, 49).

❖ *Cold in the body and cold beverages damage Lung.*

LING SHU, Chapter 4, and NAN JING, Chapter 49, show that cold injures Lung. Dryness is QI of Metal and cold is QI of Water (Metal generates Water). Lung and Kidney are sensitive to both dryness and cold. External cold or food and beverages that cool the body impair the Lung-Metal functions (Reversed Generation):
- regulation of QI flow on skin - body surface - border with the environment
- absorption of QI from the air
- descent of QI and body liquids
- evacuation of waste by Large Intestine

---

81 For the etymology of the character LU 慮 see page 128

❖ *Rage and anger* (HUI NU 恚怒) *cause upward flow of rebel QI (QI NI 氣逆) with no descent, and damage Liver.*

HUN 魂, stored in Liver, governs relations with the exterior by means of the balanced flow of JING QI 精氣 (QI which transfers JING and maintains life) upwards and towards the exterior. The upward flow of JING QI 精氣 from Lower JIAO (Kidney) to Upper JIAO (Heart, chest, throat and head) establishes the essential harmonious link between Water and Fire. Sudden or prolonged rage and anger (HUI NU 恚怒, caused by frustration, conflicts and misunderstandings in relationships with people, with the environment or with oneself) provoke the exaggerated ascent towards Upper JIAO - rebel QI (QI NI 氣逆). As a result, Liver is unable to link Water-Kidney and Heart-Fire. Rebel QI (QI NI 氣逆) resulting from anger is expressed as the excessive ascent of Liver YANG QI and Liver Blood, causing a disorganized overflow in the chest and head manifesting as tension in the diaphragm, thorax and head or high blood pressure, and an ensuing deficiency in the lower body (Kidney).

❖ *Drinks and food, physical fatigue* (LAO 勞) *and mental exhaustion* (JUAN 倦) *damage Spleen.*

The function of Spleen is the absorption of Nourishing QI (RONG/YING 榮/營), flavors and liquids from food and beverages which enter Stomach:

- Nourishing QI (RONG/YING 榮/營) flows in meridians, participates in blood production and nourishes the body,
- The five flavors build the body tissues,
- Body liquids irrigate the body.

Spleen is injured by:
- Overeating and overdrinking, or unsuitable food and beverages,
- Physical fatigue (LAO 勞) following overuse of the four limbs (which are controlled by Spleen),
- Mental exhaustion (JUAN 倦) following excessive thinking, overuse of memory and intent (YI 意).

Injury to Spleen causes insufficient absorption, which damages the nourishment of the body and the four limbs, and also injures the balance maintained by Spleen and Stomach between clear (QING 清 - food ingredients which can be used directly - Nourishing QI, flavors, water) and turbid (ZHOU 濁 - complex food ingredients which need to be transformed to be used or to be excreted).

SU WEN, Chapter 29, describes the damage to Spleen and Stomach:
When the spleen has a disease and the four limbs do not function, how is that?" Qi Bo: "All the four limbs are supplied with qi by the stomach, but [the stomach qi] is unable to reach the conduits [directly]. It is only because of the spleen that the [four limbs] get their supplies. Now, when the spleen has a disease and is unable to move the body liquids on behalf of the stomach, the four limbs are not supplied with the qi of water and grain. [Their] qi weakens day by day; the vessel paths are no [longer] passable. The sinews and the bones, the muscles and the flesh, none of them has qi to live. Hence, they do not function."[82]

SU WEN, Chapter 21, also describes damage to Spleen and Stomach:

故	GU	thus	搖	YAO	move
飲	YIN	drink	體	TI	body
食	SHI	food	勞	LAO	fatigue
飽	BAO	to eat till full	苦	KU	suffering, bitterness
甚	SHEN	much	汗	HAN	sweat
汗	HAN	sweat	出	CHU	comes
出	CHU	comes	於	YU	from
於	YU	from	脾	PI	spleen
胃	WEI	stomach			

Indeed, overeating causes sweat which comes out of Stomach.
Moving the body with fatigue and suffering (hard work) *causes sweat which comes out of Spleen.*

---

82 Translation by Unschuld, P. U. and Tessenow, H.

According to SU WEN, Chapter 21, overeating damages Stomach, while suffering and fatigue resulting from hard work damage Spleen. A sign of damage to the organ is 'empty' sweat, caused by deficiency of Defensive QI (WEI QI 衛氣), which can no longer maintain the flow of body liquids beneath the skin.

❖ *Sitting for a long time on damp ground and forcing oneself to enter* (cold) *water damage Kidney.*

Sitting for a long time on damp ground allows the cold dampness to penetrate the body through the bottom of the pelvis and the perineum. Dampness is the QI of Spleen-Soil. Dampness-Soil 'over-controls' Water and damages Kidney.

Kidney is particularly sensitive to cold water which slows QI flow in the body. The body is a person's responsibility, but it does not belong to the person. Life is based on JING 精 storage by Kidney. Forcing oneself to enter cold water requires overuse of will (ZHI 志) and therefore disturbs the balance of JING 精 storage and damages Kidney.

4

LING SHU, Chapter 8, *Roots of* SHEN (BEN SHEN 本神)
Life stages and development of Consciousness

LING SHU, Chapter 8, *Roots of* SHEN (BEN SHEN 本神), starts with an explanation of the importance of SHEN 神 in acupuncture, and continues with thirteen entities of human existence, presented in a specific order. These thirteen fundamental entities of Chinese philosophy are difficult to translate, but they may be compared with concepts in modern psychology and neurology. This chapter investigates Man according to the Trinity of Powers (SAN CAI 三才) - Heaven, Earth and Man (see Figure 12):

- Man on the subtle (non-material) level of Heaven (Upper Level) is represented by five aspects/roots of SHEN 神 (BEN SHEN 本神) - the organizers of human life,
- Man at the level of Man (Middle Level), links the subtle influence of SHEN 神 with 'substantial forms' and is expressed by means of the five emotions.
- Man at the level of Earth, the level of 'substantial forms' (Lower Level) is represented by the functions of the five ZANG 臟, which form the body by means of QI, Blood, five flavors and liquids.

A. *The first step in the art of acupuncture is rooting in* SHEN 神, LING SHU, Chapter 8-1

黃	HUANG	yellow	凡	FAN	usually
帝	DI	emperor	刺	CI	needle
問	WEN	ask	之	ZHI	auxiliary word
於	YU	of	法	FA	law
岐	QI		先	XIAN	before
伯	BO		必	BI	necessary
曰	YUE	say	本	BEN	root
			于	YU	of
			神	SHEN	

The Yellow Emperor asked QI BO saying: *The first law in the art of acupuncture is the necessity of rooting in* SHEN (BEN YU SHEN 本于神).

LING SHU, Chapter 8-1,[83] starts with the Yellow Emperor's question to his teacher QI BO about the first law of acupuncture, described as 'rooting' or 'anchoring' in SHEN (BEN YU SHEN 本于神).

In the art of acupuncture, SHEN 神 directs all stages of the encounter between the therapist and his patient, from the first meeting of eyes to the insertion and removal of the needles. Every treatment is based on the relationship between SHEN 神 of the therapist and SHEN 神 of the patient, and in this meeting SHEN 神 of the relationship is born, providing the understanding of the patient's *Roots of SHEN* (BEN SHEN 本神). The importance of SHEN 神 in Chinese medicine is emphasized also in SU WEN, Chapters 13, 27 and 54.

- SU WEN, **Chapter 13**. SHEN 神 is the acme of the art of therapy
According to SU WEN, Chapter 13, SHEN 神 is Unity/oneness (YI 一) to which the therapist must aspire in his contact with the patient in order to treat successfully by means of Chinese medicine.

岐 QI				岐 QI			
伯 BO	帝 DI	emperor	伯 BO		帝 DI	emperor	
曰 YUE	say	曰 YUE	say	曰 YUE	say	曰 YUE	say
治 ZHI	treatment	何 HE	what	一 YI	one	奈 NAI	how
之 ZHI	auxiliary word	謂 WEI	called	者 ZHE	is	何 HE	what way
極 JI	top	一 YI	one	因 YIN	cause		
於 YU	at			得 DE	obtain		
一 YI	one			之 ZHI	this		

QI BO said: *The priority of the art of therapy is oneness* (YI 一).
The emperor said: *What is oneness* (YI 一)?
QI BO said: *Oneness* (YI 一) *is to be obtained.*
The emperor said: *How* (is this oneness obtained)?

---

83 This paragraph of LING SHU, Chapter 8, *Roots of SHEN* (BEN SHEN 本神) is referred to in this book as LING SHU, Chapter 8-1

岐	QI		數 SHU	often	
伯	BO		問 WEN	ask	
曰	YUE	say	其 QI	of	
閉	BI	close	情 QING	emotions	
戶	HU	door	以 YI	in order to	
塞	SAI	block	從 CONG	follow	
牖	YOU	window	其 QI	his	
系	XI	connect	意 YI	ideas, intents	
之	ZHI	to			
病	BING	sick, disease			
者	ZHE	comma			

得 DE	obtain	
神 SHEN		
者 ZHE	is	
昌 CHANG	good	
失 SHI	lose	
神 SHEN		
者 ZHE	is	
亡 WANG	perish, death	

QI BO *said: close the doors and block the windows, relate to the patient.*

Ask (the patient) *about his emotions* (QING 情) *in order to know his state of mind* (intent) (YI 意).

Obtaining (contact) *with his* SHEN 神 *is good; losing his* SHEN 神 *is to perish.*

• SU WEN, **Chapter 27**: keeping SHEN 神 inside the body in acupuncture
It is important to 'close the acupuncture point' (press on the point with the finger) after pulling the needle out, to keep SHEN inside the body. SHEN is present in all acupuncture points.

外	WAI	outside	以 YI	to	
引	YIN	acupuncture point	閉 BI	close	
其	QI	his	其 QI	his	
門	MEN	door	神 SHEN		

From the outside, close the door of the acupuncture point to enclose SHEN 神.

• SU WEN, **Chapter 54**. The state of mind of the practitioner of acupuncture

SU WEN, Chapter 54, states that the practitioner of acupuncture should be in a state of mind *as if one looked down into a deep abyss,'* that is, do not dare to be careless....the hand [must be strong] *as if it held a tiger*;[84] and also later emphasizes that the eye contact between physician and patient is of the utmost importance, since it allows communication between SHEN 神 of the physician and SHEN 神 of the patient, enabling the required treatment.

必 BI	need	欲 YU	desire	制 ZHI	adjust	氣 QI	
正 ZHENG	rectitude	瞻 ZHAN	look	其 QI	his	易 YI	easy
其 QI	his	病 BING	sick	神 SHEN		行 XING	circulate
神 SHEN		人 REN	man	令 LING	control	也 YE	period
者 ZHE	comma	目 MU	eye				

When (the patient's) SHEN 神 *needs to be rectified*, (the physician) *should look into his eyes.*
When (the patient's) SHEN 神 *has been regulated, QI can flow easily.*

B. The Yellow Emperor's questions, LING SHU, Chapter 8-1

After emphasizing the importance of 'rooting' in SHEN 神 in all therapeutic communication, the Yellow Emperor's questions were about:

- The six vital aspects necessary for the function of the five ZANG 藏/臟
- The injury to BEN SHEN 本神 resulting from an inappropriate lifestyle
- How to define the thirteen fundamental entities concerning the existence of Man

The six vital aspects are stored in the five ZANG 藏/臟:
1. XUE 血, Blood
2. MAI 脈, blood vessels and conduits
3. YING 營, Nourishing QI
4. QI 氣, all functions of five ZANG
5. SHEN 神, Individual Spirit, Individual Consciousness
6. JING 精, fundamental vitality

---

84 Translation by Unschuld, P. U. and Tessenow, H.

血	XUE	blood	至	ZHI	concern	何	HE	which	何	HE	which
脈	MAI	vessels	其	QI	its	因	YIN	cause	謂	WEI	called
營	YING	nourish	淫	YIN		而	ER	is	德	DE	virtue
氣	QI		泆	YI	lechery	然	RAN	such	氣	QI	
精	JING		離	LI	separate	乎	HU	?	生	SHENG	life
神	SHEN		藏	ZANG	organs	天	TIAN	heaven	精	JING	
此	CI	that	則	ZE	so	之	ZHI	comma	神	SHEN	
五	WU	5	精	JING		罪	ZUI	crime	魂	HUN	
藏	ZANG	organs	失	SHI	lost	與	YU	?	魄	PO	
之	ZHI	that is	魂	HUN		人	REN	man	心	XIN	consciousness
所	SUO	what	魄	PO		之	ZHI	of	意	YI	intent
藏	CANG	store	飛	FEI	fly	過	GUO	error	志	ZHI	will
			揚	YANG	scatter	乎	HU	?	思	SI	thought
			志	ZHI					智	ZHI	wisdom
			意	YI					慮	LU	contemplation
			恍	HUANG	confuse				請	QING	please
			亂	LUAN	disorder				問	WEN	ask
			智	ZHI	wisdom				其	QI	its
			慮	LU	contemplation				故	GU	cause
			去	QU	leave						
			身	SHEN	body						
			者	ZHE	comma						

Blood (XUE 血) *and blood vessels* (MAI 脈), *Nourishing* (QI) (YING 營) *and QI* 氣, *JING* 精 *and SHEN* 神 *these are what the five ZANG* 藏 *store. However, a life full of luxury and exaggeration depletes ZANG, and so JING* 精 *is lost, HUN* 魂 *and PO* 魄 *fly away and scatter, YI* 意 *and ZHI* 志 *are in confusion and disorder, wisdom* (ZHI 智) *and contemplation* (LU 慮) *disappear from the body.*

What is the reason for all this? Is this the crime of Heaven? Is Man at fault?

What are DE 德, QI 氣, *life* (SHENG 生), JING 精, SHEN 神, HUN 魂, PO 魄, *Heart-Consciousness* (XIN 心), YI 意, ZHI 志, *thought* (SI 思), *wisdom* (ZHI 智), *contemplation* (LU 慮)? *May I ask you about the reason for this?*

Nourishing QI (YING 營) and Blood (XUE 血) distributed by conduits-meridians and blood vessels (MAI 脈) nourish the five ZANG 藏/臟,

allowing their function and communication with each other and the environment. The Three Treasures (SAN BAO 三寶: JING, QI and SHEN) are the basic condition for the existence of every living creature, and of the five ZANG 藏/臟:

- The accumulation of JING 精 in ZANG 藏/臟 is the condition for their formation and function
- Each of the five ZANG 藏/臟 has its QI 氣 which defines its function
- SHEN 神 is BEN SHEN 本神 stored in each ZANG 臟

Myself-body exists and functions by the laws of Heaven and Earth. A luxurious lifestyle injures vital reservoirs of ZANG 藏/臟: JING 精 and BEN SHEN 本神: there is no willpower, there is confusion of ideas and a loss of contact with reality. The Yellow Emperor wants to know whether the reason for this deterioration is in Heaven or in the errors of man. He also wants to understand the meaning of the thirteen fundamental entities of man's existence. We shall follow the explanations and development of these thirteen entities in the order in which they appear in the text, and interpret them using the TAI JI symbol.

The thirteen entities of man's existence are:
1. DE 德, virtue, the mandate of life
2. QI 氣, energy, all types of movement
3. SHENG 生, life
4. JING 精, fundamental vitality
5. SHEN 神, Individual Spirit, Individual Consciousness
6. HUN 魂, Wood aspect of SHEN, related to father and birth
7. PO 魄, Metal aspect of SHEN, related to mother, body and fetal life
8. XIN 心, Heart-Consciousness
9. YI 意, Soil aspect of SHEN, intent, ideas
10. ZHI 志, Water aspect of SHEN, will, determination
11. SI 思, thought, thinking process
12. LU 慮, contemplation
13. ZHI 智, intelligence, wisdom

C. QI BO replies.
The first phase. Entities 1, 2, 3: DE 德, QI 氣, **life** (SHENG 生).
Spontaneous eruption of individualized life guided by Heaven and Earth (Figure 28)

岐 QI					
伯 BO					
答 DA answer					
曰 YUE say					
天 TIAN heaven	地 DI earth	德 DE virtue
之 ZHI auxiliary word	之 ZHI auxiliary word	流 LIU flow down
在 ZAI inside	在 ZAI inside	氣 QI
我 WO me	我 WO me	薄 BO abundance
者 ZHE comma	者 ZHE comma	而 ER and
德 DE virtue	氣 QI	生 SHENG life
也 YE period	也 YE period	也 YE period

QI BO *answered and said: Heaven* (TIAN 天) *in me* (WO 我) *is* DE 德, *Earth* (DI 地) *in me* (WO 我) *is* QI 氣.
DE 德 *flows downwards,* QI *blooms and this is life* (SHENG 生).

Figure 28. Heaven in me is DE 德, **Earth in me is** QI 氣.
DE **flows downwards,** QI **blooms and this is life.**

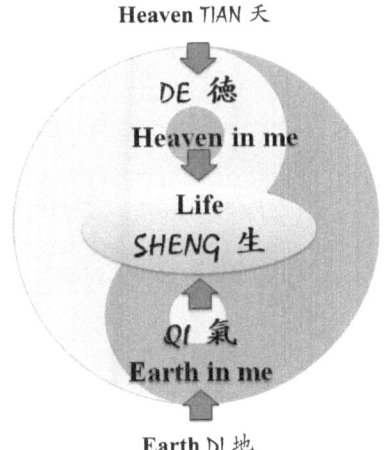

The first entity, DE 德 - Heaven in Man

Heaven (TIAN 天) in me (WO 我) is DE 德 - describes DE 德 (virtue, mandate of life, permission to live) as the link between Universal-Heaven-DAO 道 and individual-Man-myself. Heaven is not only above Man, it is everywhere around him and inside him. According to the Daoist treatise XI MING:

At the origin of the great emptiness there is the name of Heaven[85] *(YOU TAI XU ER TIAN ZHI YOU MING 由太虛而天之有名)*

Heaven is the source of the spontaneous natural movement (ZI RAN 自然) of every being from birth to death, and of all things from appearance to disappearance. Man is the witness of the vast reality - Universe. However, to be myself is to be in conflict. The character WO 我 'me, myself' shows 扌 'hand holding' 戈 'a spear', symbolizing a conflict.[86]

Figure 29. The character DE 德 **'virtue', 'efficiency', link from** DAO 道 **to Man, in ancient seal and classical script**

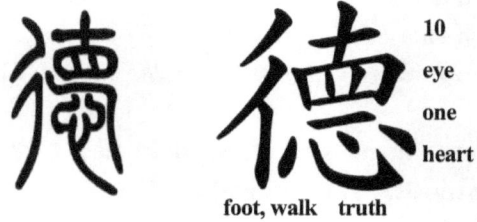

DE 德 is the direct link from Heaven (oneness-DAO 道) to Man, permission to exist which man receives from Heaven constantly throughout his lifetime. The character DE 德 shows the radical 彳 'left foot', 'a walk'. The phonetic 悳 'truth' or 'morality' shows 直 'integrity' or 'standing erect' above 心 'heart'. The character 直 'integrity' shows 十 'ten' 目 'eyes' (horizontal version) that see YI 一 'the One', 'the Unity', 'oneness' (Figure 29).[87] DE 德 is 'walking the path of truth, virtue, righteousness, efficiency'.

---

85 Quoted from ZHANG ZAI 張載 (SONG dynasty, 1020-1077) - ZHENG MENG, TAI HE BIEN DI YI, Chapter 1
86 Weiger, Lesson 71
87 Weiger, Lesson 10

Heaven interacts with Man and with all beings and things through DE 德. Every entity, every living being without exception, has DE 德. ZHUANG ZI, Chapter 12, describes DE 德 as continuous personal contact (without-rupture) of all beings with the oneness - the Universe:

泰 TAI	Supreme	一 YI	one	物 WU	being
初 CHU	Beginning	之 ZHI	auxiliary word	得 DE	obtain
有 YOU	to have, to be	所 SUO	this	以 YI	particle
無 WU	negation, void	起 QI	start	生 SHENG	life
無 WU	negation, void	有 YOU	has	謂 WEI	called
有 YOU	to have, to be	一 YI	one	之 ZHI	auxiliary word
無 WU	negation, void	而 ER	and	德 DE	
名 MING	name	未 WEI	negation		
		形 XING	substantial form		

In the Grand Beginning (of all things) there is nothing (YOU WU 有無), there is no being (WU YOU 無有) and no name (WU MING 無名). From there emerges oneness (YI 一). There is oneness, but there are no 'substantial forms' (XING 形).
Beings and things receive (oneness) and are born. This is called DE 德.

DE 德 has no tension, no contradiction and no conflict; it is initial, personal and permanent throughout a lifetime, a beneficent flow from Heaven, like water, as in DAO DE JING, Chapter 8:
The highest excellence is like (that of) water. The excellence of water appears in its benefiting all things ... without striving (to the contrary).[88]

The second entity, QI 氣 - Earth in Man

Earth (DI 地) in me (WO 我) is QI 氣 (Figure 28). Earth represents a multitude of 'substantial forms'. In ancient Chinese thought there was no contradiction between QI (movement and transformation) and 'substantial forms' (matter). DE 德 flows from Heaven which is without 'substantial forms' and connects Man with DAO 道. QI 氣 is unstable, continuous movement without a rupture, constantly changing direction (ascending and descending, scattering and gathering),

---

88 Translation by Legge.,J

creating and destroying 'substantial forms'. QI-movements, which unify or separate, are expressed either simultaneously or alternating, either in a single life form or among different life forms.

The Daoist treatise ZUN SHENG BA JIAN presents QI as the source of body (TI 體): QI is the *plentitude of body* (TI 體).[89]
(QI ZHE TI ZHI CHONG YE 氣者體之充也).

Once I have received my mandate to live (DE 德) from Heaven, my QI 氣, coming from Earth, flows in me, creates my body and directs my destiny (MING 命). Kidney YANG, called the Gate of Destiny (MING MEN 命門),[90] directs the expression of all body QI with the help of Source QI (YUAN QI 原氣/元氣).

According to ZHUANG ZI, Chapter 12:

未	WEI	negation	且	QIE	this
形	XING	substantial forms	然	RAN	thus
者	ZHE	of	無	WU	negation
有	YOU	make	間	JIAN	interval
分	FEN	split, separation	謂	WEI	called
			之	ZHI	auxiliary word
			命	MING	destiny

In the absence of 'substantial forms' (XING 形) separation is formed. Thus appears 'without-rupture', which is called destiny (MING 命).

ZHUANG ZI, Chapter 12, defines destiny (MING 命) as *'without-rupture'* and does not use the character QI 氣. However, destiny (MING 命) appears in this text after the beginning of separation, which is change, movement (QI 氣).

DE 德 flows down from oneness (YI 一), which is neither QI nor 'substantial form'. A separation occurs in this oneness. This separation can be compared to a crack in a vase. The vase does not lose its shape,

---

89 *Eight Discourses on the Art of Living*, ZUN SHENG BA JIAN 遵生八牋, GAO LIAN 高濂, 16th century
90 See page 44

and does not fall apart, but it has a crack. Destiny (MING 命), this crack, 'rupture-without-rupture', is the creation and modulation of 'substantial forms'. Destiny (MING 命) is a process of the personal expression of QI, of my life. Throughout life, every change in the direction and intensity of QI flow is a separation *'without-rupture'*.

According to the Daoist treatise XI MING, transformations and metamorphoses of QI are guided by DAO 道: *At the source of QI 氣 transformation* (HUA 化) *there is the name of DAO 道*.[91]
(YOU QI HUA YOU DAO ZHI MING 由氣化有道之名)

The third entity, life (SHENG 生)

DE 德 flows downwards, QI 氣 blooms and this is life (SHENG 生) (Figure 28). The character SHENG 生 shows 'a plant rising from the ground',[92] and is translated as 'birth', 'creation', 'generation', 'life'.

DE 德 represents the link between each living being and oneness (YI 一). Life (a continuum of change and transformation) is a meeting between DE 德 and QI 氣. DE 德 is the personal contact with oneness (YI 一) and QI 氣 brings life to 'substantial forms'-bodies and allows self-expression, conditioned by the laws of the Universe (renewal, expression, decline and storage).

ZHUANG ZI, further on in Chapter 12, relates destiny (MING 命) to Intimate Nature (XING 性); the character XING 性 includes the radical 生 'life'.[93] LING SHU, Chapter 8-1, uses the character SHENG 生, and does not use the character XING 性.

An example of the personal contact with oneness (YI 一) is presented by the Chinese landscape painter GU GUA 苦瓜 in his book *Treatise on the Philosophy of Painting*:[94] All things may be contained in the one

---

91 Quoted from ZHANG ZAI 張載 (SONG dynasty, 1020-1077) - ZHENG MENG, TAI HE BIEN DI YI, Chapter 1
92 Weiger, Lesson 79. SHENG 生 is also the name of the Law of Generation of Five Modalities
93 See page 61
94 GU GUA 苦瓜 (Bitter Gourd), also called SHI TAO (Stone Wave - 石涛) Treatise on the Philosophy of Painting, translated by LIN YUTANG

stroke (YI HUA 一畫). In the painting *'the one stroke'* refers to QI 氣 transmitting the impulse of life to the Myriad beings, allowed by DE 德 - the link to oneness (YI 一).

D. QI BO replies.
The second phase. Entities 4, 5: JING 精 **and** SHEN 神.
Self-identity is based on impersonal support (JING 精) **in space and time (Figure 30).**

故 GU	thus	兩 LIANG	both
生 SHENG	life	精 JING	
之 ZHI	auxiliary word	相 XIANG	mutually
來 LAI	comes	薄 BO	grasp, embrace, confront
謂 WEI	called	謂 WEI	called
之 ZHI	auxiliary word	之 ZHI	auxiliary word
精 JING		神 SHEN	

Thus, life (SHENG 生) *comes from what is called* JING 精.
Confrontation between the two (aspects of) JING 精 (of the father and of the mother) *is called* SHEN 神.

Figure 30. Life comes from what is called JING 精. **Confrontation between the two (aspects of)** JING 精 **is called** SHEN 神.

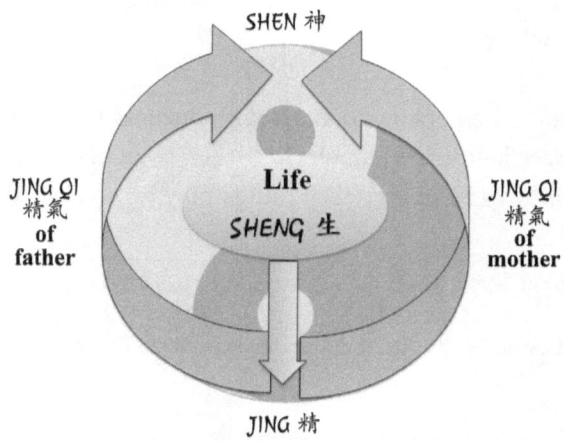

The fourth entity, JING 精 – fundamental vitality

LING SHU, Chapter 8-1, continues to define life, passing from the personal immediate Consciousness to the history of life: *Life (SHENG 生) comes from what is called* JING 精. The character JING 精 (Figure 31) shows the radical 米 'grain of rice', which symbolizes the transfer of inheritance from generation to generation and the basic support of all 'substantial forms'. The character QI 氣 also includes the same radical 米. The phonetic 青 shows 生 'a plant emerging from the soil', the lower stroke representing the surface; below the surface, there is DAN 丹/月 'cinnabar', 'the red alchemist stone', denoted by the alchemist's 'furnace of transformation'.[95] The red cinnabar symbolizes YANG, source of transformation, hidden deep in the soil and covered by plants, which symbolize YIN. The character 青 is translated as 'blue-green-turquoise' or 'dark-black';[96] it represents the dominant color of nature in non-desert areas: sky, plants and water - the blue of the sky, the green of the forest or dark green of the deep water. The character QING 情, 'emotions', includes the same phonetic 青.[97]

Figure 31. The character JING 精 'fundamental vitality' in classical and ancient seal script

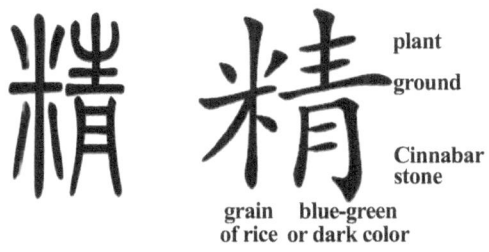

Life emerges from the background canvas which supports Heaven and Earth. There is no entity similar to JING 精 in Western languages. JING 精 is translated as 'essence', 'extract', 'semen', 'sperm', 'refined, extremely fine', 'essence of life'.[98] In textbooks of traditional Chinese

---

95 Weiger, Lesson 115
96 http://zhongwen.com/d/186/x235.htm,
97 See page 49 for the character QING 情
98 Eyssalet, J.M., *Les Cinq Chemins du Clair et de l'Obscur*

medicine, JING is usually translated as 'essence' or 'essences',[99] but in Greek philosophy the term 'essence', used by Plato and Aristotle, is the attribute or set of attributes that make an entity or substance what it is, and which it has by necessity, and without which it loses its identity.[100] Thus the Western concept 'essence' does not correspond to the message transmitted by the character JING 精, referred to in this book as 'fundamental vitality':

- JING 精 is impersonal, invisible, 'non-determined' background, without any intent, movement or direction, supporting life and all its expression in nature, hidden and revealed. JING 精 is 'action without action', 'effortless doing', supporting the Universe and life without intention and without purpose. JING 精 determines while itself being non-determined; JING is non-active background for existence.
- JING 精 is 'subtle' but 'concrete'. JING 精 is non-personal but is the basis of all personal expression of beings and things. Acquired JING 精 is transmitted by air, water and the five flavors (sour, bitter, sweet, pungent and salty). These five specified, non-personal flavors carry non-specified, non-personal JING but are the basis of personal body formation.
- JING 精 of the man's sperm cells and of the woman's blood (egg cell) is the basis of the child's genome. SHEN 神 is the meeting between Source QI (YUAN QI 原氣/元氣) which transfers the mother's Source JING (YUAN JING 原精/元精) (egg cell) and the father's Source QI which transfers Source JING 精 (sperm).

The association of the characters JING QI 精氣 may be translated as 'vital energy, QI carrying, moving, directing JING'. JING is motionless support, a necessary condition for life. JING is 'without determination', but enables the countless changes of QI. QI is always changing, thus providing multiple variations and directions of JING QI – 'life movement', 'passage of heredity'; JING QI may be expressed as *'Blowing the myriad differences'* (吹萬不同)[101] (ZHUANG ZI, Chapter 2).

---

99 Macioccia, G., *The Foundations of the Chinese Medicine*
100 Wikipedia - *Essence*
101 Translation by Legge, J.

FENG SHUI 風水 describes the effect of changes made by wind (FENG 風) and water (SHUI 水) on Earth QI, creating regions of influence, reservoirs of life, culminating points and dangerous areas which cause disorder or suffering. JING 精 can be likened to a lake with a completely calm surface, with trees, mountains and stars reflected on motionless water. JING QI 精氣 can be likened to the wind blowing, moving the water in the lake, causing the emergence of SHEN 神. SHEN 神 is an individual viewpoint on the world which governs all mechanisms of internal and external aspects of human life (intent, organization and change).

The fifth entity, SHEN 神 - Individual Spirit

LING SHU, Chapter 8-1, defines SHEN 神 with the help of JING 精: *Confrontation (BO 薄) between two (aspects of) JING 精 is called SHEN.*[102] The character BO 薄 describes 'a confrontation', 'a struggle', 'an embrace' between the JING 精 of the father and of the mother. The origin of my Individual Spirit (SHEN 神) is actualized by the confrontation of my parent's QI (desire) carrying JING (without desire), comparable to the coexistence of '*having desires* (YOU YU 有欲)' and '*without desires* (WU YU 無欲)', in LAO ZI, Chapter 1.

The passion of parents allows the meeting between two aspects of JING in time and space, and anchors SHEN, creating life and bodily form. This meeting between the two aspects of JING continues to exist in man to the end of his life. SHEN is also a constant interaction between heredity and environment – the meeting between Source JING (YUAN JING 原精/元精) and acquired JING.

SHEN 神 is the source of listening, introspection and personal identity, enabling a relationship between a man and the world, the other and himself. According to SU WEN, Chapter 66, SHEN does not depend on the rules of YIN YANG: *That which cannot be fathomed in [the alternation of] YIN and YANG, it is called spirit* (SHEN 神).[103]

---

102 See page 13 for the character SHEN 神
103 Translation by Unschuld and Tessenow

E. QI BO replies.
The third phase. Entities 6, 7: HUN 魂, PO 魄. Putting into motion and accompaniment of SHEN 神

隨	SUI	follow	並	BING	together
神	SHEN		精	JING	
往	WANG	go and come	而	ER	and
來	LAI		出	CHU	comes out
者	ZHE	auxiliary word	入	RU	comes in
謂	WEI	called	者	ZHE	auxiliary word
之	ZHI	auxiliary word	謂	WEI	called
魂	HUN	follow	之	ZHI	auxiliary word
			魄	PO	

Following SHEN 神 going away and coming back, that is called HUN 魂. Together with JING 精 exiting and entering, that is called PO 魄.

The sixth entity, HUN 魂 (Figure 32)

In ancient Chinese thought HUN 魂 was considered to be the power of initiation, creating and structuring all relationships in life, including self-image and perception of the world in space and time. In ancient China when the *Book of Songs* (SHI JING 詩經)[104] (7-11 BC) was composed, boys and girls met in spring at the convergence of rivers to play singing and dancing games. The exciting and ritualized atmosphere allowed for free and productive meetings and this was the occasion to address HUN 魂 – Spirits of 'Yellow Sources' - waiting to be reincarnated in new SHEN 神.

LING SHU, Chapter 8-1, after presenting JING as the source of life, and the emergence of SHEN through the desires of the parents, explains *Roots of SHEN* (BEN SHEN 本神) starting with HUN 魂,[105] Wood Modality, which communicates with the environment: *Following*

---

104 It is one of the "*Five Classics*" traditionally said to have been compiled by Confucius
105 See page 31 for the character HUN 魂

SHEN 神 *as it goes away and comes back, that is called* HUN 魂. HUN 魂 can be represented on the horizontal plane of the TAI JI symbol (Figure 32), and compared to the behavior of territorial animals which go away and come back along the same path every day (wolves, lions), or of migratory birds and fish following regular annual routes. HUN governs constantly or periodically, depending on the needs and desires, all modes of cyclic movement. The mechanism of HUN - *going away and coming back* - may be considered as adaptation, passion, curiosity or dream, and is expressed as journeys, walks, language, writing, paintings, music, dance.

Figure 32. *Following* SHEN 神 *going away and coming back, that is called* HUN 魂

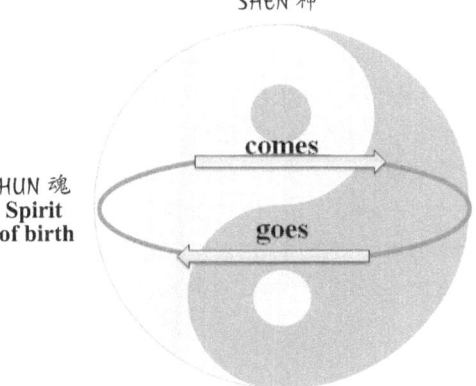

HUN 魂 directs the consciousness towards being open to the world, through presence, awareness and anticipation (intuition) with regard to life cycles and the cycles of time.

HUN 魂 is present in the fetus from conception and is related to childbirth (the passage from a liquid to an air environment). According to Daoist and medical texts, HUN is especially active in the fetus in the third and seventh months of the ten lunar months of pregnancy. In the third lunar month of pregnancy HUN of the fetus *sees through the eyes of his mother*, and therefore is affected by what she sees.[106]

---

106 Eyssalet, J.M., *Le Secret de la Maison des Ancêtres* pp.104-106, 137-141

HUN 魂 and ethics

The Earth spirit (GUI 鬼) of the five Intimate Natures (XING 性) is called HUN 魂 and it is masculine (WU XING DA YI, Chapter 18).[107]

These five Intimate Natures (XING 性), governed by HUN are: humanity, justice, observance of ritual, wisdom and loyalty. In The *Big School* in ancient China one of the three blessings was: *to illuminate in oneself the bright virtues that nature meets in the soul (HUN 魂) of each one.*[108]

HUN 魂, the first name and transmission between generations

In ancient China, a man was given his first name by his father at birth, and this name represented his HUN 魂. At death, after the last breath, HUN of the deceased was called three times. HUN 魂 follows SHEN and represents the path of communication with the Spirit of the deceased; therefore in ancient China the name (representing HUN 魂) of the deceased was carved on the wooden ancestral tablet. HUN-Wood, rooted in Kidney YANG (MING MEN 命門) -Water, transmits between generations what was not said, or said too much: family secrets, suicides, guilt, family myths, resistance to arbitrary and tyrannical laws. Balance between HUN and SHEN is based on adjustments between communication and transmission of the ancestral lines of the father and mother, which prepared our existence and the transmission to our children.

HUN 魂 and adaptation to the changing environment

HUN 魂-Liver and ZHI 志-Kidney YANG govern the production of Defensive QI (WEI 衛) in Lower JIAO.[109] Liver distributes WEI QI 衛氣 to the skin, eyes, sensory organs and tendino-muscular system, governs thermoregulation and body movements, and adjusts the rhythm of sleeping and waking, of feelings, passion, drives and sexuality. HUN 魂 and ZHI 志 through WEI QI 衛氣 allow the adaptation of the individual genome (Source QI, stored in Kidney) to the changing environment. It may be possible to relate evolution to HUN 魂.

---

107 See page 70
108 Eyssalet, J.M., *Le Secret de la Maison des Ancêtres* pp.421-426, 459-462
109 See pages 42, 45

HUN 魂 and neurology

SU WEN, Chapter 8: *Liver is the official functioning as General* (JIÀNG JUN 將軍). *Planning and contemplation originate in it* (MU LU 謀慮). It is possible to relate HUN 魂 to the neo-cortex since, in humans, the neo-cortex is involved in higher functions such as sensory perception, generation of motor commands, spatial reasoning, conscious thought and language.[110] The neo-cortex consists of six layers. Upper layers II and III, pyramidal neurons which project their axons, providing associative pathways to other areas of the neo-cortex, coordinating between them, may be related to HUN 魂.

The seventh entity, PO 魄 (Figure 33)

LING SHU, Chapter 8-1, relates HUN 魂 to SHEN (Wood-HUN ascends and generates Fire-SHEN on the left-YANG side of the TAI JI symbol), and relates PO 魄 to JING 精 (Metal-PO descends and generates Water-JING on the right-YIN side of the TAI JI symbol). PO 魄 is associated with body formation, fetal life and the mother.[111] In human development HUN 魂 and PO 魄 always function together, but at different stages of life one dominates the other. PO activity dominates embryo development. Both must be active to maintain a person's life.

Figure 33. *Together with* JING 精, *exiting and entering, that is called* PO 魄

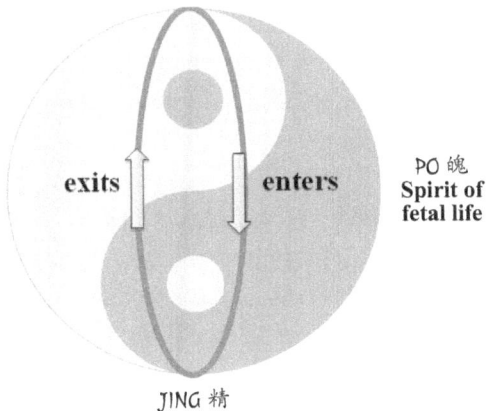

---

110 Wikipedia, Neo-cortex
111 See page 29 for the character PO 魄

Together (BING 並) *with* JING 精 *exiting and entering, that is called* PO 魄. The character BING 並 'standing together as one',[112] emphasizes that PO is inseparable from JING 精 - the background for body formation which is directed by PO. Metal-PO generates Water-Kidney-JING. During pregnancy PO 魄 of the fetus helps Kidney to distribute Source JING (YUAN JING 原精/元精):

- JING 精 originating from the father's sperm and the mother's egg cell at conception;
- JING 精 transmitted through the placenta to the fetus, absorbed from the mother's food, beverages and the air she breathes.

PO 魄 exiting and entering with JING 精 may be represented on the vertical plane of the TAI JI symbol (Figure 33) and may be seen as a metaphor for transmission of nutrients between the roots and branches of a tree:

- PO 魄 exits with Kidney JING - transmission from roots to branches. Kidney - roots of the body - organizes the structure and function of the pelvis and all bones, bone marrow, nervous and hormonal systems; it governs the ascent and distribution of Source QI (YUAN QI 原氣/元氣) carrying Source JING in Eight Extraordinary Meridians, especially in Conception Vessel (REN MAI 任脈), Governing Vessel (DU MAI 督脈) and CHONG MAI 衝脈.
- PO 魄 *enters with* JING - transmission from branches to roots. After birth, PO 魄 continues to direct the absorption of acquired JING from the air by Lung (respiratory system) and from food and beverages by Stomach and Spleen (digestive system), and transfers acquired JING downwards to Kidney.

PO 魄, the autonomic nervous system and the hypothalamus

PO 魄 may be related to the function of the autonomic nervous system (sympathetic and parasympathetic) and the hypothalamus. The autonomic nervous system is regulated by the hypothalamus.[113] The autonomic nervous system is a control system that acts largely

---

112 Wieger, Lesson 60
113 Wikipedia. *Autonomic Nervous System*

unconsciously and regulates bodily functions such as heart rate, digestion, respiratory rate, pupillary response, urination, and sexual arousal. In general, autonomic nervous system functions can be divided into sensory (afferent – 'enters') and motor (efferent – 'exits') subsystems.

Gellhorn[114] developed the theory of autonomic-somatic integration from the earlier theoretical formulations by the biologist Hess.[115] According to Gellhorn's model, the system in our body that controls adaptation and development is actually comprised of two complementary (sometimes antagonistic) systems, each of which organizes functions located at every level of the nervous system:
- The ergotropic system, which denotes those mechanisms, as well as the functional status of the nervous system, that favor the organism's capacity to **expend** energy.
- The trophotropic system which promotes rest and **reconstitution** of energy stores.

The balance between ergotropic and trophotropic nervous mechanisms corresponds in large part to that between the sympathetic and parasympathetic subdivisions of the autonomic nervous system.

The principle function of the ergotropic system is the control of short-range, moment-by-moment adaptation to events in the environment - fight-or-flight response. Anatomically, the ergotropic system incorporates the functions of the sympathetic nervous system, certain of the endocrine glands, portions of the reticular activating system in the brain stem, the posterior hypothalamus, and portions of the limbic system and frontal cortex.

The trophotropic system is responsible for regulating the vegetative functions, such as repair and growth of cells, digestion, relaxation, sleep. Anatomically, the trophotropic system incorporates the

---

114 Gellhorn 1967; Gellhorn and Loofbourrow 1963
115 Hess W.R. 1925

functions of the parasympathetic system, various endocrine glands, other portions of the reticular activating system, the anterior hypothalamus, and other portions of the limbic system and frontal cortex. PO 魄 (associated with JING) may be compared to trophotropic mechanisms assuring economy (slowing down cardiac rhythm) and internalization (digestion and sleep).

Interactions between HUN 魂 and PO 魄

HUN 魂 and PO 魄 together organize the existential consciousness of body and mind. PO with JING assures 'vegetative' existence: body maintenance, homeostasis and adaptation to the **stable** environment through the nervous and endocrine systems. HUN *follows* SHEN and directs opening outwards: adaptation to the **changing** environment, creativity and dreams.

Seventh Year of Duke ZHAO describes the interaction between PO and HUN as follows:[116]

> *When the child's body begins to elaborate, the soul that gives* (the body) *its physical shape is called* PO 魄. *After* PO 魄 *has given shape, the spiritual soul, called* HUN 魂 *appears. By the use of multiple activities* (drink, food) *the subtle elements are multiplied and* PO 魄 *and* HUN 魂 *become strong. They continue in this way growing in etherealness and brightness until they become spiritual wisdom.*

In emergency situations (stress provoking hypertension, or ejaculation) PO 魄 moves JING outwards and represents the YANG-HUN aspect of PO 魄.

Aggressiveness of the subconscious is the PO 魄 aspect of HUN 魂. Archaic and obscure aggressiveness, brutal and primitive ancient anger, for instance the rage of a bear brutally awakened during hibernation, represents the PO 魄 aspect of HUN 魂.

---

116 *Spring and Autumn Annals* (CHUN QIU ZUO ZHUAN 春秋左傳), covering a period from 722 to 468 BC. Partially based on translation by Legge, J, p. 618 and Couvreur, p. 142,

According to Damasio, there are three levels of consciousness: Protoself, Core Consciousness, and Extended Consciousness:

1. Protoself – a non-conscious state situated on the "ancient" brain, hypothalamus, *a coherent collection of neural patterns, which map moment-by-moment the state of the physical structure of the organism*[117] - is the most basic level of awareness signified by a collection of neural patterns which are representative of the body's internal state. The function of protoself is to constantly detect and record, moment by moment, the internal physical changes which affect the homeostasis of the organism. Protoself may be considered to be related to PO 魄.

Damasio describes "non-conscious creatures", which may be considered to be dominated by the influence of PO 魄:

Nonconscious creatures are capable of regulating homeostasis internally and equally capable of breathing the air and finding the water and transforming the energy required for survival within the sort of environment to which they are suitably matched by evolution.[118]

2. Core consciousness is the awareness of feelings associated with changes occurring to the internal bodily state, and the ability to recognize that one's thoughts and emotions are one's own. Core consciousness develops a momentary sense of self, as the brain continuously builds representative images, based on communications received from the protoself. The brain continues to present nonverbal narrative sequences of images in the mind of the organism, based on its relationship to objects - anything from a person, to a melody, to a neural image. Thoughts are formulated from the core consciousness perspective, concerned only with the present moment, the here and now. Core consciousness may be considered as a collaboration between PO 魄 and HUN 魂.

---

117 Damasio, A. R., *The Feeling of What Happens*, p.154
118 Damasio, A. R., *The Feeling of What Happens*, p. 201

3. Extended consciousness moves beyond the here and now. This level could not exist without protoself and core consciousness but, unlike them, requires a vast use of conventional memory. Extended consciousness may be related to SHEN 神 - the collaboration between PO 魄, HUN 魂, YI 意 and ZHI 志 as presented in LING SHU, Chapter 8-1.

Damasio presents the advantages of consciousness:
consciousness is good for extending the mind's reach and, in so doing, improving the life of the organism whose mind has that higher reach[119]...

Interaction between PO 魄 and HUN 魂 may be compared to the advantages of consciousness presented by Damasio:
Creatures with consciousness have some advantages over those that do not have consciousness. They can establish a link between the world of automatic regulation (the world of basic homeostasis that is interwoven with the proto-self)[120] *and the world of imagination (the world in which images of different modalities can be combined to produce novel images of situations that have not yet happened)*[121]. *The world of imaginary creations—the world of planning, the world of formulation of scenarios and prediction of outcomes—is linked to the world of the proto-self. The sense of self links forethought, on the one hand, to preexisting automation, on the other.*[122]

---

119 Damasio, A. R., *The Feeling of What Happens*, p. 200
120 Possible to compare with PO 魄
121 Possible to compare with HUN 魂 and YI 意
122 Damasio, A. R., *The Feeling of What Happens*, p. 201

F. QI BO replies.

The fourth phase. Entities 8, 9, 10: Heart-Consciousness (XIN 心), intent (YI 意), ability to realize life (ZHI 志). Consciousness gathers messages from the interior and from the environment to realize life (Figure 34)

所	SUO	that which	心	XIN	heart	意	YI	intent
以	YI		有	YOU	has	之	ZHI	auxiliary word
任	REN	receive	所	SUO	this	所	SUO	which
物	WU	things, beings	憶	YI	reminiscence	存	CUN	stabilized
者	ZHE	comma	謂	WEI	called	謂	WEI	called
謂	WEI	called	之	ZHI	auxiliary word	之	ZHI	auxiliary word
之	ZHI	auxiliary word	意	YI	intent	志	ZHI	
心	XIN	Heart-Consciousness						

That which receives (REN 任) things and beings (WU 物) is called Heart-Consciousness (XIN 心),

When Heart-Consciousness (XIN 心) has reminiscences (YI 憶), this is called YI 意 *(intent, ability to create and store ideas, images; memories),*

When YI 意 *is stabilized (CUN 存), this is called* ZHI 志 *(ability to realize life, determination).*

The eighth entity, Heart-Consciousness (XIN 心) [123]

That which receives/supports (REN 任) things and beings (WU 物) is called Heart-Consciousness (XIN 心)

The character REN 任 shows 亻'a man standing', in front of whom 壬 'a heavy weight is falling', or 'a man carrying a burden on a bamboo pole'[124] and is translated as 'trust', 'appoint', 'rely on', 'take charge of', 'receive' and also as 'support'.[125] In the name REN MAI 任脈, one of the eight Extraordinary Meridians, REN 任 is translated as 'conception'.

---

123 See page 38
124 Wieger, Lesson 82
125 Larre C., Rochat de la Vallee, E. *Rooted in Spirit: The Heart of Chinese Medicine*

Figure 34. When Heart-Consciousness (XIN 心) has reminiscences, this is called YI 意**. When** YI 意 **is stabilized this is called** ZHI 志

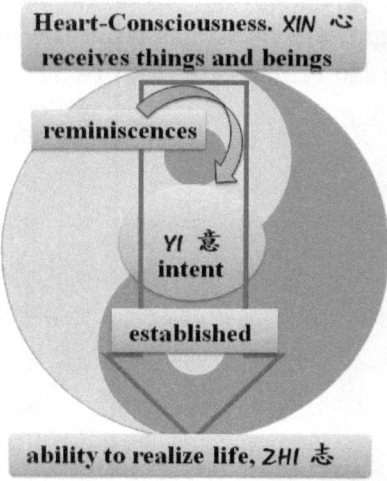

The character WU 物 'beings', 'creatures', 'objects', 'things' shows the radical 扌/牛 'bull' and 勿 'flags swaying in the wind'.[126] The bull denotes a dense 'substantial form'. The movement of flags in the wind represents QI. Therefore it may be said that within Heart-Consciousness (XIN 心), WU 物 – beings, things and objects - are both 'substantial forms' and movement (QI 氣).

Reception of things and beings (WU 物) is a free, inclusive, non-interrupted flow of listening by Heart-Consciousness to messages coming from the sense organs about phenomena (things and beings WU 物). WU 物 in Heart-Consciousness become the objects of Consciousness, which means that Consciousness is listening to **itself**.

Heart-Consciousness (XIN 心) represents the radiance of SHEN (SHEN MING 神明) (SU WEN, Chapter 8). Heart-Consciousness '*supports*'- listens to things and beings from a unique and individual perspective which allows their *reception*. Reception of things and beings (WU 物) is the ability of Heart-Consciousness to be a witness by means of a

---

[126] Wieger, Lesson 101

process of differentiation and adjustment between what is received and the receiver during a flowing, functional interaction. Heart-Consciousness-SHEN is an open perspective on the world, which re-organizes each moment of life as a part of a picture in constant motion.

The Chinese *Art of Heart* (*Art of Life*) was to empty Heart: to develop an ability to receive beings and things and let them pass freely without obstruction, while at the same time questioning them.

The ninth entity, intent, ideas (YI 意)

When Heart-Consciousness (XIN 心) has reminiscences (YI 憶), this is called YI 意 (Figure 34).

In quiet and empty Heart-Consciousness there are traces, reminiscences of what happened in the body and in the outside world. The character YI 意 describes 'sounds, vibrations of Heart-Consciousness', 'intent', 'ability to form and store ideas and images' (Figure 17).[127] YI 意 dwells in Spleen-Soil, located in the center of the TAI JI symbol, and represents the center of SHEN 神.

The character YI 憶 shows the radical 心 'heart' in its vertical version 忄 and the phonetic YI 意 'intent' (Figure 17). In the character YI 憶, the radical 忄/心 'heart' appears twice; on the left side of the character, and as the lower component of 意. YI 憶 is translated as 'reminiscences', 'traces'. YI 憶 are traces in Heart-Consciousness which animate externalized (expressed, spoken) and internalized (unexpressed) intent (YI 意). Traces (YI 憶) are sounds of Heart-Consciousness, subtle traces of memories imprinted in Heart-Consciousness (comparable to engram in neurolinguistics), which bring 'color' to intent (YI 意) and direct SHEN 神.

Intent (YI 意) appears in LING SHU, Chapter 8-1, after PO 魄 and HUN 魂. YI 意 records all traces of organization directed by SHEN 神: 'operative' traces of HUN 魂 and 'constructive' traces of PO 魄. YI 意 records reminiscences, traces and memories, and is therefore the basis

---

127 See page 34 for the character YI 意

of 'the structure of the mind' and the self-image of the person. SHEN 神 is the composer, conductor and orchestra. YI 意, with the help of HUN 魂, records, maintains, restores and changes all the information (sounds, words, images, smells, tastes) from the outside world. *Reception of things and beings* by Heart-Consciousness is recorded with the help of traces, memories and emotions. Emotions evoke sounds, words, imprinted memories and all aspects of records.

YI 意 records globally, inaccurately and subjectively with no division between body and mind, and precedes thoughts. Our life is based on YI 意 - recording of subtle impressions as a personal history and also as an expression of forms of Consciousness at each moment. YI 意 in LING SHU, Chapter 8-1, is close to the "*background feelings*" of Damasio:

> *I am postulating another variety of feeling which I suspect preceded the others* (Feelings of Basic Universal Emotions and Feelings of Subtle Universal Emotions) *in evolution. I call it background feeling because it originates in "background" body states rather than in emotional states. It is not the Verdi of grand emotion, nor the Stravinsky of intellectualized emotion but rather a minimalist in tone and beat, the feeling of life itself, the sense of being.*[128]

The tenth entity: the ability to realize life, determination (ZHI 志)

When YI 意 *is stabilized (finds its place)* (CUN 存) *this is called* ZHI 志 (Figure 34).

The character CUN 存 shows 才 'ability to produce' 子 'progeny, child',[129] and may be translated as 'establish', 'stabilize', 'maintain', 'exist', 'find a place' or 'store'. Among BEN SHEN only the characters YI 意 and ZHI 志 include the radical 心 'heart'. ZHI 志 is translated as 'determination', 'will', 'judgment', 'decisions', 'ability to realize life', but also as 'passions', 'emotions' (Figure 16).[130]

---

128 Damasio, A. R., Descartes' *Error: Emotion, Reason, and the Human Brain*, p. 150
129 Wieger, Lesson 97
130 See page 33 for the character ZHI 志

Damasio makes a connection between decisions and emotions (both of which may be translated as ZHI 志):

> ... work from my laboratory has shown that emotion is integral to the processes of reasoning and decision making, for worse and for better.[131]

Heart-Consciousness together with YI 意 and ZHI 志 organize memories. According to LING SHU, Chapter 8-1:
1. XIN 心, Heart-Consciousness receives things and beings (WU 物)
2. XIN 心, Heart-Consciousness organizes reminiscences and traces of things and beings (WU 物)
3. YI 意, the library of intent, ideas and images, is stabilized
4. ZHI 志 appears

Association between YI 意 and ZHI 志
Soil - the center of the other four Modalities on the TAI JI symbol, receives, maintains, slows and balances the complementary opposites: Fire and Water, Wood and Metal.

Figure 35. YI 意 and ZHI 志, Center-North axis of the TAI JI symbol

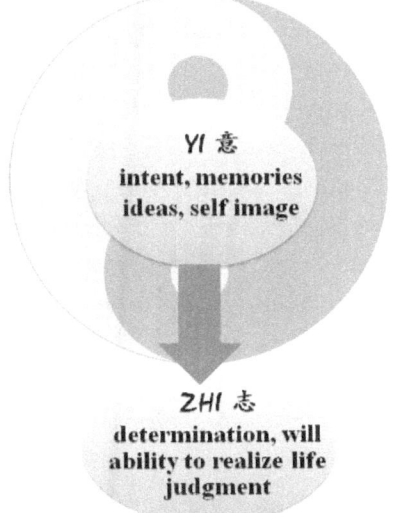

---

131 Damasio, A. R., *The Feeling of What Happens*, p. 28

Therefore, Soil-YI 意 records and coordinates the four other BEN SHEN (SHEN, PO, HUN, ZHI). Fire-South represents Heaven, Water-North represents Earth. Soil 'is anchored' in Water according to the Law of Control. Fire generates Soil, so Heart-Consciousness (Fire) in the process of organizing emotions and all traces of life becomes (generates) YI 意. Therefore YI 意 'represents' Fire-Heaven which needs to be stabilized by ZHI 志 which 'represents' Water-Earth. ZHI 志-judgment adjusts YI 意-intent to reality, life. The pair YI-ZHI represents the axis uniting Center on the TAI JI symbol to North (bottom) (Figure 35).

YI 意 - ZHI 志 and modern theories of memory

According to the Atkinson and Shiffrin model, human memory consists of three reservoirs:[132]
1. Sensory memory
2. Short-term memory and Working memory[133]
3. Long-term memory - Procedural (implicit) memory

Procedural memory (long-term memory) is not based on the conscious recall of information, but on implicit learning, and is primarily employed in learning motor skills. According to Chinese thought, inborn motor skills are governed by Kidney-ZHI 志; knowing how to do things is associated with recording by YI 意.

Dispositional representations, presented by Damasio, may be compared to traces/reminiscences (YI 憶) in LING SHU, Chapter 8-1:

Unlike our environment, whose constitution does change, and unlike the images we construct relative to that environment, which are fragmentary and conditioned by external circumstance, background feeling is mostly about body states. Our individual identity is anchored on this island of illusory living sameness against which we can be aware of myriad other things that manifestly change around the organism.[134]

---

132 Wikipedia. Memory
133 For Short-term memory and Working memory, see Wikipedia. *Working memory*
134 Damasio, A. R. *Descartes' Error: Emotion, Reason, and the Human Brain*, p. 155

This illusory permanence of body is conditioned by genetics and brain function and is called *dispositional representations*:

> *Dispositional representations constitute our full repository of knowledge, encompassing both innate knowledge and knowledge acquired by experience. Innate knowledge is based on dispositional representations in hypothalamus, brain stem, and limbic system. You can conceptualize it as commands about biological regulation which are required for survival (e.g., the control of metabolism, drives, and instincts)...*
>
> *Acquired knowledge is based on dispositional representations in higher-order cortices and throughout many gray-matter nuclei beneath the level of the cortex. Some of those dispositional representations contain records for the imageable knowledge that we can recall and which is used for movement, reason, planning, creativity; and some contain records of rules and strategies with which we operate on those images.*[135]

These *dispositional representations*, which may be compared to Yi 意, are inscribed in the cortex.

> *...there seem to be no permanently held pictures of anything, even miniaturized, no microfiches or microfilms, no hard copies. Given the huge amount of knowledge we acquire in a lifetime, any kind of facsimile storage would probably pose insurmountable problems of capacity...*
>
> *We all have direct evidence that whenever we recall a given object, or face, or scene, we do not get an exact reproduction but rather an interpretation, a newly reconstructed version of the original...*
>
> *These recalled images tend to be held in Consciousness only fleetingly, and although they may appear to be good replicas, they are often inaccurate or incomplete. I suspect that explicit recalled*

---

135 Damasio, A. R. *Descartes' Error: Emotion, Reason, and the Human Brain*, pp. 104-105

> *mental images arise from the transient synchronous activation of neural firing patterns largely in the same early sensory cortices where the firing patterns corresponding to perceptual representations once occurred.*[136]

Concepts in works of Damasio may be compared with entities in LING SHU, Chapter 8-1:
- *Dispositional representations* may be related to traces/reminiscences (YI 憶), necessary for Heart-Consciousness to generate intent (YI 意)
- Innate knowledge may be related to ZHI 志
- Acquired knowledge may be related to YI 意
- Ability to learn may be related to ZHI 志
- *Inborn regulation representations* may be related to PO 魄 and ZHI 志
- Use of convergence areas in brain may be related to a function of HUN 魂
- Initiators and determinators of language may be related to HUN 魂 and SHEN 神

The relationship between the genome (inborn) and the environment (acquired) in Chinese and in Western philosophy

According to Damasio, core consciousness is under gene control and therefore may be related to ZHI 志 and Kidney, which store Source QI.

> *Core consciousness is the process of achieving a neural and mental pattern which brings together, in about the same instant, the pattern for the object, the pattern for the organism, and the pattern for the relationship between the two.*[137]

> *...I would venture that virtually all of the machinery behind core consciousness and the generation of core self is under strong gene control... the genome puts in place the appropriate body-brain*

---

136 Damasio, A. R. *Descartes' Error: Emotion, Reason, and the Human Brain*, pp. 100-101
137 Damasio, A. R., *The Feeling of What Happens*, p.129

linkages, both neural and humoral; lays down the requisite circuits, and, with help from the environment, allows the machinery to perform in reliable fashion for an entire lifetime.[138]

The autobiographical self (YI 意) is based on core consciousness (ZHI 志) and represents the inscribed influence of the environment (individual history, society, culture). The following citation from Damasio on the autobiographical self echoes the relationship between YI 意 and ZHI 志:

The development of the autobiographical self is a different matter. To be sure, the connection between core self and the structures which support the development of autobiographical memory is organized under genomic control. So are the processes on the basis of which learning can take place and modeling of cortical and subcortical circuits can occur so that convergence zones and their dispositions are put in place. In other words, autobiographical memory develops and matures under the looming shadow of an inherited biology. However, unlike the core self, much will occur in the development and maturation of autobiographical memory that is not just dependent on, but is even regulated by the environment. For instance, the schedules of reward and punishment offered to developing infants, children, and adolescents do vary among different home, school, and social environments; the shaping of the events which constitute the historical past of an individual and his or her anticipated future is controlled in no small measure by the environment; the rules and principles of behavior governing the cultures in which an autobiographical self is developing are under the control of the environment; likewise for the knowledge according to which individuals organize their autobiography, which ranges from the models of individual behavior to the facts of a culture.[139]

YI 意 which finds its anchor in ZHI 志 may be compared to *autobiographical memory… organized under genomic control.*

---

138 Damasio, A. R., *The Feeling of What Happens*, p.153
139 Damasio, A. R., *The Feeling of What Happens*, p.153

The French biophysicist and philosopher Atlan[140] proposes concepts that may be compared with entities discussed in LING SHU, Chapter 8,
- Consciousness is *"presence of the known"* and *"presence of the past"* and may be compared to YI 意;
- 'Will is unconscious may be compared' to ZHI 志;
- 'The *"presence of the past"* develops into the vaster consciousness' may be compared to contribution of YI 意 to SHEN.

According to LING SHU, Chapter 8, an inappropriate way of life puts YI and ZHI *in confusion and disorder*,[141] since YI 意 and ZHI 志 through communication between the inborn and acquired enable body-formation, organization of Consciousness and organization of self-identity:
- ZHI 志 by means of Kidney directs Source QI (YUAN QI 原氣/元氣) - the genome
- YI 意 by means of Spleen, Stomach and SAN JIAO organizes:
  - absorption of acquired QI from food, beverages and air
  - production and distribution of Nourishing QI (RONG/YING 榮/營氣) and Blood
- Kidney YANG-ZHI 志 and Liver-HUN 魂 govern the production of Defensive QI (WEI QI 衛氣) in Lower JIAO.

YI 意 conserves all 'traces', maintains and responds, but does not act. ZHI 志 is the force of life, an inborn, unconscious ability for action and transformation of the person. ZHI 志 determines decisions and interactions with the Universe, and represents the ability for global and spontaneous adaptation to the changing environment. ZHI 志 is related to DAO 道 (the movement of the Universe) as expressed by:
- SAN GUO ZHI 三國志:[142] ZHI 志 *unites with* DAO 道 (ZHI TONG DAO HE 志同道合).

---

140 Atlan, H., *Entre le cristal et la fumée: Essai sur l'organisation de vivant*, pp. 140-141
141 See page 41, the beginning of Chapter 8
142 Cited from CHEN SHOU 陳壽 (third century AD), SAN GUO ZHI, *Records of the Three Kingdoms*, a Chinese historical text, which covers the history of the late Eastern Han dynasty (184–220 AD) and the Three Kingdoms period (220–280 AD).

- HUAI NAN ZI 淮南子, Chapter 2,¹⁴³ showing a link between ZHI 志 and DAO 道: *When ZHI 志 is obtained, DAO 道 moves* (ZHI DE DAO XING 志得道行).
- HUAI NAN ZI 淮南子, Chapter 1,¹⁴⁴ showing a link between ZHI 志 and SHEN 神: *When ZHI 志 finds its place, SHEN 神 has its anchor* (ZHI YOU SUO ZAI ZE SHEN YOU SUO XI 志有所在則神有所繫).

G. QI BO replies:
The fifth phase. Entity 11: thought (SI 思) (Figure 36)

因	YIN	when
志	ZHI	ability to realize life
而	ER	auxiliary word
存	CUN	exist, stabilize
變	BIAN	transform
謂	WEI	is called
之	ZHI	auxiliary word
思	SI	thought, thinking

When ZHI 志 is stabilized (finds a place) *(CUN 存) and transforms (BIAN 變), this is called thought (SI 思).*

In Chinese medicine, the thinking process (SI 思) is seen as an **emotion** (called obsessive thinking when intense or long-lasting) related to Spleen-Soil-YI 意. ZHI 志 is stabilized (finds a place) (CUN 存) and provides basic but effective judgments regarding desires and passions, which determine the position of each man in the Universe, then it transforms and thoughts (SI 思)¹⁴⁵ emerge. Thinking is a process of changing attitudes. In the process of thinking, thoughts take shape and transform, just as in the walking process one leg has to be placed on the ground before moving the other; in the Peripatetic school in Ancient Greece, philosophy was taught while walking.¹⁴⁶

---

143 http://www.100jia.net/texte/huainanzi/
144 http://www.100jia.net/texte/huainanzi/
145 See page 56 for the character SI 思
146 Aristotle was the founder of the Peripatetic school of philosophy

The 'changing attitudes' of ZHI 志 have to be stabilized to create a person's self-image and image of the world. Logical thinking (reason) is the product of ZHI 志 (related to Kidney Source QI – genome) which is what allows adaptability to the environment.

Figure 36. When ZHI 志 **is stabilized and transformed this is called** SI 思

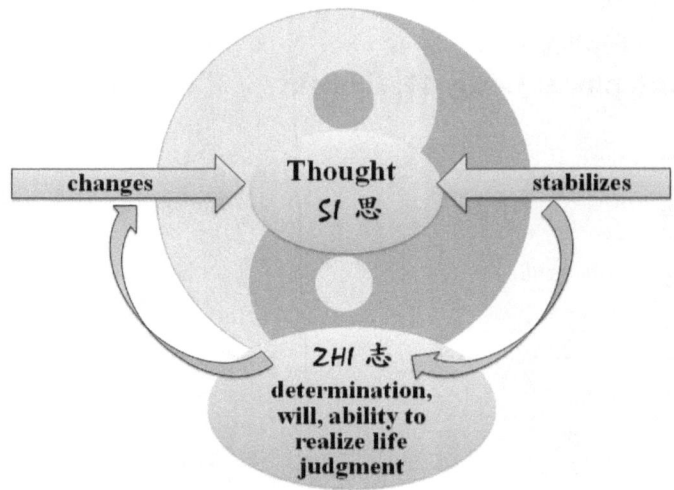

LING SHU, Chapter 8-1, explains the thinking process:

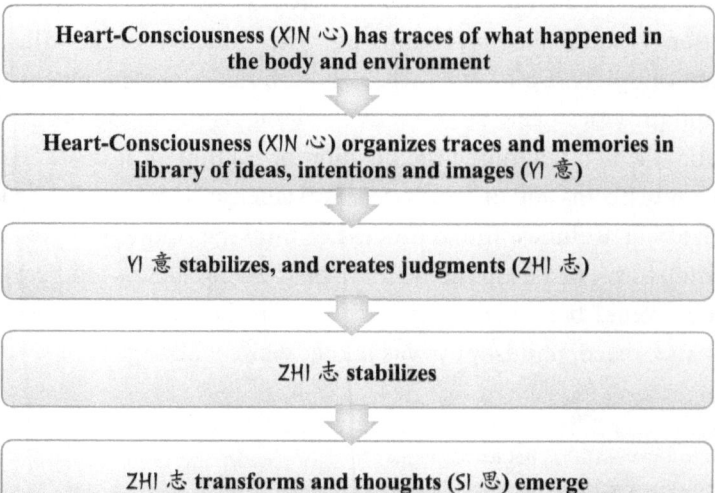

Damasio calls feelings about the body "somatic markers"; the process in which "somatic markers" appear is similar to the process in which ZHI 志 is stabilized (CUN 存) and transformed (BIAN 變):

When the bad outcome connected with a given response option comes into mind, however fleetingly, you experience an unpleasant gut feeling. Because the feeling is about the body, I gave the phenomenon the technical term somatic state ("soma" is Greek for body); and because it "marks" an image, I called it a marker. Note again that I use somatic in the most general sense (that which pertains to the body) and I include both visceral and nonvisceral sensation when I refer to somatic markers.

What does the somatic marker achieve? It forces attention on the negative outcome to which a given action may lead, and functions as an automated alarm signal which says: Beware of danger ahead if you choose the option which leads to this outcome. The signal may lead you to reject, immediately, the negative course of action and thus make you choose among other alternatives. The automated signal protects you against future losses, without further ado, and then allows you to choose from among fewer alternatives. There is still room for using a cost / benefit analysis and proper deductive competence, but only after the automated step drastically reduces the number of options...

In short, **somatic markers are a special instance of feelings generated from secondary emotions. Those emotions and feelings have been connected, by learning, to predicted future outcomes of certain scenarios.** *When a negative somatic marker is juxtaposed to a particular future outcome the combination functions as an alarm bell. When a positive somatic marker is juxtaposed instead, it becomes a beacon of incentive.*[147]

The partnership between so-called cognitive processes and processes usually called "emotional" should be apparent.[148]

---

147 Damasio, A. R. *Descartes' Error: Emotion, Reason, and the Human Brain*, pp. 173-174

148 Damasio, A. R. *Descartes' Error: Emotion, Reason, and the Human Brain*, p. 175

Damasio also shows that reason (logical thinking) and decisions are connected with feelings and the body. Reason may be regarded as thought resulting from the process of transformation of the stabilized ZHI 志.

> *Reason does seem to depend on specific brain systems, some of which happen to process feelings. Thus there may be a connecting trail, in anatomical and functional terms, from reason to feelings to body. It is as if we are possessed by a passion for reason, a drive that originates in the brain core, permeates other levels of the nervous system, and emerges as either feelings or non conscious biases to guide decision making. Reason, from the practical to the theoretical, is probably constructed on this inherent drive by a process which resembles the mastering of a skill or craft.*[149]

H. QI BO replies:
The sixth phase. Entities 12 and 13: LU 慮 and ZHI 智. Development of thought: contemplation and wisdom

因	YIN	therefore	因	YIN	therefore
思	SI	thought	慮	LU	contemplation
而	ER	auxiliary word	而	ER	auxiliary word
遠	YUAN	far off	處	CHU	settle, handle, arrange
慕	MU	admire, consider	物	WU	things, beings, objects
謂	WEI	is called	謂	WEI	is called
之	ZHI	auxiliary word	之	ZHI	auxiliary word
慮	LU	contemplation	智	ZHI	wisdom, intelligence, knowledge

So the thought (SI 思) *which considers* (the situation) *from afar is called contemplation* (LU 慮).

So contemplation (LU 慮) *which arranges things and beings* (WU 物) *is called wisdom* (ZHI 智).

---

149 Damasio, A. R. *Descartes' Error: Emotion, Reason, and the Human Brain*, p. 245

The twelfth entity: contemplation (LU 慮) (Figure 37)

Thoughts (the thinking process) appear *when ZHI 志 is stabilized and transformed. The thought (SI 思) which considers the situation from afar is called contemplation* (LU 慮) (Figure 37). When thought reflects the situation without being emotionally involved it is called LU 慮, translated as 'contemplation', 'reflection', 'consideration' but in pathology it manifests as 'concern', 'worry'.

Figure 37. The thought (SI 思) which considers the situation from afar is called contemplation (LU 慮)

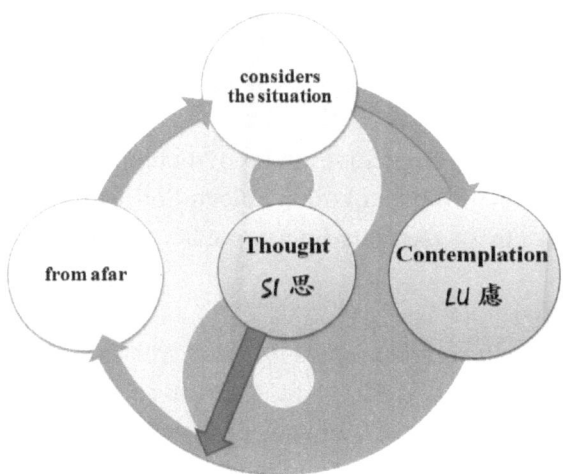

The character LU 慮 (Figure 38) shows 思 'thought'[150] and 虍 'tiger'.[151] The character XU 虛 'emptiness', 'void' also includes the character 虍 'tiger', as well as 'two people sitting back to back'[152] - the emptiness is created by a tiger that devours everything. In the character LU 慮, Soil-thought (SI 思) is subject to the tension and the open space-emptiness created by the tiger (虍). White Tiger is a symbol of Metal-West, but tiger also possesses the qualities of Wood-East: creation of the open space allowing wind to blow. The smooth flow of QI without

---

150 See page 56 for the character SI 思
151 Radical 141.
152 Wieger, Lesson 27

obstruction, similar to wind blowing in emptiness, represents a proper function of Liver-Wood. LU 慮 is the tiger of the thinking process, penetrating deeply into the entire situation in order to understand it, evaluate the results of action and plan further actions.

Figure 38. The character LU 慮 'contemplation' in classical and ancient seal script

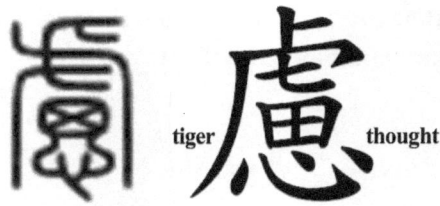

Spleen-Soil produces repetitive circles of thoughts in order to stabilize the center. Liver-Wood controls Spleen-Soil, and transforms the repetitive circles of thoughts into unpredictable and adaptive spiral movements.

Planning and contemplation of the situation (MU LU 謀慮) is considered to be the quality of Liver-HUN 魂, the Army General of the human body (SU WEN, Chapter 8). In ancient China, war strategy required that the general 'contemplate from the distance' (LU 慮) to predict the outcome of the battle. The general observed (with eyes-Liver) stars, planets and landscape, and contemplated in order to choose the right time and place to enable victory. Liver-eyesight creates visual images (main theme of the story) which after contemplation return illuminated and transformed. Contemplation (LU 慮) may be considered to be a preverbal process.

Damasio describes *preverbal neural representations which can become images*:
> *Brains can have many intervening steps in the circuits mediating between stimulus and response, and still have no mind, if they do not meet an essential condition: the ability to display images internally and to order those images in a process called thought.*

(The images are not solely visual; there are also "sound images," "olfactory images," and so on.) ...

My view then is that having a mind means that an organism forms neural representations which can become images, be manipulated in a process called thought, and eventually influence behavior by helping predict the future, plan accordingly, and choose the next action. Herein lies the center of neurobiology as I see it: the process whereby neural representations, which consist of biological modifications created by learning in a neuron circuit, become images in our minds; the process that allows for invisible microstructural changes in neuron circuits (in cell bodies, dendrites and axons, and synapses) to become a neural representation, which in turn becomes an image we each experience as belonging to us.[153]

Let me make clear what I mean by making a narrative or telling a story. The terms are so connected to language that I must ask you again not to think of them in terms of words. I do not mean narrative or story in the sense of putting together words or signs in phrases and sentences. I do mean telling a narrative or story in the sense of creating a non languaged map of logically related events.[154]

I believe the imaged, nonverbal narrative of core consciousness is swift, that its unexamined details have eluded us for a long time, that the narrative is barely explicit, so half hinted that its expression is almost like the emanation of a belief.[155]

Wordless storytelling is natural. The imagetic representation of sequences of brain events, which occurs in brains simpler than ours, is the stuff of which stories are made. A natural preverbal

---

153 Damasio, A. R., *Descartes' Error: Emotion, Reason, and the Human Brain*, pp. 89-90
154 Damasio, A. R., *The Feeling of What Happens*, p.122
155 Damasio, A. R., *The Feeling of What Happens*, p.124

occurrence of storytelling may well be the reason why we ended up creating drama and eventually books, and why a good part of humanity is currently hooked on movie theaters and television screens. Movies are the closest external representation of the prevailing storytelling that goes on in our minds. What goes on within each shot, the different framing of a subject that the movement of the camera can accomplish, what goes on in the transition of shots achieved by editing, and what goes on in the narrative constructed by a particular juxtaposition of shots is comparable in some respects to what is going on in the mind...[156]

From the ancient Chinese perspective, the thinking process (SI 思):
- originates in Spleen-YI 意
- its automatic function emerges from PO 魄
- its unconscious regulation emerges from ZHI 志
- its effectiveness emerges from the life force, desires and imagination of Liver-HUN 魂

Spleen and Liver (YI 意 and HUN 魂) provide subtle 'substantial forms' to Heart-Consciousness, enabling the anticipation of change and the adaptation of responses ("advantages of consciousness"). Damasio expresses "advantages of consciousness" in neurological terms:

...devices in the brain stem and hypothalamus can coordinate, non consciously and with great efficiency, the jobs of the heart, lungs, kidneys, endocrine system, and immunological system such that the parameters that permit life are maintained within the adequate range, while the devices of consciousness handle the problem of how an individual organism may cope with environmental challenges not predicted in its basic design such that the conditions fundamental for survival can still be met.[157]

Creatures with consciousness have some advantages over those that do not have consciousness. They can establish a link

---

[156] Damasio, A. R., *The Feeling of What Happens*, p.125
[157] Damasio, A. R., *The Feeling of What Happens*, p.200

between the world of automatic regulation (the world of basic homeostasis that is interwoven with the proto-self) and the world of imagination (the world in which images of different modalities can be combined to produce novel images of situations that have not yet happened). The world of imaginary creations—the world of planning, the world of formulation of scenarios and prediction of outcomes—is linked to the world of the proto-self.[158]

The thirteenth entity: wisdom, intelligence, use of knowledge (ZHI 智)

The last entity, the final development of the thinking process in LING SHU, Chapter 8-1, is wisdom (ZHI 智). So contemplation (LU 慮) which arranges things and beings (WU 物) is called wisdom (ZHI 智) (Figure 39).

Figure 39. Contemplation (LU 慮) **which arranges things and beings is called wisdom** (ZHI 智)

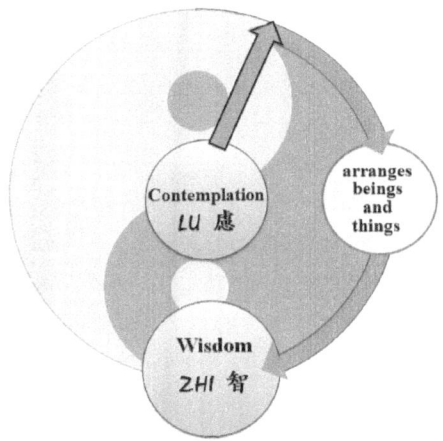

The character ZHI 智 includes two mouths, 口 'an open mouth' and 曰 'a mouth with a tongue inside' and 矢 'an arrow which hits its target'.[159] ZHI 智 signifies 'using words precisely', like 'an arrow which hits its target' and which may signify 'language'; it is translated as 'wisdom',

---

158 Damasio, A. R., *The Feeling of What Happens*, p.201
159 For the character ZHI 智 see page 65. The characters ZHI 智 and ZHI 志 have identical PINYIN letters but differ in tones

'intelligence', 'knowledge', 'knowing how', 'common sense', 'discerning between good and evil'. ZHI 智, the virtue attributed to Kidney,[160] is a vast intuitive, visionary contemplation contributing to the interaction with society and the environment, 'nourishing life' to achieve longevity. It is rooted in ZHI 志 'ability to realize life', 'the inborn will to live'.

When contemplation (LU 慮) is adjusted to the problems of existence, to what happens in society and the environment (things and beings), it becomes ZHI 智. ZHI 智 is personal intelligence, wisdom and knowledge, the wisdom of the body, the wisdom of constant adjustment of the relationship with nature, with the seasons, with life cycles, with society and beings. ZHI 智 also includes memories and traces of the past.

Knowledge and intelligence in the works of Damasio
According to Damasio, consciousness, which centers knowledge (*the creation of novel responses*), is a problem-solver in the changing environment, and is the latest development in evolution; it may be compared to ZHI 智:

> *I would say that consciousness, as currently designed, constrains the world of imagination to be first and foremost about the individual, about an individual organism, about the self in the broad sense of the term. I would say that the effectiveness of consciousness comes from its unabashed connection to the non conscious proto-self. This is the connection that guarantees that proper attention is paid to the matters of individual life by creating a concern. Perhaps the secret behind the efficacy of consciousness is selfness. In short, the power of consciousness comes from the effective connection it establishes between the biological machinery of individual life regulation and the biological machinery of thought. That connection is the basis for the creation of an individual concern which permeates all aspects of thought processing, focuses all problem-solving activities, and inspires the*

---

160 See page 65

ensuing solutions. Consciousness is valuable because it centers knowledge on the life of an individual organism.[161]

Consciousness is not the sole means of generating adequate responses to an environment and thus achieving homeostasis. Consciousness is just the latest and most sophisticated means of doing so, and it performs its function by making way for the creation of novel responses in the sort of environment which an organism has not been designed to match, in terms of automated responses.[162]

According to Damasio, extended consciousness is not intelligence (ZHI 智) but intelligence is its basic condition:

Memory, language, and intelligence make the difference, not emotion. The same probably applies to consciousness. Extended consciousness occurs in minds endowed with core consciousness, but only when those minds can rely on superior memory, language, and intelligence, and when the organisms which construct those minds interact with suitable social environments.[163]

I regard the problem of consciousness as a combination of two intimately related problems. The first is the problem of understanding how the brain inside the human organism engenders the mental patterns we call, for lack of a better term, the images of an object. By object I mean entities as diverse as a person, a place, a melody, a toothache, a state of bliss; by image I mean a mental pattern in any of the sensory modalities, e.g., a sound image, a tactile image, the image of a state of wellbeing... Quite candidly, this first problem of consciousness is the problem of how we get a "movie-in-the-brain"...

Now, for the second problem of consciousness. This is the problem of how, in parallel with engendering mental patterns for an object, the brain also engenders a sense of self in the act of knowing...

The sensory images of what you perceive externally, and the related images you recall, occupy most of the scope of your mind, but not

---

161 Damasio, A. R., *The Feeling of What Happens*, p.201
162 Damasio, A. R., *The Feeling of What Happens*, p.201
163 Damasio, A. R., *The Feeling of What Happens*, p.206

all of it. Besides those images there is also this other presence that signifies you, as observer of the things imaged, owner of the things imaged, potential actor on the things imaged. There is a presence of you in a particular relationship with some object... I shall propose that the simplest form of such a presence is also an image, actually the kind of image that constitutes a feeling.[164]

*The neural patterns and images necessary for consciousness to occur are those which constitute proxies for the organism, for the object, and for the relationship between the two. Placed in this framework, understanding the biology of consciousness becomes a matter of discovering how the brain can map **both** the two players **and** the relationships they hold.*[165]

The contents of the autobiographical self — the organized, reactivated memories of fundamental facts from an individual's biography — are prime beneficiaries of core consciousness. Whenever an object X provokes a pulse of core consciousness (which is under gene control) and the core self emerges relative to object X, selected sets of facts from the implicit autobiographical self are also consistently activated as explicit memories and provoke pulses of core consciousness of their own... Without such autobiographical memories we would have no sense of past or future, there would be no historical continuity to our persons.[166]

When we are aware of an object, there is an activation of previous memories (*contemplation which arranges things and beings*):

...recall of an object and deployment of its image in mind is accompanied by the reconstruction of at least some of the images which represent those pertinent aspects. Reconstructing that collection of organism accommodations for the object you recall generates a situation similar to the one that occurs when you perceive an external object directly.[167]

---

164 Damasio, A. R., *The Feeling of What Happens*, pp.9-10
165 Damasio, A. R., *The Feeling of What Happens*, p.16
166 Damasio, A. R., *The Feeling of What Happens*, p.145
167 Damasio, A. R., *The Feeling of What Happens*, p.122

...the consciousness of apprehending something is the same, whether perceived or recalled.[168]

Speech, storytelling and communication

The character ZHI 智 'wisdom', 'intelligence' describes the precise use of words emerging from the mouth and may be seen as precise use of language.[169] From the ancient Chinese perspective, language is considered to be a complex product of the drive to communicate, related to HUN 魂. HUN finds the images necessary for communication in YI 意, which receives, encodes and stores images. Images are not immediately available and ready to be used. Memorized images become available as a review of imprints organized by HUN 魂 and inscribed by YI 意.

Inscriptions of inner states of consciousness and exterior expressions through gestural language are the function of Spleen, which stores YI 意 and is responsible for the four limbs. Communication through gestural language widens the 'territorial consciousness' (the associative network that comprises the complexity of the brain cortex).

According to Damasio, the organization and construction of images began early in human evolution. Consciousness arises when the brain can tell a story without words. A repeated story is the beginning of knowledge. Damasio relates *imagetic representation of sequences* to the origin of language:

The entire construction of knowledge, from simple to complex, from nonverbal imagetic to verbal literary, depends on the ability to map what happens over time, inside our organism, around our organism, to and with our organism, one thing followed by another thing, causing another thing, endlessly.

Telling stories, in the sense of registering what happens in the form of brain maps, is probably a brain obsession and probably begins relatively early both in terms of evolution and in terms of the

---

168 Damasio, A. R., *The Feeling of What Happens*, p.122
169 see page 65

complexity of the neural structures required to create narratives. Telling stories precedes language, since it is, in fact, a condition for language, and it is based not just in the cerebral cortex but elsewhere in the brain and in the right hemisphere as well as the left.[170]

The *imagetic representation of sequences* are traces arranged according to life events, and the relationships between the traces are reminiscent of the function of Defensive QI (WEI 衛), and especially its role in the arrangement of dreams.[171]

Consciousness begins when brains acquire the power, the simple power I must add, of telling a story without words, the story that there is life ticking away in an organism, and that the states of the living organism, within body bounds, are continuously being altered by encounters with objects or events in its environment, or, for that matter, by thoughts and by internal adjustments of the life process. Consciousness emerges when this primordial story—the story of an object causally changing the state of the body—can be told using the universal nonverbal vocabulary of body signals. The apparent self emerges as the feeling of a feeling. When the story is first told, spontaneously, without it ever having been requested, and forevermore after that when the story is repeated, knowledge about what the organism is living through automatically emerges as the answer to a question never asked. From that moment on, we begin to know.[172]

The language explanation of consciousness is improbable and we need to go behind the mask of language to find a more plausible alternative. Curiously, the very nature of language argues against it having a primary role in consciousness. Words and sentences denote entities, actions, events, and relationships. Words and

---

170 Damasio, A. R., *The Feeling of What Happens*, p.125
171 Eyssalet, J.M., *La Rumeur du Dragon et l'Order du Tigre.*, pp.373-375
172 Damasio, A. R., *The Feeling of What Happens*, pp.23-24

sentences translate concepts, and concepts consist of the non language idea of what things, actions, events, and relationships are. Of necessity, concepts precede words and sentences in both the evolution of the species and the daily experience of each and every one of us. The words and sentences of healthy and sane humans do not come out of nowhere, cannot be the de novo translation of nothing before them. So when my mind says "I" or "me," it is translating, easily and effortlessly, the non language concept of the organism that is mine, of the self that is mine. If a perpetually activated construct of core self were not in place, the mind could not possibly translate it as "I," or as "me,"...

*One could argue, in fact, that the consistent content of the **verbal** narrative of consciousness—regardless of the vagaries of its form—permits one to deduce the presence of the equally consistent **nonverbal, imaged** narrative that I am proposing as the foundation of consciousness.*

The narrative of the state of the proto-self being changed by the interaction with an object must first occur in its non language form if it is ever to be translated by suitable words.[173]

The first statement of QI BO's reply starts with exploring 'I'-'me' (WO 我): *Heaven **in me** (WO 我) is* DE 德 - *Earth **in me** (WO 我) is* QI 氣.[174] 'I'-'me' is between Heaven - the ability to exist, and Earth - the ability to create 'substantial forms'.

YI 意, images (XIANG 象) and words (YAN 言) according to WANG BI 王弼

In Chinese thought, the emergence of words (language) was considered as both a natural and a precious outcome of a series of events in the organization of the body.

---

173 Damasio, A. R., *The Feeling of What Happens*, p. 123
174 See page 10

WANG BI 王弼[175] (226–249), of the Daoist school of thought, presents the process of the emergence of speech using the following entities:
- images - XIANG 象
- ideas (intent) - YI 意
- words (speech) - YAN 言
- names (MING 名) which create 'forms' to express images

WANG BI - Part 1:

言 YAN	word	象 XIANG	image	盡 JIN	express	盡 JIN	express
生 SHENG	born	生 SHENG	born	意 YI	idea	象 XIANG	image
於 YU	from	於 YU	from	莫 MO	none	莫 MO	none
象 XIANG	image	意 YI	idea	若 RUO	like	若 RUO	like
				象 XIANG	image	言 YAN	word

Words (YAN 言) are born from images (XIANG 象).
Images (XIANG 象) are born from ideas (YI 意).
To explain an idea (YI 意) there is nothing like an image (XIANG 象).
To explain an image (XIANG 象) there is nothing like words (YAN 言).

- WANG BI: *Words (YAN 言) are born from images (XIANG 象). Images are born from ideas (YI 意).*

Words (speech, language) (YAN 言) emerge from images (XIANG 象). The character XIANG 象, translated as 'image', 'phenomenon', shows a cave painting of an elephant.[176] In ancient China there were no elephants, so it was presumed that the ancestors used the image of an elephant found in a cave painting to describe an unusual phenomenon. The cave painting of an elephant is the consequence of an emotion expressed outwardly as a painted message, a reference to an impression for those who had seen an elephant, and also to prepare those who had not. XIANG 象 represents an imprint, a trace, the emotional shock of the meeting with an elephant externalized by the painter. XIANG 象 becomes an image of the relationship between the painter and the elephant, and this becomes a reference which helps to understand the situation.

---

175 WANG BI JI JIAO SHI, *Critical Edition of Wang Bi's Collected Works*
176 http://www.zhongwen.com/

The images (XIANG 象) can be compared with cognitive maps.[177] *Images are born from* YI 意 – the library of intent and ideas.

According to Damasio, the use of "preverbal images" is essential for core consciousness:

> *The hypothesis states that core consciousness occurs when the brain forms an imaged, nonverbal, second-order account of how the organism is causally affected by the processing of an object.*[178] *Core consciousness is generated in pulselike fashion, for each content of which we are to be conscious. It is the knowledge that materializes when you confront an object, construct a neural pattern for it, and discover automatically that the now-salient image of the object is formed in your perspective, belongs to you, and that you can even act on it. You come by this knowledge, this discovery as I prefer to call it, instantly: there is no noticeable process of inference, no out-in-the-daylight logical process that leads you there, and no words at all — there is the **image of the thing** and, right next to it, is the sensing of its possession by you.*[179]

> *...core consciousness has a major influence on those other cognitive processes. Core consciousness focuses and enhances attention and working memory; core consciousness favors establishment of memories; core consciousness **is indispensable for the normal operations of language;** and core consciousness enlarges the scope of the intelligent manipulations we call planning, problem solving, and creativity.*[180]

> *In core consciousness, the sense of self arises in the subtle, fleeting feeling of knowing, constructed anew in each pulse.*[181]

---

177 Two brain areas are especially important in cognitive maps: the prefrontal cortex and the paralimbic cortex, both connected with the limbic system. See Triune Brain, Wikipedia
178 Damasio, A. R., *The Feeling of What Happens*, p.128
179 Damasio, A. R., *The Feeling of What Happens*, p. 85
180 Damasio, A. R., *The Feeling of What Happens*, p. 84
181 Damasio, A. R., *The Feeling of What Happens*, p.130

- WANG BI: *To explain an idea* (YI 意) *there is nothing like an image* (XIANG 象).

The explanation of ideas is related to knowledge and to the extended consciousness. According to Damasio, extended consciousness allows connection to ideas (information and knowledge) recorded in the brain as preverbal images:

> *Extended consciousness goes beyond the here and now of core consciousness, both backward and forward.*[182]

> *...extended consciousness is the precious consequence of two enabling contributions: First, the ability to learn and thus retain records of myriad experiences, previously known by the power of core consciousness. Second, the ability to reactivate those records in such a way that, as objects, they, too, can generate "a sense of self knowing," and thus be known.*[183]

The records of myriad experiences (Damasio) can be compared to images (XIANG 象).

> *Extended consciousness is, then, the capacity to be aware of a large compass of entities and events, i.e., the ability to generate a sense of individual perspective, ownership, and agency, over a larger compass of knowledge than that surveyed in core consciousness. The sense of autobiographical self to which this larger compass of knowledge is attributed includes unique biographical information.*[184]

The autobiographical self[185] corresponds to the traces of Heart-Consciousness and participates in the formation of ideas (YI 意), and also of knowledge (ZHI 智). According to Damasio:

> *The sustained display of autobiographical self is the key to extended consciousness. Extended consciousness occurs when working memory holds in place, simultaneously, **both** a particular object **and** the autobiographical self, in other words, when*

---

182 Damasio, A. R., *The Feeling of What Happens*, p.129
183 Damasio, A. R., *The Feeling of What Happens*, p.130
184 Damasio, A. R., *The Feeling of What Happens*, p.131
185 See page 121

both *a particular object* **and** *the objects in one's autobiography simultaneously generate core consciousness.*[186]

The key elements of our autobiography that need to be reliably activated in a nearly permanent fashion are those that correspond to our identity, to our recent experiences, and to the experiences that we anticipate, especially those in the near future. I propose that those critical elements arise from a continuously reactivated network based on convergence zones which are located in the temporal and the frontal higher-order cortices, as well as in subcortical nuclei such as those in the amygdala. The coordinated activation of this multisite network is paced by thalamic nuclei, while the holding of the reiterated components for extended periods of time requires the support of prefrontal cortices involved in working memory. In short, the autobiographical self is a process of coordinated activation and display of personal memories, based on a multisite network.[187]

- WANG BI: *To explain an image* (XIANG 象) *there is nothing like words* (YAN 言).

The relationship between idea (YI 意), image-phenomenon and word-language proceeds continually and simultaneously without rupture and may be related to the basis of conscience as described by Damasio:

...the nonconscious neural signaling of an individual organism begets the **proto-self** *which permits* **core self** *and* **core consciousness**, *which allow for an* **autobiographical self**, *which permits* **extended consciousness**. *At the end of the chain,* **extended consciousness** *permits* **conscience**.[188]

The real marvel, as I see it, is that autobiographical memory is architecturally connected, neurally and cognitively speaking, to the nonconscious proto-self and to the emergent and conscious core self of each lived instant.[189]

---

186 Damasio, A. R., *The Feeling of What Happens*, p.148
187 Damasio, A. R., *The Feeling of What Happens*, pp.147-148
188 Damasio, A. R., *The Feeling of What Happens*, p.154
189 Damasio, A. R., *The Feeling of What Happens*, p.114

WANG BI - Part 2

				有 YOU	have		
				形 XING	form		
夫 FU	so			夫 FU	so	夫 FU	so
象 XIANG	image	言 YAN	word	形 XING	form	名 MING	name
者 ZHE	comma	者 ZHE	comma	也 YE	comma	以 YI	which
出 CHU	come out	明 MING	light	者 ZHE	so	定 DING	fix
意 YI	idea	象 XIANG	image	物 WU	being	形 XING	form
者 ZHE	auxiliary word	者 ZHE	auxiliary word	之 ZHI	of		
也 YE	period	也 YE	period	累 LEI	limit		
				也 YE	period		

So images (XIANG 象) emerge from ideas (YI 意). Words illuminate images.
There are 'substantial forms' (XING 形).
So 'substantial forms' are boundaries of things and beings (WU 物).
So names (MING 名) stabilize 'substantial forms' (XING 形).

WANG BI continues to investigate the relationship between images, ideas, words and names (MING 名), which create boundaries and stabilize 'substantial forms' (XING 形):

- Images (XIANG 象) surge from YI 意, 'library of intent, ideas and images'. Images, which may be compared to a cognitive map, are gathered in YI 意 non-consciously, in a haze.
- Speech externalizes thoughts (based on images) with the help of words (YAN 言), and thus transfers images from consciousness, illuminates them.
- Names (MING 名) stabilize (fix) boundaries, they define 'substantial forms' (XING 形) - beings and things.

Damasio quotes the seventeenth-century French philosopher Malebranche:

It is through light and through a clear idea that the mind sees the essence of things, numbers, and extensions. It is through a vague idea or through feeling that the mind judges the existence of creatures and that it knows its own existence.[190]

Damasio also defines the neurobiological problems of consciousness:
*...problem of how the movie-in-the-brain is generated, and the problem of how the brain also generates the sense that there is an owner and observer for that movie. The two problems are so intimately related that the latter is nested within the former. In effect, the second problem is that of generating the **appearance** of an owner and observer for the movie **within the movie**...*[191]

WANG BI - Part 3
Further investigation of image, idea and words by WANG BI recalls the non-conscious:

忘	WANG	forget	忘	WANG	forget
言	YAN	words	象	XIANG	image
者	ZHE	auxiliary word	者	ZHE	auxiliary word
乃	NAI	so	乃	NAI	so
得	DE	attain	得	DE	attain
象	XIANG	image	意	YI	intent, idea
者	ZHE	auxiliary word	者	ZHE	auxiliary word
也	YE	period	也	YE	period

Forgetting (WANG 忘) *the words* (YAN 言), *one attains images* (XIANG 象), *Forgetting the images, one attains the idea* (YI 意).

The character WANG 忘 shows 亡 'death', 'loss', 'perish' and the radical 心 'heart', giving the meaning 'a loss of heart', and is translated 'to forget'[192]. To forget here is not a negative loss, but the expanding of attention to objects on the second plane - the background, and the third plane - beyond the horizon. This process is similar to looking

---

190 Damasio, A. R., *The Feeling of What Happens*, p.207
191 Damasio, A. R., *The Feeling of What Happens*, p.11
192 http://zhongwen.com/d/167/x209.htm

at a painting: first you look at the central figure in the painting, then you move your attention to the background of the picture and then to the frame. In Daoism the character WANG 忘 is used to express liberty and freedom:
- WANG QING 忘情 - to forget your desires, to be free from attachment,
- WANG XING 忘形 - to forget 'substantial forms', to be beyond the appearance.

Forgetting the words, dropping out of awareness, allows attainment of the image-phenomenon, the living imprint (similarly to representations which become the cognitive maps in the brain). The image-phenomenon becomes a symbol in the non-consciousness. After the word is forgotten, the idea (YI 意) of the image surges out and manifests instantly in the consciousness.

WANG BI - Part 4
WANG BI quotes ZHUANG ZI, Chapter 26, to prove his statements.

得 DE	attain	得 DE	attain	得 DE	attain
兔 TU	rabbit	魚 YU	fish	意 YI	intent, idea
而 ER	then	而 ER	then	而 ER	then
忘 WANG	forget	忘 WANG	forget	忘 WANG	forget
蹄 TI	snare	荃 QUAN	net	言 YAN	word

Snares are employed to catch hares, but when the hares are got, men forget the snares.
Fishing-stakes are employed to catch fish; but when the fish are got, the men forget the stakes.
Words (YAN 言) are employed to convey ideas (YI 意); but when the ideas are apprehended, men forget the words.[193]

The propositions made by WANG BI and ZHUANG ZI are a practical invitation to explore reality, to understand myself, and "the feeling of what happens". Contemplation of ideas (YI 意) is performed through

---

193 Translated to English by Legge, J.

one's Heart-Consciousness (XIN 心), or Intimate Nature (XING 性).[194] XING 性 brings a man close to DE 德 - link to the Unity, oneness. In the Unity there is no difference between the individual and the universal. In global listening, with no attention to anything specific, an image-phenomenon from the non-consciousness brings out feelings. Feelings emerge through the senses: vision, hearing, smell, taste, touch. This inner contemplation, which may be called spiritual or meditative, is founded on dynamic observation of the world and of oneself which enables the maintaining, organizing and refining of personal life. In this inner contemplation, all personal knowledge, based on personal or ambient images and words (which construct language and culture) melts, is 'forgotten', and gives place to a feeling of existence and of listening to oneself. Common knowledge must be forgotten from time to time. Listening to oneself is listening to YI 意 'the source of images-phenomena' and to SHEN 神, which rules and organizes the sense of words and images.

The tea ceremony, TAI JI QUAN, the martial arts, the art of flower arrangement, calligraphy, painting and poetry all come from this deep, quiet and relaxed contemplation and listening.

In the Chinese *Art of Nourishing Life* (YANG SHENG 養生), the listening without-action was very important in everyday life. This approach is different from the conventional Western desire to act which takes us away from ourselves.

The listening without-action occurs during sleep. During the deep phase of sleep, the brain is not active, it rests and recuperates - there is a suspension of knowledge and consciousness (YI 意 is inactive), which is reminiscent of the forgetting of words and images in WANG BI. During the paradoxical (Rapid Eye Movements R.E.M.) phase of sleep the brain is active (YI 意 is active) producing dreams filled with images and scenarios; at the same time, there is low muscle tone throughout the body.

---

[194] See page 61

I. LING SHU, Chapter 8-1, continues:

Thus wisdom (ZHI 智) is the nourishment of life (YANG SHENG 養生).
Do not fail to observe the four seasons and to adapt to heat and cold,
To harmonize joy and anger (XI NU 喜怒) and to be calm in activity as in rest,
To regulate the YIN-YANG and to balance the hard and the soft,
In this way, having deflected the perverse influences,
Therefore will be long life (CHANG SHENG 長生) and everlasting visions (JIU SHI 久視).[195]

故智者之養生也，必順四時而適寒暑，和喜怒而安居處，節陰陽而調剛柔，如是，則僻邪不至，長生久視

---

[195] translated by Rochat de la Vallee

5

Interaction between the Three Levels of Man according to LING SHU, Chapter 8-2, and SU WEN, Chapter 62

LING SHU, Chapter 8-2, and SU WEN, Chapter 62, refer to the functions and pathology of the five ZANG 臟, expressed at Three Levels of Man:[196]
- Man at the subtle non-material level of Heaven - Five Roots of SHEN, (BEN SHEN 本神): SHEN 神, HUN 魂, PO 魄, YI 意 and ZHI 志
- Man at the level of Man - expression of the five emotions-desires-passions
- Man at the level of Earth - level of 'substantial forms' - the five ZANG 臟 (Liver, Heart, Spleen, Lung and Kidney) which create and maintain the body

LING SHU, Chapter 8-2, describes for each of the five ZANG the aspect of body function which it controls, its BEN SHEN 本神, and the effects of its pathology (QI deficiency and excess) on the physical body or mental state. According to LING SHU, Chapter 8-2:
- XUE 血 'Blood' is related to Liver function and HUN 魂
- YING 營 'Nourishing QI' is related to Spleen function and YI 意
- MAI 脈 'blood vessels and conduits' are related to Heart function and SHEN 神
- QI 氣 is related to Lung function and PO 魄
- JING 精 is related to Kidney function and ZHI 志

SU WEN, Chapter 62, describes physical and mental pathologies (deficiencies and excesses) of the five vital aspects (related to the five ZANG):
- SHEN 神 is related to Heart function, which it governs
- QI 氣 is related to Lung function and PO 魄
- XUE 血 'Blood' is related to Liver function and HUN 魂

---

196 See page 26

- XING 形 'body-substantial forms' and ROU 肉 'flesh' are related to Spleen function and YI 意
- ZHI 志 is related to Kidney function, which it governs

A. The influence of QI excess and QI deficiency on the functioning of the five ZANG 臟 according to LING SHU, Chapter 8-2[197]

1. Liver, Blood and HUN 魂, LING SHU, Chapter 8-2

肝 GAN	liver	血 XUE	blood	肝 GAN	Liver	實 SHI	excess
藏 CANG	store	舍 SHE	dwell	氣 QI		則 ZE	then
血 XUE	blood	魂 HUN		虛 XU	deficiency	怒 NU	anger
				則 ZE	then		
				恐 KONG	fear		

Liver stores Blood (XUE 血). Blood is the dwelling of HUN 魂. When Liver QI is deficient there is fear (KONG 恐). (When Liver QI) is in excess there is anger (NU 怒).

Blood - 'moving body tissue' - is governed by Liver YANG and HUN 魂, and by Heart YANG and SHEN 神. Liver, the Army General,[198] stores Blood, which 'carries' SHEN 神.[199] Blood flows to different body parts as needed and protects, nourishes and cleanses. Blood syndromes manifest first in mental states, and then in body function.

Liver QI deficiency

Liver QI deficiency, expressed as an emotion of Kidney - fear (KONG 恐), may result from:
- Blood loss which causes Liver QI deficiency. Liver QI deficiency depletes Kidney QI (by reversed generation) causing fear
- Kidney QI/YANG deficiency, expressed as fear, causes Liver QI deficiency (generation)

---

197 LING SHU, Chapter 8, Phrases 12-16
198 SU WEN, Chapter 8
199 LING SHU, Chapter 8

Liver QI deficiency causes an insufficient flow of blood to the upper part of the body. Blood deficiency is especially harmful to Heart and brain (the heart needs adequate blood pressure and the brain needs glucose). The signs of Liver QI deficiency are: hypotension, headache, dizziness, cold sweat, restlessness with body weakness, hypoglycemia and panic, accompanied by trembling legs and a feeling of loss of support.

Liver QI excess

Liver QI excess causes anger (NU 怒) - excessive movement of QI and Blood upwards to the heart, brain and face with the following signs: red face and eyes, restlessness, shouting, violence, headache, bleeding of gums and nose, high blood pressure. Most cases of HBP are the result of continuous, even moderate, Liver QI excess resulting from anger that is not expressed outwardly.

2. Spleen, Nourishing QI (YING 營) **and** YI 意, LING SHU, Chapter 8-2

脾	PI	spleen	脾	PI	spleen	實	SHI	excess
藏	CANG	store	氣	QI		則	ZE	then
營	YING	Nourishing QI	虛	XU	deficiency	腹	FU	abdomen
營	YING	Nourishing QI	則	ZE	then	脹	ZHANG	inflate
舍	SHE	dwell	四	SI	4	經	JING	way
意	YI		肢	ZHI	limbs	溲	SOU	urine
			不	BU	not	不	BU	not
			用	YONG	use	利	LI	function
			五	WU	5			
			臟	ZANG				
			不	BU	not			
			安	AN	peaceful			

Spleen stores Nourishing QI (YING 營). *Nourishing* QI *is the dwelling of* YI 意.
When Spleen QI *is deficient it is impossible to use the four limbs and the five* ZANG 臟 *are agitated.*
(*When Spleen* QI) *is in excess there is abdominal swelling and dysfunction of the urinary tract.*

In Middle JIAO Spleen absorbs simple components from the food entering Stomach: flavors, liquids and Nourishing QI (YING 營), and raises Nourishing QI to Upper JIAO (chest). In Upper JIAO, Nourishing QI:
- becomes part of ZONG QI 宗氣 ('QI of the rhythm of breath and Blood flow', 'QI of the chest')
- participates in blood production and blood flow
- flows in Twelve Meridians (the flow in Twelve Meridians starts from Lung Meridian, which originates in the chest), on the surface of the skin and inside the body, sustaining life and communication between Spirit-mind-body. It can be influenced by activating the acupuncture points located on meridians (all meridians pass through the four limbs, which are governed by Spleen)

Nourishing QI (YING 營):
- participates together with Defensive QI (WEI 衛) in exterior body protection and thermoregulation
- directs the flow of Blood and body liquids
- assures ZANG-FU 臟腑 (all body functions, including hormonal and nervous systems unknown in ancient China)
- nourishes limbs and joints
- nourishes brain
- regulates emotions, especially the ability to think

YI 意 dwells in Spleen. YI 意 is the library of memories of sensations, images, words and all types of messages and knowledge (including flavors and QI). YI and Spleen break down what they have absorbed from the outside world into simpler units, change and use them according to need and personal ability for physical and emotional functioning. YI 意 with the help of Nourishing QI connects and activates self-awareness, self-image, and the individual's image of the world.

According to *The Secret Canon of the Golden Flower*, Chapter 2:
usually people generate their bodies (personality) (SHEN 身) *using Intentionality* (YI 意).[200]

---

[200] *The Secret of the Golden Flower*, Wilhelm; Translated from German by Baynes

The character SHEN 身[201] is translated as 'body', 'personality', 'I' or *'sense of self'*, since in Chinese thought there was no separation between Spirit-Mind-Body. According to Damasio, there is a connection between *'sense of self'* and body (physiological regulation):[202]

> ...the organism, as represented inside its own brain, is a likely biological forerunner for what eventually becomes the elusive sense of self. The deep roots for the self, including the elaborate self which encompasses identity and personhood, are to be found in the ensemble of brain devices which continuously and nonconciously maintain the body state within the narrow range and relative stability required for survival.[203]

Spleen QI deficiency
Spleen represents the entire gastrointestinal tract, including Stomach, Small Intestine and Large Intestine. Malnutrition or inappropriate food cause deficiency of Spleen QI and Nourishing QI (YING 營) expressed as: Blood deficiency, fatigue and exhaustion, and lack of supply of Nourishing QI to the four limbs (causing difficulty in limb movement) and to the five ZANG 臟, which become 'agitated' (for example agitation in hypoglycemia or in fasting).

Spleen QI excess
Overeating and overconsumption of sweet or greasy food cause Spleen QI excess - food congestion in the stomach or intestines interfering with absorption of Nourishing QI (YING 營), flavors and substances, expressed as: intestinal (abdominal) swelling, and problems with urination resulting from disturbance of the absorption and raising of liquids. Congested Spleen does not raise liquids to Lung, and Lung does not send liquids down to Kidney and Bladder, resulting in *dysfunction of the urinary tract*.

---

201 The characters SHEN 身 'body' and SHEN 神 'Spirit' have identical PINYIN letters but differ in tones
202 See page 13
203 Damasio, A. R., *The Feeling of What Happens*, p.18

3. Heart, conduits and blood vessels (MAI 脈) and SHEN 神, LING SHU, Chapter 8-2

心	XIN	heart	心	XIN	heart		
藏	CANG	store	氣	QI		實	SHI excess
脈	MAI	conduits, blood vessels	虛	XU	deficiency	則	ZE then
脈	MAI	conduits, blood vessels	則	ZE	then	笑	XIAO laugh
舍	SHE	dwell	悲	BEI	sorrow	不	BU not
神	SHEN					休	XIU rest

Heart stores conduits and blood vessels (MAI 脈). *Conduits and blood vessels are the dwelling of SHEN* 神.
When Heart QI is deficient there is sorrow (BEI 悲).
(When Heart QI) is in excess there are uncontrollable giggles.

Heart stores conduits and blood vessels (MAI 脈). The character MAI 脈 shows the radical 肉/月 'flesh' (body) and the phonetic 辰 'water flow'.[204] MAI can be written as 脉 which also shows the radical 肉/月 'flesh' (body) and 永 'water flow'[205] or 'longevity'.[206] The characters MAI 脈/脉 represent the nourishing flow in the flesh-body, and are translated as 'conduits', 'meridians', 'vessels', 'blood vessels' (arteries, veins), 'Blood circulation or pulse' – active aspect of the Blood. MAI 脈/脉 is one of six Organs of Extraordinary Longevity (QI HENG ZHI FU 奇恒之腑), which store JING 精. Blood (XUE 血) flows in blood vessels (DONG MAI 動脈). Arteries are called XUE MAI 血脈. Nourishing QI (YING 營/RONG 榮) flows in conduits-meridians (JING MAI 經脈).

Liver stores Blood and Spleen stores Nourishing QI. Heart is responsible for the flow of Blood in blood vessels and for the flow of Nourishing QI in meridians. Balance in life is organized by Heart-SHEN. Heart maintains the balance between Blood and QI. SHEN 神 maintains the balance between the interior of the body and the environment,

---

204 Wieger, Lesson 125
205 Wieger, Lesson 125
206 Eyssalet, *La Rumeur du Dragon et l'Ordre du Tigre*

between 'substantial forms' and QI, and between 'substantial forms' and BEN SHEN 本神, with the help of the meridians and blood vessels.

ZHUANG ZI, Chapter 11, calls this balance in life the *'central way'* (ZHONG DAO 中道), which is harmed by excessive joy and anger (XI NU 喜怒):

人 REN	man	陰 YIN		其 QI	this	居 JU	support
大 DA	big	陽 YANG		反 FAN	return	處 CHU	place
喜 XI	joy	并 BING	together	傷 SHANG	harm	無 WU	not
邪 YE	period	毗 PI	damage	人 REN	man	常 CHANG	constant
毗 PI	damage	四 SI	4	之 ZHI	of	思 SI	thought
於 YU	to	時 SHI	season	形 XING	form	慮 LU	contemplation
陽 YANG		不 BU	not	乎 HU	!	不 BU	not
大 DA	big	至 ZHI	come	使 SHI	make	自 ZI	spontaneous
怒 NU	anger	寒 HAN	cold	人 REN	man	得 DE	obtain
邪 YE	damage	署 SHU	heat	喜 XI	joy	中 ZHONG	center
毗 PI		之 ZHI	of	怒 NU	anger	道 DAO	
於 YU	to	和 HE	harmony	失 SHI	lose	不 BU	not
陰 YIN		不 BU	not	位 WEI	stability	成 CHENG	accomplish
		成 CHENG	accomplish			章 ZHANG	composition

Are men exceedingly joyful (XI 喜)? *- they will do damage to the YANG (element).*
Are men exceedingly angry (DA NU 大怒)? *- they will do damage to the YIN.*
And when both YANG and YIN are damaged, the four seasons will not come as they should, heat and cold will fail to achieve their proper harmony.
This in turn will do harm to the bodies of men. It will make men lose a proper sense of joy and anger (XI NU 喜怒).[207]
(Man) *loses stability. His thoughts and contemplations are not expressed spontaneously. The 'central way'* (ZHONG DAO 中道) (Heart) *cannot realize itself completely.*

---

207 Translated by B. Watson, https://terebess.hu/english/chuangtzu.html

HUN 魂 dwells in Blood (Liver) and follows SHEN 神[208] - Consciousness and emotions. Therefore disorders of Liver and Heart are expressed as emotions.

Heart QI deficiency
Heart QI deficiency causes sorrow (BEI 悲). The character BEI 悲 shows a denial of Heart, sudden strong pain.[209] Heart QI deficiency is also expressed as Heart's loss of ability to control the blood vessels and meridians.

Sorrow closes the chest and impairs Lung function. Lung does not move body liquids down and there is an accumulation of cold mucus (TAN YIN 痰飲) in the chest, causing depression (DIAN 癲),[210] expressed by passive and negative behavior, a pale complexion, stupor, prostration and reluctance to talk.

Heart QI excess
Heart QI excess increases the flow in blood vessels and meridians. QI excess in a healthy Heart is expressed by smiling. Joy and amused surprise cause passing Heart QI excess expressed by laughter.

Uncontrollable giggles and nonstop laughing for no reason are caused by the ascent of YANG (*Heart fire*) towards the head, damaging YIN (Heart Blood flow), and are accompanied by a red-face, insomnia, lack of concentration, palpitation, restless dreams and memory loss. *Heart fire* also impairs the flow of body liquids causing *phlegm-fire* (TAN HUO 痰火), expressed as restlessness and manic behavior (KUANG 狂).[211]

---

208 See page 13, for LING SHU, Chapter 8-1
209 See page 52
210 See page 352
211 See page 352

4. Lung, breath (QI 氣) and PO 魄, LING SHU, Chapter 8-2

肺 FEI	lung	肺 FEI	lungs	實 SHI	excess
藏 CANG	store	氣 QI		則 ZE	then
氣 QI		虛 XU	deficiency	喘 CHUAN	wheezing
氣 QI		則 ZE	then	喝 HE	cough
舍 SHE	dwell	鼻 BI	nose	胸 XIONG	chest
魄 PO		塞 SAI	block	盈 YING	full
		不 BU	not	仰 YANG	raise the head
		利 LI	function	息 XI	respiration
		少 SHAO	shallow		
		氣 QI	breath		

Lung stores breath-QI 氣. QI is the dwelling of PO 魄.
When Lung QI is deficient, the nose is congested; there is difficulty in breathing and shortness of breath.
(When Lung QI) is in excess there is breathing with wheezing, coughing, chest congestion, and the head has to be lifted to breathe.

Lung and PO 魄 are related to acquired QI flow in man:
- DA QI 大氣, QI of the Universe, of the air, Great QI, which enters through the orifice of Lung - the nose.
- RONG/YING QI 榮/營氣, Nourishing QI flows in Twelve Meridians. The daily circuit of Nourishing QI flow in Twelve Meridians starts from Lung Meridian.
- ZONG QI 宗氣, 'QI temple of the Universe', 'QI of the chest', 'the rhythm of QI and Blood flow',[212] which originates from DA QI (absorbed by Lung) and Nourishing QI.
- WEI QI 衛氣, Defensive QI, which circulates on the skin surface (Lung body tissue) and transports body liquids below the skin.

Lung QI deficiency
Lung QI deficiency causes an inadequate supply of DA QI 大氣 and provokes ZONG QI 宗氣 deficiency in the chest, and QI deficiency in

---

[212] Eyssalet, J.M.. *Emergence et Immersion du Souffle et du Desir*

the whole body. Lung is the first victim of QI deficiency: respiratory rhythm and the descent of body liquids are damaged. Signs of Lung QI deficiency are congested nose and shortness of breath (dyspnea).

Lung QI excess
Lung QI excess in LING SHU, Chapter 8-2, is 'false excess' syndrome of Lung, caused by *Liver YANG rising* (reversed control) or by *Heart YANG rising* (over-control). YANG (fire or heat) rising prevents Lung lowering and dispersing body liquids which cool and clean the body. Stagnant liquids in Lung become *phlegm-fire* (TAN HUO 痰火) or edema, expressed by shortness of breath, wheezing, coughing and a feeling of chest congestion. This shortness of breath may be expressed as an asthma attack or pulmonary edema resulting from chronic heart failure.

In an asthma attack accompanied by wheezing and dry cough, lifting the head releases the region above the sternum (REN MAI, points CV22, CV23) and allows breathing by 'pushing' QI of REN MAI towards the face.

5. Kidney, JING 精 and ZHI 志, LING SHU, Chapter 8-2

腎 SHEN	kidney	精 JING		腎 SHEN	kidney	實 SHI	excess
藏 CANG	store	舍 SHE	dwell	氣 QI		則 ZE	then
精 JING		志 ZHI		虛 XU	deficiency	脹 ZHANG	swelling
				則 ZE	then		
				厥 JUE	exhaustion		

Kidney stores JING 精. JING is the dwelling of ZHI 志.
When Kidney QI is deficient there is exhaustion.
(When Kidney QI) is in excess there is swelling.

Kidney stores JING 精, the dwelling of ZHI 志 - 'determination', 'judgment', 'ability to realize life', 'ability to make decisions', which anchors the body.

According to NAN JING, Chapter 34: *Kidney stores JING* 精 *together with ZHI* 志 (SHEN CANG JING YU ZHI YE 腎藏精與志也).
ZHI 志 and Kidney YIN govern the reservoir of JING 精 by means of Source QI (YUAN QI 原氣). ZHI 志 and Kidney YANG (Gate of Destiny, MING MEN 命門) represent Original Fire, which raises JING QI 精 氣 (QI carrying JING).[213] ZHI 志 (Water Modality) functions together with YI 意 (Soil Modality), which directs the absorption of substances necessary to form the body.[214]

According to a Daoist saying, ZHI, SHEN, QI and body substance are connected:
ZHI 志 *represents the spirit* (SHEN 神) *of QI* 氣. *QI* 氣 *represents the abundance of body substances* (TI 體). (ZHI ZHE QI ZHI SHEN YE QI ZHE TI ZHI CHONG YE 志者氣之神也 氣者體之充也)

Destiny is shaped by SHEN 神, the composer. SHEN 神 through ZHI 志 administrates Source QI (YUAN QI 原氣). ZHI 志 through activation of Kidney YANG (MING MEN 命門), allows the expression of the genome, and by means of YUAN QI 原氣 directs *the abundance of body substances* (TI 體), thereby facilitating body formation according to heredity and adaptation to the changing environment.

Kidney QI deficiency
Kidney QI deficiency depletes JING 精 and provokes JING QI 精氣 deficiency in the entire body, impairing its function, and causing a feeling of exhaustion and fatigue.

Kidney QI excess
Kidney QI excess is described as edema - a 'false excess' of body liquids. Kidney QI **deficiency** prevents the excretion of body liquids as urine and also their movement upwards to Lung, causing edema in lower abdomen and legs. When Kidney QI deficiency damages Spleen (reversed control) there may be edema in the entire body.

---

213 See page 37
214 See page 117

B. The five vital aspects stored in the five ZANG 臟, and their pathologies expressed in the body and the mind according to SU WEN, Chapter 62

SU WEN, Chapter 62, *Discourse on Regulating the Conduits* (Meridians) (TIAO JING LUN 調經論),[215] completes the information given by LING SHU, Chapter 8-2, and describes:

1. The five vital aspects, each related to one of the five ZANG 臟:
   - SHEN 神 – is related to Heart function, which it governs
   - QI 氣 – is related to Lung function and PO 魄
   - XUE 血 'Blood' – is related to Liver function and HUN 魂
   - XING 形 'body-substantial forms' and flesh (ROU 肉) – are related to Spleen function and YI 意
   - ZHI 志 – is related to Kidney function, which it governs
2. The influence of the pair ZHI-YI 志意 on man (complemented by the description in LING SHU, Chapter 47)
3. Signs of deficiency and excess of these five vital aspects of man (10 pathologies)

1. The five vital aspects and the five ZANG 臟, SU WEN, Chapter 62

神 SHEN	氣 QI	血 XUE blood	形 XING form	志 ZHI
有 YOU have	有 YOU have	有 YOU have	有 YOU have	有 YOU have
餘 YU excess	餘 YU excess	餘 YU excess	餘 YU excess	餘 YU excess
有 YOU have	有 YOU have	有 YOU have	有 YOU have	有 YOU have
不 BU not	不 BU not	不 BU not	不 BU not	不 BU not
足 ZU enough	足 ZU enough	足 ZU enough	足 ZU enough	足 ZU enough

SHEN 神 *has excess and deficiency;*
QI 氣 *has excess and deficiency;*
Blood (XUE 血) *has excess and deficiency;*
'Substantial forms' (XING 形) *have excess and deficiency;*
ZHI 志 *has excess and deficiency.*

---

215 Characters 62-334-4 - 62-335-4

凡 FAN	其 QI	皆 JIE	all
此 CI in all	氣 QI	生 SHENG	originate
十 SHI 10	不 BU not	於 YU	from
者 ZHE comma	等 DENG similar	五 WU	5
	也 YE period	藏 ZANG	organs functions

In each of the ten cases there are different flows of QI.
All (these ten cases) originate from the five ZANG.

夫 FU						而 ER	and
心 XIN	肺 FEI	肝 GAN	脾 PI	腎 SHEN	此 CI		all these
藏 CANG	藏 CANG	藏 CANG	藏 CANG	藏 CANG	成 CHENG		achieve
神 SHEN	氣 QI	血 XUE	肉 ROU	志 ZHI	形 XING		form

So Heart stores SHEN 神.
Lung stores QI 氣.
Liver stores Blood (XUE 血).
Spleen stores flesh (ROU 肉).
Kidney stores ZHI 志.
And all these accomplish 'substantial forms' (XING 形).

The five vital aspects and the five ZANG 臟 according to LING SHU, Chapter 8-2 and SU WEN, Chapter 62:

ZANG 臟	LING SHU, Chapter 8-2	SU WEN, Chapter 62
Liver	Blood (XUE 血)	Blood (XUE 血)
Heart	SHEN 神	Blood vessel and conduits (MAI 脈)
Spleen	Nourishing QI (YING 營)	Flesh (ROU 肉), body-'substantial forms' (XING 形)
Lung	QI 氣	QI 氣
Kidney	ZHI 志	JING 精

SHEN, QI, Blood, flesh and ZHI 志 generate 'substantial forms'-body (XING 形). The character XING 形, translated as 'body', 'substances',

'substantial forms', may also represent forms of consciousness.[216]
There are three differences (shaded in the table above) between LING SHU, Chapter 8-2 and SU WEN, Chapter 62:

1. 'Blood vessels (MAI 脈)' replace 'SHEN 神'. However, Blood which flows in MAI 脈 transfers SHEN 神.
2. 'Flesh' (ROU 肉) and 'substantial forms' (XING 形) replace 'Nourishing QI', which builds them.
3. 'JING 精' (SU WEN, Chapter 62) replaces 'ZHI 志' (which governs JING 精).

2. YI 意 and ZHI 志, and the five ZANG 臟, SU WEN, Chapter 62

志 ZHI		五 WU	5	血 XUE	blood	是 SHI	to be
意 YI		藏 ZANG	organs	氣 QI		故 GU	so
通 TONG	communicate	之 ZHI	of	不 BU	not	守 SHOU	receive
內 NEI	inside	道 DAO	pathway	和 HE	harmony	經 JING	meridian
連 LIAN	link	皆 JIE	all	百 BAI	100	隧 SUI	conduit
骨 GU	bones	出 CHU	exit	病 BING	disease	焉 YAN	this
髓 SUI	marrow	於 YU	by	乃 NAI	then		
而 ER	and	經 JING	meridian	變 BIAN	change		
成 CHENG	achieve	隧 SUI	conduit	化 HUA	metamorphosis		
身 SHEN	body	以 YI	so that	而 ER	and		
形 XING	form	行 XING	circulate	生 SHENG	generate		
五 WU	5	血 XUE	blood				
藏 ZANG	organs	氣 QI					

ZHI 志 and YI 意 *communicate and provide a connection between bones and bone marrow inside the body, and accomplish the body* (SHEN 身), '*substantial forms*' *(of mind)* (XING 形) *and the five* ZANG. *All pathways of the five* ZANG *exit as meridians and conduits* (JING SUI 經隧) *to circulate Blood and* QI.

When Blood and QI *are not harmonized, changes and metamorphoses are produced, and one hundred diseases are generated.*

Hence, guard meridians and conduits.

---

216 See page 116

SU WEN, Chapter 62, introduces two BEN SHEN 本神 pairs:
- SHEN 神 and ZHI 志 (Fire-Water - the central axis of the TAI JI symbol), are among the five vital aspects of man;
- ZHI 志 and YI 意 (Water-Soil)[217] which accomplish 'substantial forms' (body and mind) of the five ZANG.

Kidney and ZHI 志 govern inborn Source QI (YUAN QI 原氣) which stores JING 精 in bones and marrow. Spleen-YI governs acquired QI production. The pair ZHI and YI, which together generate 'substantial forms' of the physical body and mind and allow the function of the five ZANG, may in modern terms represent the integration between the neural and endocrine systems and the brain.

The five ZANG govern the circulation in meridians and conduits (JING SUI 經隧). Good function of the five ZANG is expressed by a balanced QI flow in meridians (JING 經) and blood flow in conduits (SUI 隧).

The character SUI 隧 'tunnel'[218] or 'passage' of 豕 'pigs'[219] (pigs symbolize life), may also be translated as 'underground passage' or 'conduit'.

Another way of considering SUI 隧 is as the vascular and nervous systems of the muscles and tendons, in the area of the trajectories of the Twelve Meridians and their acupuncture points. Some of these points are located on arteries on which pulses can be felt. For example, the radial pulse is felt on the radial artery, on the Lung Meridian pathway, points LU9, LU8, LU7. The peripheral pulse on the common carotid artery on the Stomach Meridian pathway, point ST9, indicates the condition of YANG in the entire body. The peripheral pulse on the posterior tibial artery on Kidney Meridian, posterior to the point K3, indicates the condition of Source QI and of the Extraordinary Meridian CHONG MAI 衝脈.

---

217 See page 117 for ZHI 志 and YI 意
218 http://zhongwen.com/d/192/x71.htm
219 Wieger, Lesson 69

Evaluation of the balance between ZHI and YI by means of evaluation of Blood and QI flow of the five ZANG in meridians and conduits (JING SUI 經隧) is important to prevent 100 (all) diseases.

3. YI 意 and ZHI 志, and the five ZANG 臟, LING SHU, Chapter 47

志 ZHI							
意 YI	intent						
者 ZHE	comma						
所 SUO							
以 YI	which						
御 YU	conduct	收 SHOU	gather	適 SHI	adapt	和 HE	harmonize
精 JING		魂 HUN		寒 HAN	cold	喜 XI	joy
神 SHEN		魄 PO		溫 WEN	heat	怒 NU	anger
						者 ZHE	
						也 YE	period

ZHI 志 and YI 意 conduct JING SHEN 精神 (SHEN carrying JING, Vital Spirits),
Gather HUN 魂 and PO 魄,
Adapt to cold and heat,
Harmonize joy and anger (XI NU 喜怒).

志 ZHI	則 ZE	then	魂 HUN		悔 HUI	regret	五 WU	5
意 YI	intent	精 JING	魄 PO		怒 NU	anger	藏 ZANG	organs
和 HE	harmony	神 SHEN	不 BU	not	不 BU	not	不 BU	not
		專 ZHUAN	circulate	散 SAN	disperse	起 QI	arise	受 SHOU	receive
		直 ZHI	right				邪 XIE	pernicious
							矣 YI	period

When ZHI 志 and YI 意 are balanced, JING SHEN 精神 (SHEN carrying JING, Vital Spirits) follow the right direction.
HUN 魂 and PO 魄 are not dispersed. Regret and anger (HUI NU 悔怒) do not arise.
So the five ZANG are not affected by pernicious influences (XIE 邪).

LING SHU, Chapter 47, provides complementary information on the importance of the BEN SHEN pair ZHI-YI 志意, Water and Soil, as a source of balance in man, which also influence another BEN SHEN pair: HUN-PO 魂魄, Wood and Metal.

The pair ZHI-YI 志意, a source of balance in man, influence:
- Distribution of JING SHEN 精神 (SHEN carrying both Source and acquired JING 精, potential of personal development). JING SHEN 精神 (Water and Fire) here replace the pair SHEN-ZHI 神志 in SU WEN, Chapter 62, which also represent Water and Fire.
- Coordination between another pair, HUN 魂 and PO 魄 (Wood and Metal). HUN 魂 follows SHEN (horizontal plane of TAI JI symbol), and PO 魄 is linked with JING (ZHI 志) (vertical plane of TAI JI symbol).[220]
- Emotional balance (joy-SHEN 神, anger-HUN 魂, regret-PO 魄).
- Proper function of the five ZANG, when there is emotional balance. The five ZANG are the source of Blood and QI circulation which provide:
  - Thermoregulation (adaptation to cold and heat)
  - Defense against pernicious (XIE 邪) external influences

4. Signs of deficiencies and excesses of the five vital aspects of man, SU WEN, Chapter 62

SU WEN, Chapter 62, presents signs of deficiencies and excesses of the five vital aspects, related to ZANG 臟: SHEN 神, QI 氣, Blood (XUE 血), body-'substantial forms' (XING 形) and ZHI 志.

This is identical to LING SHU, Chapter 8-2, with the exception of excess of ZHI 志-Kidney described here in SU WEN, Chapter 62, as *abdominal swelling and diarrhea* (enteritis with abdominal pain and cramping). LING SHU, Chapter 8-2, describes a stagnation of Kidney YIN (water retention which results in abdominal swelling). SU WEN, Chapter 62, describes a release of this stagnation by means of Kidney YANG through 'hot diarrhea' with abdominal pain and cramps.

---

220 See pages 107 LING SHU, Chapter 8-1

SU WEN, Chapter 62:

神 SHEN		氣 QI		血 XUE	blood	形 XING	body	志 ZHI	
有 YOU	has	有 YOU	has	有 YOU	has	有 YOU	has	有 YOU	has
餘 YU	excess	餘 YU	excess	餘 YU	excess	餘 YU	excess	餘 YU	excess
則 ZE	this	則 ZE	this	則 ZE	this	則 ZE	this	則 ZE	this
笑 XIAO	laugh	喘 CHUAN	wheeze	怒 NU	anger	腹 FU	belly	腹 FU	belly
不 BU	not	欬 KE	cough	不 BU	not	脹 ZHANG	swell	脹 ZHANG	swell
休 XIU	rest	上 SHANG	up	足 ZU	enough	經 JING	way	飧 SUN	diarrhea
不 BU	not	氣 QI		則 ZE	this	溲 SOU	urine	泄 XIE	
足 ZU	enough	不 BU	not	恐 KONG	fear	不 BU	not	不 BU	not
者 ZHE	comma	足 ZU	enough			利 LI	function	足 ZU	enough
悲 BEI	sorrow	則 ZE	this			不 BU	not	則 ZE	this
		息 XI	breath			足 ZU	enough	厥 JUE	exhaust
		利 LI	function			則 ZE	this		
		少 XIAO	small			四 SI	4		
		氣 QI				肢 ZHI	limbs		
						不 BU	not		
						用 YONG	use		

When SHEN 神 is in excess there are uncontrollable giggles. (When SHEN 神) is deficient there is sorrow (BEI 悲).

When QI is in excess there is breathing with wheezing, coughing and QI flows upwards. (When QI) is deficient there is difficulty in breathing and shortness of breath.

When Blood (XUE 血) is in excess there is anger (NU 怒). (When Blood) is deficient there is fear (KONG 恐).

When 'substantial forms' (XING 形) are in excess there is abdominal swelling and dysfunction of the urinary tract. (When 'substantial forms') are deficient it is impossible to use the four limbs.

When ZHI 志 is in excess there is abdominal swelling and diarrhea. (When ZHI 志) is deficient there is exhaustion.

6

The nine fluctuations of QI flow expressed as emotions, SU WEN, Chapter 39

SU WEN, Chapter 39, *Discourse on Origin of Pain* (舉痛論), begins with a statement made by the Yellow Emperor:[221]

余	YU	I
知	ZHI	know
百	BAI	100
病	BING	disease
生	SHENG	generate
於	YU	from
氣	QI	
也	YE	period

I know that a hundred diseases (all diseases) are generated by QI 氣.

The Yellow Emperor presents the nine types of QI, and QI BO explains the effects of each. These nine types of QI include six emotions/passions (QI of internal origin) and three types of QI of external origin (cold, heat, exhaustion), and appear in the following order:

1. Anger (NU 怒)
2. Joy (XI 喜)
3. Sorrow (BEI 悲)
4. Fear (KONG 恐)
5. Cold (HAN 寒)
6. Heat (JIONG 炅)
7. Panic (JING 驚)
8. Exhaustion (LAO 勞)
9. Thought / excessive thinking (SI 思)

---

221 SU WEN, 39-221-5 - 39-222-4

怒 NU anger	喜 XI joy	悲 BEI sorrow	恐 KONG fear	寒 HAN cold
則 ZE this	則 ZE this	則 ZE this	則 ZE this	則 ZE this
氣 QI	氣 QI	氣 QI	氣 QI	氣 QI
上 SHANG raise	緩 HUAN slow	消 XIAO vanish	下 XIA down	收 SHOU gather

Anger (NU 怒) moves QI upwards.
Joy (XI 喜) slows QI.
Sorrow (BEI 悲) depletes QI.
Fear (KONG 恐) moves QI downwards.
Cold (HAN 寒) contracts QI.

灵 JIONG heat	驚 JING panic	勞 LAO fatigue	思 SI think	九 JIU 9
則 ZE this	則 ZE this	則 ZE this	則 ZE this	氣 QI
氣 QI	氣 QI	氣 QI	氣 QI	不 BU not
泄 XIE disperse	亂 LUAN disorder	耗 HAO consume	結 JIE knot	同 TONG similar
				病 BING disease
				之 ZHI of
				生 SHENG generate

Heat (JIONG 灵) disperses QI.
Panic (JING 驚) causes disorder of the QI flow.
Exhaustion following hard work (LAO 勞) consumes QI.
Thinking (SI 思) knots QI.
These nine QI are different from each other, which illnesses do they generate?

The effects of these nine types of QI on man are:

1. Anger (NU 怒) moves QI and Blood upwards to the head and chest. According to LING SHU, Chapter 8-2,[222] and SU WEN, Chapter 62,[223] excess of Liver QI and Blood causes anger.

2. Joy (XI 喜) is the expression of Heart QI excess. Joy expands the flow in meridians and Blood vessels, slowing down and harmonizing QI

---

222 See page 149
223 See page 159

circulation, but the change of the QI flow dynamic may provoke fatigue.

3. Sorrow (BEI 悲) closes the chest and interferes with respiration and communication with the environment. Lung does not absorb enough QI from the air and QI vanishes from the body.

4. Fear (KONG 恐) damages Kidney, the root of life and the ability to stand upright between Heaven and Earth, causing QI to flow downwards and to be lost through urinary incontinence and diarrhea.

5. Cold (HAN 寒) is QI of the winter. QI and Blood enter deep into the body from the periphery for protection. Cold contracts QI in order to maintain it inside the body. Cold may also manifest itself in emotions.

6. Heat (JIONG 灵) is QI of the summer. Heat disperses body liquids outwards to cool the body through perspiration. Which disperses QI outwards. Heat may also manifest itself in emotions.

7. Panic (JING 驚) is confusion and loss of QI flow rhythm. Ascent and descent, inward and outward movements of QI are chaotic and disorderly.

9. Thinking (SI 思) slows the activity of Spleen and interferes with Nourishing QI (RONG 榮) production in Middle JIAO. Repetitive-compulsive thinking is similar to spinning in a circle and knots the QI flow.

8. Exhaustion (LAO 勞) following excessive physical effort (overuse of muscle strength) or mental effort (concentration) consumes QI.

In his reply, QI BO presents the damage caused by each of the nine types of QI.

1. Anger (NU 怒), SU WEN, Chapter 39 (Figure 40)

怒	NU	anger	甚	SHEN	too much	故	GU	so
則	ZE	this	則	ZE	this	氣	QI	
氣	QI		嘔	OU	vomit	上	SHANG	raise
逆	NI	rebel	血	XUE	blood	矣	YI	period
			乃	NAI	up to			
			殄	SUN	food			
			泄	XIE	diarrhea			

Anger (NU 怒) causes QI to rebel (excessive QI flow upwards) (QI NI 氣逆).
Severe cases are manifested in vomiting blood and diarrhea.
So QI 氣 moves upwards.

Figure 40. Anger (NU 怒) according to SU WEN, Chapter 39

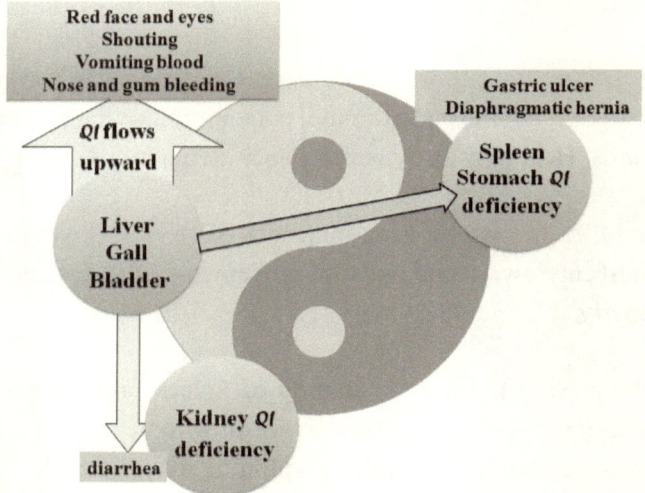

❖ SU WEN, Chapter 39: *Anger (NU 怒) causes QI to rebel (excessive flow upwards) (QI NI 氣逆).*

Anger (NU 怒),[224] expressed or non-expressed, caused by an external event or interior disorder, is a manifestation of Liver-Wood QI which is wind:

---

[224] See page 53

SU WEN, Chapter 54: *Human emotions are wind.*
SU WEN, Chapter 5: *Wind* (communicates) *with Liver.*

The natural direction of Liver-Wood QI flow is upwards, from Kidney to Heart, like wind blowing from Earth to Heaven. Wind is an expression of YANG and represents tension at the start of communication, and is the expression of a dynamic connection.

Anger is the opposite of the virtue of Liver - humanity, empathy, the ability to take the other into consideration, communication skills (REN 仁).[225]

Deviation from natural flow is called rebel (NI 逆), 治反為逆 (SU WEN, Chapter 65). Anger (NU 怒), caused by external conflict or internal imbalances, does not change the natural upward direction of Liver QI and blood flow, but increases the intensity and speed of their ascent towards the chest and head.

❖ SU WEN, Chapter 39. Anger: *Severe cases are manifested in vomiting blood...*

In anger, rebel Liver QI provokes YANG excess in the upper body: QI and Blood rise excessively towards the chest and head, and their descent to the lower body slows down, causing: reddish complexion and red eyes (eye inflammation), headache, shouting, bleeding gums and bleeding from the nose, shortness of breath, rapid heart rate, and in severe cases:

- Vomiting of blood; Liver over-controls Stomach and causes 'Stomach QI and blood to rise' (gastric ulcer, heartburn). Even now in China the popular belief is that anger provokes vomiting of blood. In Chinese movies when a hero becomes really angry he vomits blood.
- Formation of *Phlegm-dampness* or *phlegm-fire* from accumulated body liquids; Liver (reversed control) prevents Lung from moving body liquids down.

---

225 See page 64

- Tension below the diaphragm and under the ribs (hypochondrium). In severe anger QI accumulates below the ribs. This QI accumulation may push the stomach upwards towards the thorax and distend the passage of the esophagus through the diaphragm,[226] causing hiatal (diaphragmatic) hernia.

LING SHU, Chapter 4, describes damage to caused by anger to Liver and the region below the ribs (diaphragm):

若	RUO if	氣	QI	積	JI	accumulation
有	YOU has	上	SHANG ascend	於	YU	at
所	SUO like	而	ER and	脅	XIE	ribs
大	DA big	不	BU not	下	XIA	below
怒	NU anger	下	XIA descend	則	ZE	then
				傷	SHANG	damage
				肝	GAN	liver

In big anger (DA NU 大怒) QI ascends, cannot flow down, accumulates below the ribs and then damages Liver.

❖ SU WEN, Chapter 39. Anger: *Severe cases are manifested as… diarrhea.*

In anger Liver YANG rises to Upper JIAO, and this depletes QI in Middle and Lower JIAO. In Lower JIAO, anger provokes disharmony between YIN-YANG, causing Kidney QI deficiency (reversed generation), expressed as accumulation of liquids in the intestines and watery diarrhea.

In Middle JIAO, overactive Liver over-controls Spleen and Stomach, interfering with the transformation and transportation of food and provoking diarrhea with non-digested food.

Regulating QI by acupuncture in cases of anger
Use of a synergetic combination of acupuncture points enhances the desired effect. For each treatment, the relevant information on the acupuncture points used is presented:

---

226 Epiploic foramen (Winslow Hiatus)

- The name of the point.
- The traditional function of the acupuncture point:
  - the five 'antique' points (WU SHU 五輸): JING-Well 井, YING 榮, SHU 俞, JING-River 經, HE 合;
  - LUO 絡, Source-YUAN 元, MU 募, SHU 俞, XI 郄;
  - regulation of flow in Meridians, Connecting Channels (LUO 絡) and Divergent Channels (BIE 別), meeting with other meridians;
  - regulation of Eight Extraordinary Meridians;
  - regulation of the Four Seas;
  - entry or exit;
  - HUI-meeting;
  - 'knot' of one of Six Levels;
  - regulation of BEN SHEN;
  - Celestial Window.
- Relevant actions of the point on ZANG, FU, QI, Blood, body liquids, BEN SHEN and emotions.
- Synergetic combinations between the main point (shaded) and other points.
- Recommendation for the acupuncture technique: tonify, disperse, direction of the needle, moxibustion.

Anger provokes	main points	point synergy
a. QI flows upwards	LU9-LIV8-Ki7	
	LU1, BL18	
	CV18	LIV6-CV18, CV18-Ki21
	LU3	LU3-LU9-BL17, PC1-LU3
	PC8	PC8-H7-LI4-GV26, PC8-Ki7, LU10-PC8
	LIV2	LIV2-PC7-H7-GV14-ST40, LIV2-GB38, LIV2-ST40-LI4-TW6, LIV2-LU5-SP6
b. Phlegm-dampness or *phlegm-fire*	CV14	
	PC7	PC7-ST40-GV26, LIV2-LIV3-ST44-PC7
c. Diarrhea	Ki7	Ki7-SP6, LIV3-Ki7-SP6
	SP6	SP6-SP9-ST25-ST44, SP4-H7-SP6

a. Acupuncture points to move QI downwards and calm anger

name	function	action
LU9-LIV8-Ki7 calm anger		
LIV8 QU QUAN 曲泉 Spring at the Bend	HE-Water of Liver, tonify Wood	tonify Liver YIN (especially in Ki. YIN deficiency), nourish Liver Blood, clear excess heat, move dampness, regulate Lower JIAO
Ki7 FU LIU 復溜 Returning Current	JING-River-Metal of Kidney, tonify Water, enhance flow in meridians from Ki. towards M.H. (PC)	tonify Kidney YIN, brain and bone marrow, tonify Heart, reduce fire, move dampness, calm anger
LU9 TAI YUAN 太淵 Supreme Abyss	SHU-YUAN-Soil of Lung, tonify Metal, HUI-meeting of vessels	purify heat, release and tonify Lung, regulate injuries of Wood to Metal, resolve phlegm
LU1 ZHONG FU 中府 Middle Palace	MU of Lung, regulate Lung YIN, entry point, meeting with Sp. Meridian	open QI passage to Upper JIAO, disseminate and move Lung QI and rebel QI down, stop vomiting, reduce G.B. heat
BL18 GAN SHU 肝俞 Liver SHU	SHU of Liver, Liver YANG regulation	move Liver QI and Blood stagnation, move stagnant blood down from head, treat vomiting of blood and bleeding from nose and gums
CV18-LIV6 regulate QI ascent, CV18-Ki21 calm anger accompanied by chest tightness		
CV18 YU TANG 玉堂 Jade Palace	'knot' of JUE YIN	move QI down, open the chest, clear Lung, regulate breathing
LIV6 ZHONG DU 中都 Capital Center	XI of Liver	sedate and regulate Liver
Ki21 YOU MEN 幽門 Dark Door	meeting of Ki. Meridian with CHONG MAI	move Liver congestion caused by anger; calm agitation and suffering
PC8-H7-LI4-GV26 calm hysterical anger; PC8-Ki7 calm habitual anger; LU10-PC8 calm alternating anger and sorrow		
PC8 LAO GONG 勞宮 Labor Palace	RONG-Fire of Master of Heart	disperse heat from JUE YIN, purify Heart, awaken SHEN, cool Blood, purify mouth
GV26 SHUI GOU 水溝 Water Trough	open LUO channels in facial region	calm SHEN, open Heart orifices, purify head and brain; calm uncontrollable, unreasonable laughter
LI4 HE GU 合谷 Union Valley	YUAN of Large Intestine	clear channels, regulate QI, release excess YANG from head, expel wind, **needle towards PC8**
LU10 YU JI 魚際 Fish Belly	RONG-Fire of Lung	release fire from throat

b. Acupuncture points to facilitate the descent of QI, calm anger and stop vomiting

name	function	action
LU3-LU9-BL17 control Blood ascent, stop mouth bleeding; PC1-LU3 control QI ascent from Middle JIAO to head. LU1,BL18 stop vomiting		
LU3 TIAN FU 天府 Celestial Palace	Celestial Window	control QI ascent, regulate conflicts between Lung and Liver (LING SHU, Chapter 21), release Lung, clear heat, move obstructions
PC1 TIAN CHI 天池 Celestial Pool	Celestial Window	move exaggerated QI and Blood flow down from head, open and calm chest, clear Lung
BL17 GE SHU 膈俞 Diaphragm SHU	HUI-meeting of Blood	influence diaphragm, open chest, tonify and move Blood
LU1 ZHONG FU 中府 Middle Palace	MU of Lung, regulate Lung YIN, entry point, meeting with Sp. Meridian	enhance QI passage to Upper JIAO, disseminate and move Lung QI down, move rebel QI down, stop vomiting, reduce G.B. heat
BL18 GAN SHU 肝俞 Liver SHU	Liver SHU, Liver YANG regulation	move Liver QI and blood stagnation, move stagnant blood down from head, treat vomiting of blood and bleeding from nose and gums
Ki9-GV12 treat anger accompanied by a desire to kill		
Ki9 ZHU BIN 築賓 Guest House	XI and start of YIN WEI MAI, start of Ki.-Bl. JING BIE	cut harmful hereditary transfers (S. de Morand, p.519), purify Heart, calm SHEN, calm rage, insults, hate, swearing; calm anger in early pregnancy; dissolve mucus, relax spasms
GV12 SHEN ZHU 身柱 Body Pillar		purify Heart and Lung, calm uncontrollable hatred and desire to kill
LIV2-GB38 calm anger caused by Liver and Gallbladder fire LIV2-LU5-SP6 calm anger that harms Lung and causes bleeding		
LIV2 XING JIAN 行間 Moving Between	RONG-Fire of Liver	move YANG down, benefit Gallbladder, stop wind, calm anger, **disperse**
GB38 YANG FU 陽輔 YANG Assistance	JING-River-Fire of Gallbladder	release heat from G.B. meridian, regulate SHAO YANG, **disperse**
LU5 CHI ZE 尺澤 Cubit Marsh	HE-Water of Lung	cool Lung, release Lung QI and TAI YIN, **tonify**
SP6 SAN YIN JIAO 三陰交 Meeting of Three YIN	meeting of Sp., Liv., and Ki. Meridians	tonify and nourish Blood, QI and YIN, move YIN upwards, nourish Spleen, stop diarrhea

c. Acupuncture points to calm anger accompanied by phlegm-dampness-fire

name	function	action
PC7-ST40-GV26,[227] **CV14** calm agitation-KUANG with *phlegm-fire*, **LIV2-LIV3** harmonize JUE YIN; **LIV2-LIV3**-ST44-PC7 calm anger with agitation **LIV2**-PC7-H7-GV14-ST40 calm mental agitation caused by *Liver fire* TW6-**LIV2**-ST40-LI4 calm anger causing ascent of blood (suspicion of stroke)		
PC7 DA LING 大陵 Big Mound	SHU-YUAN-Soil of Master of Heart	calm and purify SHEN, cool Heart (palpitation), cool blood, purify RONG QI
LIV3 TAI CHONG 太冲 Great Rush	SHU-YUAN-Soil of Liver	release and harmonize Liver
CV14 JU QUE 巨闕 Great Tower Gate	MU of Heart, regulate Heart YIN	calm SHEN and Heart, dissolve phlegm, open chest, move *turbid* QI down
ST44 NEI TING 内庭 Inner Courtyard	RONG-Water of Stomach	cool and move QI of YANG MING and fire down from head, dissolve phlegm, treat hatred of noise of man, **needle in direction of** QI **flow**
H7 SHEN MEN 神門 SHEN Gate	SHU-YUAN-Soil of Heart	calm SHEN, cool Heart, open Heart orifices
GV14 DA ZHUI 大椎 Big Mallet	meeting of DU MAI with six YANG Meridians	regulate QI and YANG flow to head and heart, release excess heat and damp-heat from Upper JIAO
ST40 FENG LONG 豐隆 Bountiful Bulge	LUO of Stomach	dissolve *phlegm-fire* (heat), calm SHEN
TW6 ZHI GOU 支溝 Branch Ditch	JING-River-Fire of SAN JIAO	regulate QI of SAN JIAO, treat vomiting, **disperse**

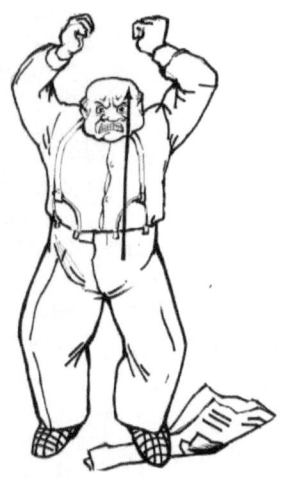

---

[227] See page 172

d. Acupuncture points to calm anger and stop diarrhea

name	function	action
SP6-Ki7 (tonify both)-LIV3 (disperse) gather YIN, calm Liver – anger, stop diarrhea SP4-H7-**SP6** (H7 needle in direction of QI flow without manipulation, **SP6** tonify, SP4 disperse) cool blood and calm SHEN, stop diarrhea accompanied by agitation and anger, SP9-**SP6** (disperse both)-ST25-ST44 cool blood, disperse phlegm		
SP6 SAN YIN JIAO 三陰交 Meeting of 3 YIN	meeting of Sp., Liv., and Ki. Meridians	tonify and nourish Blood, QI, YIN, Spleen, move YIN upwards, stop diarrhea
LIV3 TAI CHONG 太沖 Great Rush	SHU-YUAN-Soil of Liver	release and harmonize Liver, **disperse**
SP4 GONG SUN 公孫 Grandfather Grandson	open CHONG MAI, LUO of Spleen	move Spleen QI upwards through CHONG MAI
SP9 YIN LING QUAN 陰陵泉 YIN Mound Spring	HE-Water of Spleen	stop diarrhea, tonify Spleen YANG, disperse
ST25 TIAN SHU 天樞 Celestial Axis	MU of Large Intestine	dissolve phlegm, calm SHEN, **needle in direction of QI flow**

2. Joy (XI 喜), SU WEN, Chapter 39 (see Figure 41)

喜	XI	joy	榮	RONG	Nourishing QI	故 GU so
則	ZE	this	衛	WEI	Defensive QI	氣 QI
氣	QI		通	TONG	communicate	緩 HUAN slow
合	HE	harmony	利	LI	benefit, easy	矣 YI period
志	ZHI	emotion				
達	DA	express				

Joy (XI 喜) *harmonizes* (HE 合) *QI. Emotions* (ZHI 志) *are fully expressed. Nourishing QI* (RONG 榮) *and Defensive QI* (WEI 衛) *communicate easily. So (joy) slows QI* 氣.

Figure 41. Joy (XI 喜), SU WEN, **Chapter 39.** The numbers show the sequence in the text

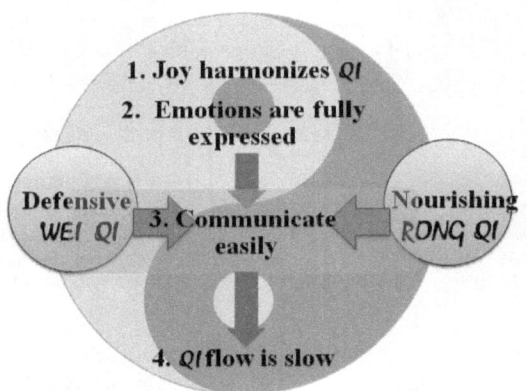

❖ SU WEN, Chapter 39. *Joy* (XI 喜) *harmonizes* (HE 合) *QI.*
   Emotions (ZHI 志) *are fully expressed.*
Joy (XI 喜) - the emotion of Heart[228] is beneficial to man. Joy opens Heart, harmonizes QI and Blood flow, and expands the expression of Consciousness, emotions and desires (ZHI 志).[229]

❖ SU WEN, Chapter 39, Joy: *Nourishing QI* (RONG 榮) *and Defensive QI* (WEI 衛) *communicate easily. So joy slows* (HUAN 緩) *QI* 氣
In joy QI flows harmoniously without obstructions. Easy communication between Nourishing QI (RONG 榮, the organized flow in meridians, governed by Lung-Metal) and Defensive QI (WEI 衛, adaptive flow, related to Liver-Wood), is a sign of good SAN JIAO function. Joy emerges from Center of Chest (TAN ZHONG 膻中) (SU WEN, Chapter 8), and is related to Master of Heart, the communication system of Heart (XIN XI 心系).

Joy harmonizes and slows (HUAN 緩) the flow of QI and Blood, especially in Upper JIAO, and is expressed as:

---

228 See page 51 for the character XI 喜
229 See page 33

- Opening of the chest (which includes Heart and Master of Heart);
- Expansion of Consciousness;
- Release of *Qi* and Blood obstructions;
- Benefit to the communication between the chest - body center and limbs - body periphery, and between the interior of the body and the environment.

Joy is beneficial to man but intense (or prolonged) joy, which causes expansion of *Qi* and outward blood flow, may be harmful and cause:
- Fatigue;
- Loss of anchor of Heart in Kidney, leading to *Heart empty fire*.

In sudden joy *Qi* flow opens violently, intensifies Heart function and damages Heart YANG. Frail or elderly people may die from sudden, unexpected joy.

Joy is closely related to pleasure and happiness, but the ending of pleasure may cause suffering. Some philosophers have hypothesized that feelings of pain (suffering) and pleasure are part of a continuum. Emerging evidence from pain and reward research points to extensive similarities in the anatomical substrates of painful and pleasant sensations. There is strong evidence of connections between the neurochemical pathways used for the perception of both pain and pleasure.[230]

This is especially true in cases of addiction (alcohol, drugs, sex, eating, games, control), in which cessation of the pleasure causes suffering.

In Buddhist tradition there are Five *Skandas*[231] (WU YUN 五蘊), the five functions or aspects that constitute sentient beings. One of these Five Skandas is 'sensation' or 'feeling' (vedanā,[232] XING YUN 行蘊): sensing an object as pleasant or unpleasant, which leads to change

---

230 Leknes, S.; Tracey, I.
231 Pāli; Sanskrit
232 Pāli; Sanskrit

of states between joy (pleasure) and misery (lack of pleasure). Craving for and attachment to vedanā (sensations) leads to suffering. Awareness and liberation of *Five Scandas* may lead to enlightenment and the extinction of the causes of suffering.

Regulating QI by acupuncture in cases of excessive joy

excessive joy causes	main points	points synergy
a. *Heart fire*	H5-PC7	H5-PC7-GV24
		H5-PC7-ST40-ST44-GV26
b. *Heart fire* with giggles	H7-SI5	H7-SI5-CV13-GV26
	PC8-PC7	
c. Euphoria and agitation (difficult cases)	PC3	ST25-ST36-PC3-H7-CV13-ST40-ST44
	H9, SI4	
d. Slowing down of RONG QI and WEI QI	ST36-SP6	
e. Heart weakness, disturbance of QI and Blood flow		CV14-CV17-BL43

a. Acupuncture points to calm excessive joy expressed as *Heart fire*

name	function	action
H5-PC7-GV24 calm *Heart fire* causing excessive joy		
H5 TONG LI 通里 Penetrating the Interior	LUO of Heart	purify Heart, calm SHEN, release QI congestion in throat
PC7 DA LING 大陵 Big Mound	SHU-YUAN-Soil of Master of Heart	calm and purify SHEN, cool Heart (palpitation), cool blood, purify RONG QI
GV 24 SHEN TING 神庭 SHEN Court	meeting of DU MAI with Bl. and St. Meridians	communicate between orifices, calm SHEN

b. Acupuncture points to calm excessive joy accompanied by giggles

name	function	action
H5-PC7-ST40-ST44-GV26 calm excessive joy with giggles and phlegm-heat		
GV26 SHUI GOU Water Trough 水溝	open LUO channels in facial region	calm SHEN, open Heart orifices, purify head and brain; calm uncontrollable, unreasonable laughter
ST40 FENG LONG 豐隆 Bountiful Bulge	LUO of Stomach	dissolve phlegm-fire (heat), calm SHEN
ST44 NEI TING 內庭 Inner Courtyard	RONG-Water of Stomach	cool and move QI of YANG MING and fire down from head, dissolve phlegm
PC8-PC7 or **H7-SI5**-GV26 calm uncontrollable laughter **H7-SI5**-CV13 calm uncontrollable laughter accompanied by joy and agitation		
PC8 LAO GONG 勞宮 Labor Palace	RONG-Fire of Master of Heart	clear JUE YIN heat, purify Heart and mouth, awaken SHEN, cool blood
H7 SHEN MEN 神門 SHEN Gate	SHU-YUAN-Soil of Heart	calm SHEN, cool Heart, open Heart orifices
SI5 YANG GU 陽谷 YANG Valley	JING-River-Fire of Small Intestine	clear heat, calm SHEN, **disperse**
CV13 SHANG WAN 上脘 Upper Venter	meeting of REN MAI with St. and S.I. Meridians	move QI downwards

c. Acupuncture points to calm euphoria and agitation (difficult cases)

name	function	action
PC3-H7-CV13-ST40-ST44-ST25-ST36 cool and purify damp-heat causing KUANG		
PC3 QU ZE 曲澤 Marsh at the Crook	HE-Water of Master of Heart	dissipate heat from Upper JIAO, cool blood and Heart, disperse stagnant blood, disperse toxins caused by stagnation
ST25 TIAN SHU 天樞 Celestial Axis	MU of Large Intestine	disperse phlegm, calm SHEN
ST36 ZU SAN LI 足三里 Leg Three Miles	HE-Soil of Stomach, tonify QI, potentiate other points	regulate YANG deficiency above and YIN excess below, regulate WEI QI, treat lack of SHEN
SI4 WAN GU 腕骨 Wrist Bone	YUAN of Small Intestine	purify heat, calm joy with agitation
H9 SHAO CHONG 少衝 Lesser Surge	JING-well-Wood of Heart, tonify Fire	increase presence (SHEN), regulate excessive expansion of emotions

d. Acupuncture points to regulate RONG QI and WEI QI

Puncture ST36-SP6 in the direction of QI flow without needle manipulation. ST36 regulates Defensive QI (WEI 衛) and SP6 regulates Nourishing QI (RONG 榮).

e. Acupuncture points to protect Heart, QI and Blood from excessive joy

name	function	action
CV14-CV17-BL43 tonify Heart, QI and Blood flow		
CV14 JU QUE 巨闕 Great Tower Gate	MU of Heart, regulate Heart YIN	calm SHEN and Heart, dissolve phlegm, open chest, move *turbid* QI down
BL17 GE SHU 膈俞 Diaphragm SHU	HUI-meeting of Blood	influence diaphragm, open chest, tonify and move blood, **disperse**
BL43 GAO HUANG SHU 膏肓俞 SHU of liquid fat	gather JING in Upper JIAO	strengthen Source QI, Kidney, Spleen, brain and bone marrow

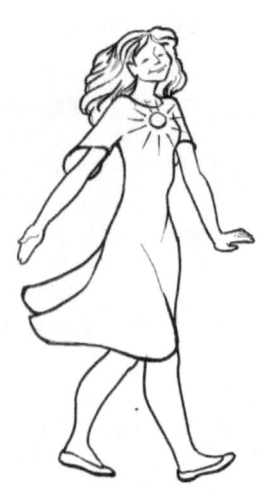

3. Sorrow (BEI 悲), SU WEN, Chapter 39 (Figure 42)

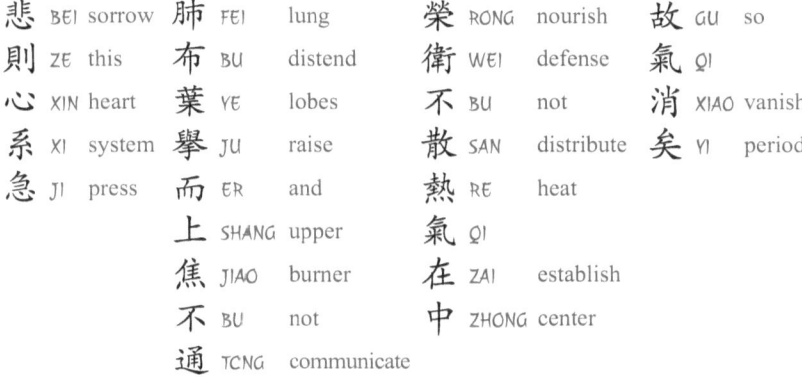

悲	BEI	sorrow	肺	FEI	lung	榮	RONG	nourish	故	GU	so
則	ZE	this	布	BU	distend	衛	WEI	defense	氣	QI	
心	XIN	heart	葉	YE	lobes	不	BU	not	消	XIAO	vanish
系	XI	system	舉	JU	raise	散	SAN	distribute	矣	YI	period
急	JI	press	而	ER	and	熱	RE	heat			
			上	SHANG	upper	氣	QI				
			焦	JIAO	burner	在	ZAI	establish			
			不	BU	not	中	ZHONG	center			
			通	TONG	communicate						

Sorrow (BEI 悲) *compresses the communication system of Heart* (XIN XI 心系).
Lung distends, lung lobes rise and Upper JIAO does not communicate. Nourishing QI (RONG 榮) and Defensive QI (WEI 衛) are not distributed, and QI of heat settles in the center. So, QI vanishes.

Figure 42. Sorrow (BEI 悲), SU WEN, **Chapter 39.** The numbers show the sequence in the text

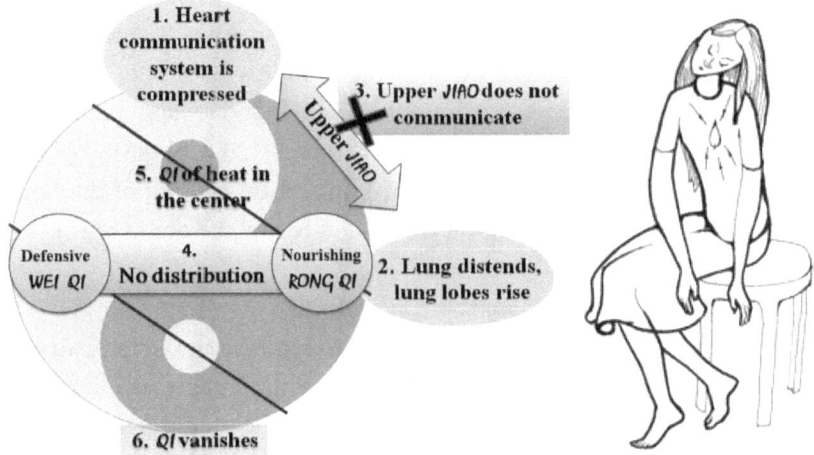

❖ SU WEN, Chapter 39, *Sorrow*: (BEI 悲) *compresses the communication system of Heart* (XIN XI 心系). *Lung distends, lung lobes rise and Upper JIAO does not communicate*

Sorrow (BEI 悲)[233] – the emotion of Lung - harms Lung function: respiration, the flow of Nourishing QI in meridians, body cooling and the descent of body liquids.

Sorrow (BEI 悲) causes compression of the communication system of Heart (XIN XI 心系), and therefore closes the chest - Upper JIAO, disturbing the function of Heart, Lung and Master of Heart. Compression of the communication system of Heart is a loss of connection with the environment, loss of ability to be happy, loss of emotional communication. Master of Heart, Heart's envoy, responsible for the communication system of Heart, is distressed by sorrow.

❖ SU WEN, Chapter 39, *Sorrow: Nourishing QI (RONG 榮) and Defensive QI (WEI 衛) are not distributed, and QI of heat settles in the center*

Nourishing QI (RONG 榮) (organized flow in meridians, governed by Lung-Metal) ascends from Middle JIAO towards Upper JIAO (chest). Defensive QI (WEI 衛) (adaptive flow, related to Liver-Wood) ascends from Lower JIAO towards Upper JIAO. In sorrow, Nourishing QI and Defensive QI cannot ascend to the compressed Upper JIAO and congests between the chest and the region above and below the diaphragm (between Upper JIAO and Middle JIAO). Congested QI and the failure of the cooling function of Lung cause heating of the body center (the chest and the region above and below the diaphragm).

❖ SU WEN, Chapter 39, *Sorrow*: *QI vanishes*.

Heating of the body center disperses QI towards the exterior, causing QI deficiency in the interior. This QI deficiency may cause collapse 'below the heart' (the region above and below the diaphragm) causing blood to flow downwards (towards Lower JIAO) and loss of blood by urine (hematuria).

---

233 See page 52 for the character BEI 悲

SU WEN, Chapter 44, describes the loss of Blood in QI deficiency following injury to communication vessels of Heart envelope (BAO LUO 胞絡) (Master of Heart) from big sorrow and grief (BEI AI TAI 悲哀太):

悲	BEI	sorrow	胞	BAO	envelope	發	FA	develop
哀	AI	grief	絡	LUO	connect	則	ZE	then
太	TAI	great	絕	JUE	exhaust, fatigue	心	XIN	heart
甚	SHEN	considerable	則	ZE	then	下	XIA	below
則	ZE	then	陽	YANG		崩	BENG	collapse
胞	BAO	envelope	氣	QI		數	SHU	often
絡	LUO	connect	内	NEI	interior	溲	SOU	urinate
絕	JUE	exhaust, fatigue	動	DONG	move, agitate	血	XUE	blood
						也	YE	period

Very big sorrow and grief (BEI AI TAI 悲哀太) *exhaust communication vessels of* (Heart) *envelope* (BAO LUO 胞絡).
The exhaustion of communication vessels of (Heart) *envelope* (BAO LUO 胞絡) *causes restlessness of* YANG QI *in the interior* (of the body), *and develops into collapse below the heart, and often into hematuria.*

Regulating QI by acupuncture in cases of sorrow

Sorrow causes	main points	points synergy
a. compression of communication system of Heart	PC4	CV18-PC4-Ki4-ST18 ST14
	PC7,H5,CV14,GV11	
	CV11-PC6, PC5	
b. rising of lung lobes	LU2	LU2-CV12
	LI5, Ki21,CV19	
c. non-communication of RONG QI and WEI QI	SP4	SP7-PC7, SP15
d. heat in the center	ST41, TW10	ST41-ST15, TW10-BL15-GV11
e. QI to vanish	CV6	CV6-BL43-CV12

a. Acupuncture points to treat sorrow which compresses communication system of Heart

name	function	action
CV18-**PC4**-Ki4-ST18, ST14 treat sorrow		
PC4 XI MEN 郄門 XI-Cleft Gate	XI of Master of Heart	open flow in channels, cool blood, calm SHEN, purify RONG QI, calm suffering and stress in sorrow
CV18 YU TANG 堂玉 Jade palace	'knot' of JUE YIN	move QI down, open the chest, clear Lung, regulate breathing
Ki4 DA ZHONG 大鍾 Big Bell	LUO of Kidney, enhance QI flow in meridians from Ki. towards M.H.(PC)	open Upper JIAO, treat *misanthropy, fear, emotionalism*, a *desire to leave the world and shut the door*, *melancholy and lack of joy* (S. de Morand,. p. 517)
ST18 RU GEN 乳根 Breast Root	passage of Stomach Great LUO	release Lung and ZONG QI, benefit QI and Blood, treat sorrow and mental pain
ST14 KU FANG 庫房 Storeroom		move rebel QI down, dissolve phlegm, unbind chest: treat shock, pressure in chest, irregular breathing
PC7, H5, CV14, GV11 treat compression of Heart		
PC7 DA LING 大陵 Big Mound	SHU-YUAN-Soil of Master of Heart	calm and purify SHEN, cool Heart (palpitation), cool blood, purify RONG QI
H5 TONG LI 通里 Penetrating the Interior	LUO of Heart	purify Heart, calm SHEN, release Heart from mourning, treat despair crisis (S. de Morand)
CV14 JU QUE 巨闕 Great Tower Gate	MU of Heart, regulate Heart YIN	calm SHEN and Heart, dissolve phlegm, open chest, move *turbid* QI down
GV11 SHEN DAO 神道 Spirit Path	communicate between LUO	dissolve phlegm, calm SHEN, clear heat, treat *melancholy, search the solitude and darkness, short breath, craving for alcohol and coffee, erroneous ideas without joy, flooding by worries* (S. de Morand,. p.636)
CV11-PC6 treat feeling of bitterness in chest, PC5- feeling of blandness in chest		
CV11 JIAN LI 建里 Established Way	*regulate Middle JIAO*	release Gallbladder and diaphragm
PC6 NEI GUAN 內關 Inner Barrier	LUO of Master of Heart, open YIN WEI MAI	release three YIN, open chest, remove congestion between pelvis and chest, regulate QI, awaken SHEN
PC5 JIAN SHI 間使 Interval Envoy	JING-River-Metal of Master of Heart-JUE YIN, Group LUO of 3 arm YIN	regulate YIN deficiency above and YIN stagnation below, open chest, calm SHEN, suffering and stop the crying, dissolve phlegm, calm SHAO YANG, treat feeling of blandness in chest and withdrawal

b. Acupuncture points to treat sorrow which causes lung distention

name	function	action
LU2-CV12, LI5, Ki21,CV19 release Lung QI outward		
LU2 YUN MEN 雲門 Cloud Gate		move *Lung* QI down, release QI of Lung and Upper JIAO outward, release heat from chest
CV12 ZHONG WAN 中脘 Central Venter	MU of Stomach, HUI-meeting of FU, 'knot' of TAI YIN, start of Lu. Meridian	dissolve phlegm, move stagnation, regulate Stomach
LI5 YANG XI 陽谿 YANG Ravine	JING-River-Fire of Large Intestine	purify heat from Metal, treat agitation-with-heat-in-chest and respiratory difficulties, calm SHEN
Ki21 YOU MEN 幽門 Dark door	meeting with CHONG MAI	calm restlessness and suffering
CV19 ZI GONG 紫宮 Purple Palace	unbind chest	purify Lung, open chest, treat stagnation from chest accompanied by sexual disorders in women

c. Acupuncture points to treat sorrow which blocks communication between RONG QI and WEI QI

name	function	action
SP4		
SP7-PC7 treat hysterical depression; SP15 - if there is cold in abdomen		
SP4 GONG SUN 公孫 Grandfather-Grandson	LUO of Spleen, open CHONG MAI	move Spleen QI upwards through CHONG MAI, externalize acquired QI through Source QI[234]
PC7 DA LING 大陵 Big Mound	SHU-YUAN-Soil of Master of Heart	calm and purify SHEN, cool Heart (palpitation), cool blood, purify RONG QI
SP7 LOU GU 漏谷 Leaking Valley		strengthen Spleen, invigorate QI and blood flow, reduce swelling, calm SHEN, cool blood, purify RONG QI, treat fatigue, sadness, hysteria
SP15 DA HENG 大横 Great Horizontal	meeting of Sp. Meridian with YIN WEI MAI	treat sorrow accompanied by cold in abdomen and problems with bowel movement

---

234 CHONG MAI is the meeting between Source and acquired QI directly and through YANG MING

d. Acupuncture points to treat sorrow accompanied by heat in the center

name	function	action
ST41-ST15 disperse heat from body center		
ST41 JIE XI 解谿 Ravine Divide	JING-River-Fire of Stomach, tonify Soil	move fire congested in Stomach, treat *sorrow and depression by shock* (S. de Morand, p. 442)
ST15 WU YI 屋翳 Roof.	release WEI QI and QI flow from inside chest towards outside	*treat repression of worries, displease, melancholy* (S. de Morand, p. 446)
TW10-BL15-GV11 treat sadness and mental confusion		
TW10 TIAN JING 天井 Celestial Well	HE-Soil of SAN JIAO, increase communication between LUO	calm SHEN, cool blood, purify heat, dissolve phlegm, treat *affliction, sadness and insomnia* (S. de Morand, p. 539)
GV11 SHEN DAO 神道 Spirit Path	communicate between LUO	dissolve phlegm, calm SHEN, clear heat
BL15 XIN SHU 心俞 Heart SHU	SHU of Heart, regulate Heart YANG	calm SHEN, move congestion of Heart blood, clear heat from Heart, **disperse**

e. Acupuncture points to treat sorrow that causes QI to vanish

name	function	action
CV6-BL43-CV12 improve QI production and flow in chronic cases		
CV6 QI HAI 氣海 Sea of QI	MU of QI	tonify QI, especially Source QI, move congested QI, treat *depression with a desire to die* (S. de Morand,. p. 615) **moxa**
CV12 ZHONG WAN 中脘 Central Venter	MU of Stomach, HUI-meeting of FU, 'knot' of TAI YIN, start of Lu. Meridian	dissolve phlegm, move stagnation, regulate Stomach, **moxa**
BL43 GAO HUANG SHU 膏肓俞 SHU of liquid fat	gather JING in Upper JIAO	strengthen Source QI, Kidney, Spleen, brain and bone marrow, **moxa**

4. Fear (KONG 恐), SU WEN, Chapter 39 (Figure 43)

恐 KONG	fear	閉 BI	close	故 GU	so
則 ZE	this	則 ZE	this	氣 QI	
精 JING		氣 QI		不 BU	not
卻 QUE	retreat	還 HUAN	turn back	行 XING	circulate
卻 QUE	retreat	還 HUAN	turn back		
則 ZE	this	則 ZE	this		
上 SHANG	upper	下 XIA	lower		
焦 JIAO	burner	焦 JIAO	burner		
閉 BI	close	脹 ZHANG	inflate		

Fear (KONG 恐 *makes* JING 精 *retreat. When* JING 精 *retreats, Upper JIAO closes.*
When (Upper JIAO) *is closed*, QI 氣 *reverses its flow* (flows down to the pelvis).
(*When* QI) *reverses its flow, Lower JIAO inflates.*
So QI 氣 *does not circulate.*

Figure 43. Fear (KONG 恐), SU WEN, **Chapter 39.** Numbers match the sequence in the text

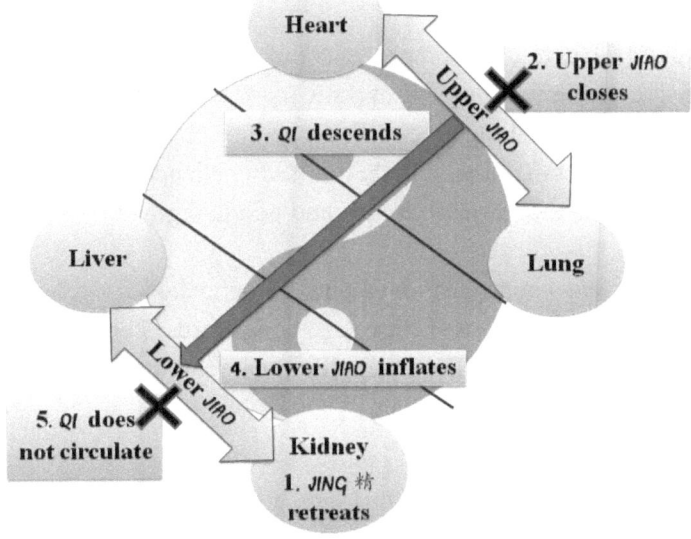

❖ SU WEN, Chapter 39: *Fear* (KONG 恐) *makes JING* 精 *retreat. When JING* 精 *retreats, Upper JIAO closes.*

Fear (KONG 恐)[235] is the emotion of Kidney, which is located in Lower JIAO. Kidney stores JING 精 with the help of Source QI (YUAN QI 原氣/元氣) and raises JING QI 精氣 (QI carrying JING) from Lower JIAO towards Upper JIAO. SAN JIAO, the envoy of Kidney Source QI (NAN JING, Difficulty 66), directs the flow of JING QI. In Upper JIAO, JING QI participates in the production of ZONG QI 宗氣 (QI of the chest, of the rhythm of breath and Blood flow) and contributes to QI flow in the meridians, which starts from the chest.

Fear causes JING 精 to 'retreat' and 'freeze' and JING QI is unable to ascend to Upper JIAO. JING QI deficiency in Upper JIAO 'closes' it - prevents it functioning.

❖ SU WEN, Chapter 39, Fear: *When* (Upper JIAO) *is closed, QI reverses its flow.* (When QI) *reverses its flow, Lower JIAO inflates.*

Nourishing QI (RONG 榮) (the organized flow in meridians, governed by Lung-Metal) ascends from Middle JIAO towards Upper JIAO. Defensive QI (WEI 衛) (adaptive flow, related to Liver-Wood) ascends from Lower JIAO towards Upper JIAO.

Fear 'closes' Upper JIAO and prevents the ascent of Nourishing QI and Defensive QI. Nourishing QI *reverses its flow* and descends towards Lower JIAO. Nourishing QI and Defensive QI congest in Lower JIAO and do not direct the flow of body liquids, which become stagnant and cause edema in the lower abdomen and pelvic region.

Anger and fear cause QI movements in opposite directions. Anger moves QI upwards and fear moves QI downwards. Fear and joy may be part of a continuum. For example, in parachuting fear is replaced with a sense of joy after landing.[236]

---

235 See page 54 for the character KONG 恐
236 Vincent J.D. Biologie des Passions

Both sorrow and fear obstruct Upper JIAO. The difference is that sorrow starts and ends with Upper JIAO congestion; fear starts and ends with Lower JIAO congestion but also obstructs Upper JIAO.

❖ SU WEN, Chapter 39, Fear: QI 氣 does not circulate.
JING QI 精氣 is obstructed in Lower JIAO and is lost through the lower orifices: incontinence, diarrhea, spermatorrhea. Therefore QI 氣 does not circulate.

Regulating QI by acupuncture in cases of fear

Fear causes	points	points synergy
a. JING QI not to ascend	Ki5 SP4 Ki7-Ki8	CV23-**Ki5** GB41-**SP4**, GV1
b. Upper JIAO to close	Ki4 LU7	H7-**Ki4**, PC4-**Ki4**, **Ki4**-BL64-PC7 **LU7**-CV14, **LU7**-K20, K26
c. QI to descend	LIV13	**LIV13**-H7-K20, **LIV13**-BL66, CV13
d. Lower JIAO to inflate	TW2	**TW2**-TW10, LI11, ST30-ST36 **TW2**-TW10-GV11-GV20 (Upper JIAO is obstructed)
e. QI not to circulate	ST34	**ST34**-BL65-BL66
f. insomnia	ST27	**ST27**-Ki6, **ST27** - CV7/CV6

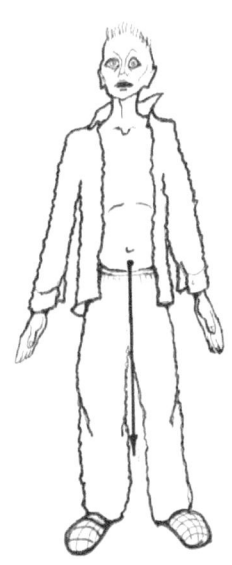

a. Acupuncture points to treat fear which prevents ascent of JING QI 精氣

name	function	action
CV23-**Ki5**,GB41-**SP4**, GV1,**Ki7-Ki8** treat fear which prevents ascent of JING QI		
Ki5 SHUI QUAN 水泉 Water Spring	XI of Kidney, regulate CHONG MAI and REN MAI	open Kidney obstruction following sudden fear
SP4 GONG SUN 公孫 Grandfather-Grandson	open CHONG MAI, LUO of Spleen	move Spleen QI upwards through CHONG MAI, treat fear (with sighs and insomnia)
CV23 LIAN QUAN 廉泉 Ridge Spring	'knot' of SHAO YIN, meeting of REN MAI with YIN WEI MAI	dissolve phlegm, obstructions and swellings, release ascent of body liquids
GB41 ZU LIN QI 足臨泣 Bend to Cry (located on foot)	SHU-Wood of Gallbladder, regulate QI of G.B, open DAI MAI	open communication between upper and lower body, dissolve phlegm, treat fear related to epilepsy in children
Ki7 FU LIU 復溜 Returning current	JING-River-Metal of Kidney, tonify Water, enhance QI flow in meridians from Ki. towards M.H. (PC)	tonify Kidney YIN, brain and bone marrow, tonify Heart, reduce fire, move dampness, improve coherence and decisiveness
Ki8 JIAO XIN 交信 Intersecting Sincerity	XI of YIN QIAO MAI	drain damp from Lower JIAO, stimulate ZHI, improve coherence, decision ability
GV1 CHANG QIANG 長強 Always Strong	LUO of DU MAI, meeting of DU MAI with REN MAI, Ki. and G.B. Meridians	treat fear (with loss of JING) in children, tonify YANG, release urinary tract

b. Acupuncture points to treat fear which closes Upper JIAO

name	function	action
H7-Ki4 calm fear accompanied by palpitations and insomnia PC4-Ki4 treat fear of people accompanied by tightness in chest, feeling of inferiority and withdrawal, PC7 'easily scared' Ki4-BL64 regulate Kidney and Bladder Meridians by YUAN-LUO points		
Ki4 DA ZHONG 大鐘 Large Bell	LUO of Kidney, start of Longitudinal LUO of Ki. towards Upper JIAO, enhance QI flow in meridians from Ki. towards M.H.(PC)	open Upper JIAO, regulate inferior orifices, treat urinary dysfunction and edema, treat fear
H7 SHEN MEN 神門 SHEN Gate	SHU-YUAN-Soil of Heart	calm SHEN, cool Heart, open Heart orifices
PC4 XI MEN 郄門 XI-Cleft Gate	XI of Master of Heart	open flow in channels, cool blood, calm SHEN, purify RONG QI
PC7 DA LING 大陵 Big Mound	SHU-YUAN-Soil of Master of Heart	calm and purify SHEN, cool Heart (palpitation), cool blood, purify RONG QI, treat 'easily scared'
BL64 JING GU 京骨 Capital Bone	YUAN of Bladder	calm SHEN
LU7-Ki20 treat fear that closes Upper JIAO with feeling of suffocation in throat LU7-CV14 treat fear accompanied by palpitation		
LU7 LIE QUE 列缺 Broken Sequence	LUO of Lung, open REN MAI	treat rebel QI and fear that closes Upper JIAO
Ki20 FU TONG GU 腹通谷 Communication Valley of Abdomen	meeting of Ki. Meridian with CHONG MAI	treat fear with a feeling of suffocation in throat
CV14 JU QUE 巨闕 Great Tower Gate	MU of Heart, regulation of Heart YIN	calm SHEN and Heart, dissolve phlegm, open chest, move turbid QI down
Ki26 YU ZHONG 彧中 Lively Center		treat suffocation caused by phlegm, release respiration

c. Acupuncture points to treat fear which causes QI to descend

name	function	action
LIV13-H7-K20[237] open chest and treat fear		
LIV13-BL66, CV13 treat tendency to long lasting fear		
LIV13 ZHANG MEN 章門 Camphor wood Gate	MU of Spleen, HUI-meeting of five ZANG, meeting of Liv., G.B., Ki., H., Sp. and Lu. Meridians	treat Upper JIAO obstruction and rebel QI which obstructs WEI QI
BL66 TONG GU 通谷 Valley of Communication	RONG-Water of Bladder	treat agitation constraining flow in head and eyes
CV13 SHANG WAN 上脘 Upper Venter	meeting of REN MAI with St. and S.I. Meridians	treat rebel QI, fear with palpitation, anxiety which ties QI below heart

d. Acupuncture points to treat fear accompanied by Lower JIAO inflation

name	function	Action
TW2-TW10, LI11 move dampness and liquids obstructed in Lower JIAO		
TW2-TW10-GV11-GV20 treat fear-with-palpitation when Upper JIAO is obstructed		
TW2 YE MEN 液門 Body Liquids Gate	RONG-Water of SAN JIAO	enhance flow of body liquids, treat fear and anxiety
TW10 TIAN JING 天井 Celestial Well	HE-Soil of SAN JIAO, increase communication between LUO	calm SHEN, cool blood, purify heat, dissolve phlegm
LI11 QU CHI 曲池 Pool at the Bend	HE-Soil of Large Intestine	balance QI and Blood, dissipate heat from upper body, treat fear with memory loss
GV11 SHEN DAO 神道 Spirit Path	communicate between LUO	dissolve phlegm, calm SHEN, clear heat
GV20 BAI HUI 百會 Hundred Meetings	meeting of DU MAI with six YANG	move YANG down through DU MAI, purify head and brain, treat restlessness-with-heavy-head
ST30-ST36 move liquids and WEI QI in Lower JIAO (LING SHU, Chapter 56) through regulation of Sea of Food		
ST36 ZU SAN LI 足三里 Leg Three Miles	HE-Soil of Stomach, tonify QI, Sea of Food point (with ST30)	regulate YANG deficiency above and YIN excess below, regulate WEI QI, treat fear, sighs, lack of SHEN
ST30 QI CHONG 氣沖 Surging QI	meeting of St. Meridian with CHONG MAI, Sea of Food point	treat fear accompanied by insomnia

---

237 See page 191 above for H7-K20

e. Acupuncture points to treat fear which prevents QI flow

name	function	action
ST34 stimulate flow in YANG MING **BL65-BL66**[238] stimulate TAI YANG (points SHU and RONG of Bladder) to accelerate flow in SHAO YIN		
ST34 LIANG QIU 梁丘 Beam Hill	XI of Stomach, relieve obstruction from YANG MING	release SHAO YIN by YANG MING, treat fear-with-hypersensitivity
BL65 SHU GU 束骨 Bundle Bone	SHU-Wood of Bladder	treat fright accompanied by nonstop talk

f. Acupuncture points to treat fear accompanied by insomnia

name	function	action
ST27-Ki6 treat fear and insomnia ST27-CV7/CV6 treat fear and insomnia by tonification of QI production and flow		
ST27 DA JU 大巨 Great Gigantic	passage of YANG from chest to abdomen	move stagnant YIN in abdomen caused by YANG deficiency, tonify Kidney and JING, treat fear with insomnia
Ki6 ZHAO HAI 照海 Shining Sea	open YIN QIAO MAI, move YIN of SHAO YIN upwards	calm SHEN, treat insomnia and dreams accompanied by fear and sadness
CV6 QI HAI 氣海 Sea of QI	MU of QI	tonify QI and especially Source QI, move congested QI
CV7 YIN QIAO 陰交 YIN Intersection	meeting of REN MAI with CHONG MAI, Command point of SAN JIAO	warm Lower JIAO, regulate SAN JIAO

---

238 See page 191 above for H7-K20

5. Cold (HAN 寒), SU WEN, Chapter 39 (Figure 44)

寒 HAN cold	氣 QI	故 GU so
則 ZE this	不 BU not	氣 QI
腠 COU lineaments	行 XING circulate	收 SHOU contract
理 LI skin		矣 YI period
閉 BI close		

Cold (HAN 寒) *closes the skin lineaments* (COU LI 腠理).
QI 氣 *does not circulate. So QI* 氣 *is contracted* (SHOU 收).

Figure 44. Cold (HAN 寒), SU WEN, **Chapter 39**. Numbers match the sequence in the text

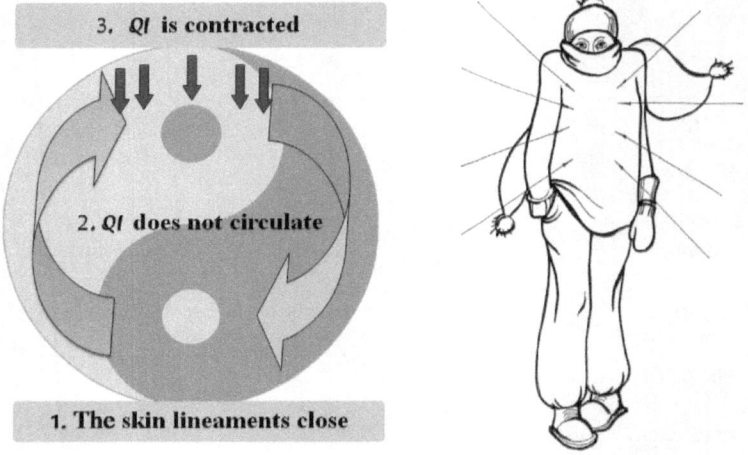

A balanced flow of Nourishing QI and Defensive QI on the body surface enables the function of the skin lineaments (COU LI 腠理) which open towards the exterior through the pores of the skin. The skin lineaments contain superficial body liquids (JIN 津). The pores are half open and moisturize the skin.

Both cold and fear, which represent Water Modality, damage Upper JIAO and cause the accumulation of body liquids in Lower JIAO. Upper JIAO directs communication with the environment – the flow of QI towards the body surface.

Cold slows down QI flow on the surface and the skin lineaments close. Body QI contracts (SHOU 收) and moves with the body liquids from the skin surface towards Lower JIAO (Kidney and Bladder). So both cold and fear provoke excessive urine production and urinary urgency.

In emotions, a lack of communication with the environment is expressed by cold: 'frozen in place', 'cold look', 'cold-blooded', 'cold heart', 'cold person' and 'frigidity'. Sometimes fear causes an emotional withdrawal accompanied by a feeling of cold, cold back or cold hands. Fear causes fight-flight or freeze (inability to move) response, a physiological reaction that occurs as a reaction to a perceived harmful event, attack, or threat to survival.

6. Heat (JIONG 炅), SU WEN, Chapter 39 (see Figure 45)

炅	JIONG	heat	榮	RONG	Nourishing QI	故	GU	so
則	ZE	this	衛	WEI	Defensive QI	氣	QI	
腠	COU	lineaments	通	TONG	communicate	泄	XIE	disperse
理	LI	skin	汗	HAN	sweat	矣	YI	period
開	KAI	open	大	DA	big			
			泄	XIE	disperse			

Heat (JIONG 炅) opens the skin lineaments (COU LI 腠理).
Nourishing QI (RONG 榮) and Defensive QI (WEI 衛) communicate with each other.
A lot of sweat disperses (evaporates) *(XIE 泄). So QI 氣 is dispersed (XIE 泄).*

Heat warms the body, enhances the flow of QI, Blood and body liquids, and activates the cooling process on the surface of the skin. Spleen raises body liquids to Lung (Upper JIAO). Lung enhances the dispersion of body liquids towards the skin. When skin lineaments (COU LI 腠理) are filled with liquids, skin pores open and there is profuse sweating.

Figure 45. Heat (JIONG 灵), SU WEN, **Chapter 39.** Numbers match the sequence in the text

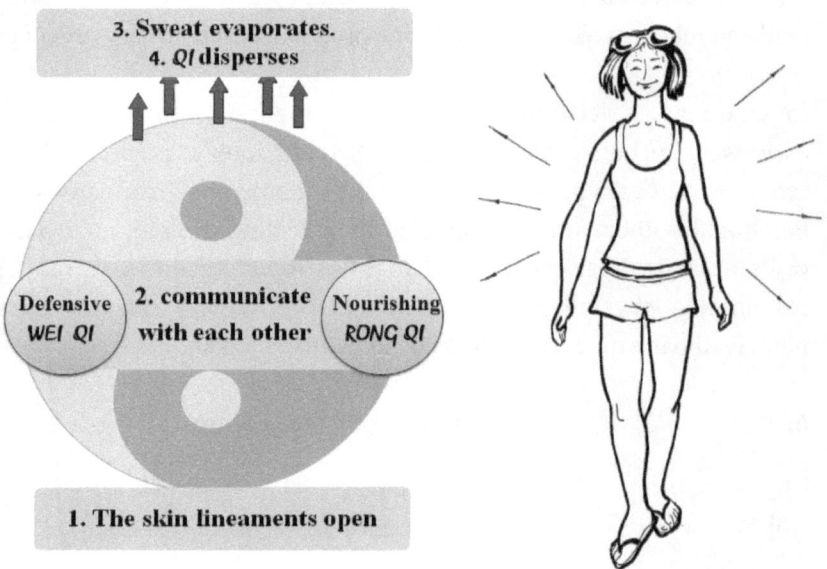

Heat causes intensive communication between Nourishing QI (RONG 榮) (organized flow in meridians, governed by Lung-Metal) and Defensive QI (WEI 衛) (adaptive flow, related to Liver-Wood) which move body liquids to the skin surface. QI exits together with body liquids through perspiration and disperses (XIE 泄) towards the exterior.

Both heat and joy belong to Fire Modality; they enhance the flow of Nourishing QI (RONG 榮) and Defensive QI (WEI 衛) towards the exterior, strengthen communication with the environment and, in excess, disperse QI. Dispersion of QI leads to a loss of JING QI 精氣 (QI carrying JING) and therefore a loss of JING 精. Lung does not move the body liquids required for nourishment and drainage downwards towards Lower JIAO (Kidney and Bladder).

In emotions, good communication with the environment is expressed by heat: 'warm regards', 'warm welcome', 'warm person', 'heart-warming'.

7. Panic (JING 驚), SU WEN, Chapter 39 (Figure 46)

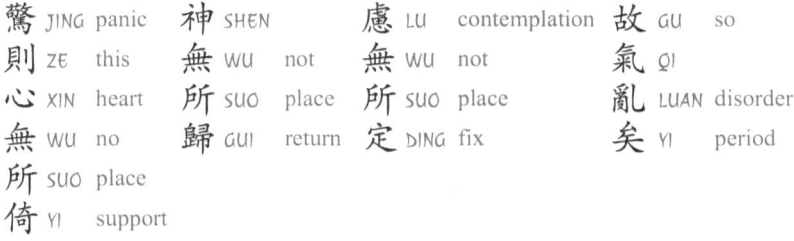

In panic (JING 驚), Heart-Consciousness (XIN 心) has no place of support,
SHEN 神 has nowhere to return to,
Contemplation (LU 慮) has no anchor (DING 定).
So (panic) causes disorder (LUAN 亂) of the QI 氣 flow.

Figure 46. Panic (JING 驚), SU WEN, **Chapter 39**. Numbers match the sequence in the text

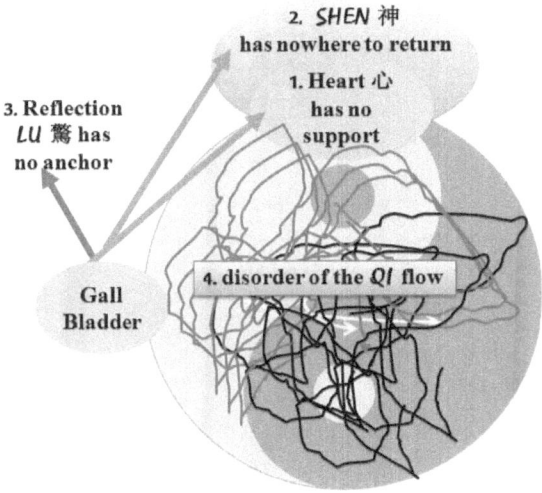

The character JING 驚 (Figure 47)[239] in the upper component has 苟 'to be like a lamb', 'give respect', and 攵 'a hand holding a stick', 'giving light blows'. The upper component depicts 敬 'to honor',

---

239 http://zhongwen.com/d/197/x229.htm

'worship', 'know your place', 'to be humble before authority'.[240] The lower component is the radical 馬 'horse'. In Ancient China, the horse was a symbol of fear and also of freedom, and training horses was considered to be against their nature.[241] The character JING 驚 shows 'a horse scared in the presence of authority', and conveys the meaning 'unexpected event' (meeting with a great personality, a significant person in life, fire or a big crowd) causing a loss of the center, vague thoughts and uncharacteristic behavior. JING 驚 is translated as 'panic', 'alarm', 'fright', 'surprise', 'to be startled'. The character JING 驚 does not contain the radical 心 'heart', found in most Chinese characters for emotions.

Figure 47. The character JING 驚 **'panic' in ancient seal and classical script**

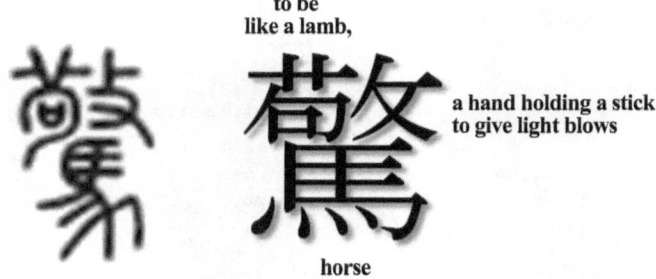

Panic (JING 驚) causes a disorder of QI flow following injury to:
- Heart-Consciousness (XIN 心)
- SHEN 神
- Contemplation (LU 慮)

❖ SU WEN, Chapter 39: *In panic (JING 驚) Heart-Consciousness (XIN 心) has no place of support*

The physical support of the heart is the diaphragm in constant motion. The diaphragm is a muscle (governed by Liver and Gallbladder), which separates the chest cavity from the abdominal cavity.

---

240 Wieger, Lesson 54
241 ZHUANG ZI, Chapter 9

Inhalation is accompanied by the active lowering of the diaphragm. In exhalation, the diaphragm rises passively through the action of the abdominal muscles. In panic the respiratory rhythm becomes irregular and Heart loses the **support** of the diaphragm.

Heart-Consciousness (XIN 心) communicates with the environment: *receives things and beings* (LING SHU, Chapter 8).[242] In panic, Heart-Consciousness (XIN 心) 'without support/anchor' loses contact with reality, provoking an uncertain self-image and image of the world around and therefore anxiety.

❖ SU WEN, Chapter 39, Panic: SHEN 神 *has nowhere to return to.*
Heart and SHEN may be seen as a YIN-YANG relationship. Heart-YIN opens up the space of Consciousness and SHEN-YANG moves Consciousness - providing it with rhythms, colors, shapes and a special point of view on the world. SHEN is 'the Spirit in motion' and has endless cycles of *'going away and coming back'. Following* SHEN 神 *going away and coming back, that is called* HUN 魂 (LING SHU, Chapter 8).[243]

Without the support of the diaphragm, Heart loses the respiratory rhythm and therefore SHEN, the YANG aspect of Consciousness, loses its rhythm, consistency and the direction of its motion, and cannot return to reality.

❖ SU WEN, Chapter 39, Panic: *Contemplation* (LU 慮) *has no anchor* (DING 定)
Contemplation arranges thoughts-Soil by activating HUN 魂-Wood.

Thought (SI 思) *which considers the situation from afar is called contemplation* (LU 慮). *So contemplation* (LU 慮) *which arranges things and beings is called wisdom* (ZHI 智) (LING SHU, Chapter 8).[244]

---

242 See page 113
243 See page 104
244 See page 131

In panic, SHEN 神 loses its rhythm and direction and contemplation (LU 慮) loses stability (DING 定). The character DING 定 is translated as 'stable' or 'to decide, determine'.²⁴⁵ When SHEN and HUN have *nowhere to return to*, contemplation loses its direction, consistency and ability to organize thoughts. Contemplation unable to organize and classify thoughts causes the loss of wisdom.

❖ SU WEN, Chapter 39: Panic *causes disorder* (LUAN 亂) *of the QI flow*

Heart-Consciousness without support, SHEN 神 unable to 'come back' to reality and contemplation incapable of organizing thoughts, result in disorder in the QI flow (LUAN 亂).

LING SHU, Chapter 40, describes LUAN 亂 as a disorder of *clear* and *turbid*. Clear (QING 清) are substances ready to use, and QI above the diaphragm. *Turbid* (ZHOU 濁) are raw substances which need to be processed in order to be absorbed, and QI below the diaphragm.

清	QING	clear	命	MING	name
濁	ZHOU	turbid	曰	YUE	called
相	XIANG	together	亂	LUAN	disorder
幹	GAN	confront	氣	QI	

When clear (QING 清) *and turbid* (ZHOU 濁) *confront, this is called disorder* (LUAN 亂) *of QI 氣 flow.*

Panic provokes a disorder (LUAN 亂) of *clear* and *turbid* and therefore injures:
- First, the function of the diaphragm, and therefore the function of Liver and Gallbladder which are located below the diaphragm, a muscle which they govern. Liver does not drain, assure the smooth flow of QI, or store Blood. Gallbladder's function as *Rectitude of the Center* (ZHONG ZHENG 中正)²⁴⁶ - regulating *clear* and *turbid* -

---

245 Wieger, Lesson 112
246 SU WEN, Chapter 8

is disturbed. Gallbladder - one of six Organs of Extraordinary Longevity (QI HENG ZHI FU 奇恒之腑) also loses its function of JING 精 storage.

• Secondly, Kidney and JING 精 storage. *Clear* and *turbid* are also regulated on the axis Fire-Water through SHAO YIN (Heart-Kidney). In panic, disorder of *clear* and *turbid* damages Heart-SHEN 神 and injures Kidney and JING 精 storage.

In SU WEN, Chapter 39, panic (JING 驚) is similar to anxiety attack in western psychiatry. Anxiety attack is described as periods of intense fear of sudden onset accompanied by at least four or more bodily or cognitive symptoms (such as heart palpitation, dizziness, shortness of breath, feeling of unreality). In panic (JING 驚) there is tension, insomnia, hyper-activity, over-reaction, inability to decide, to think rationally (Gallbladder imbalance).

Panic, which interferes with the function of Liver, Gallbladder, Heart and Kidney, corresponds to the following syndromes of Chinese Medicine:
• *Liver QI Stagnation Accompanied by Liver Blood Deficiency.*
• *Liver Blood Deficiency and the Loss of* JING 精 (Gallbladder and Kidney YIN are damaged) which damage Heart, provoking Heart fire which injures the head and Consciousness.

Regulating QI by acupuncture in cases of panic

Panic causes	main points	points synergy
a. Heart to lose its support	PC5	ST26-ST27-H6-LIV14-PC5
b. inability of SHEN to 'come back' to reality	GB24 BL44 CV14	Ki1-GB34-GB24 BL44-BL62, GV16 CV14-H7
c. contemplation to lose anchor	GB43 Ki20	GB43-GB24-GB40 Ki20-Ki21-LU7

a. Acupuncture points to treat Heart without support in panic

name	function	action
ST26-ST27-H6-LIV14-**PC5** treat lack of connection to reality, lack of belonging, feeling of heart as if suspended in emptiness		
PC5 JIAN SHI 間使 Interval Envoy (Master of Heart is an envoy of Heart and diaphragm is interval of the center)	JING-River-Metal of Master of Heart-JUE YIN, Group LUO of 3 arm YIN	regulate YIN deficiency above and YIN stagnation below, open chest, calm SHEN, calm SHAO YANG, treat apprehension, insecurity, violent hyperexcitation; nocturnal terror (S. de Morand, p. 483), feeling of blandness in chest, feeling of heart as if suspended
ST26 WAI LING 外陵 Outer Mound		feeling of emptiness below heart
ST27 DA JU 大巨 Great Gigantic	passage of YANG from chest to abdomen	move stagnant YIN in abdomen caused by YANG deficiency, tonify Kidney and JING, treat fear accompanied by insomnia
LIV14 QI MEN 期門 Cycle Gate	MU of Liver, meeting of Liv., Sp. Meridians and YIN WEI MAI	raise QI from abdomen to chest, benefit Gallbladder, calm restlessness (with arrhythmia and obsession)
H6 YIN XI 陰郄 YIN Cleft	XI of Heart	nourish YIN, calm SHEN, consolidate exterior (BIAO)

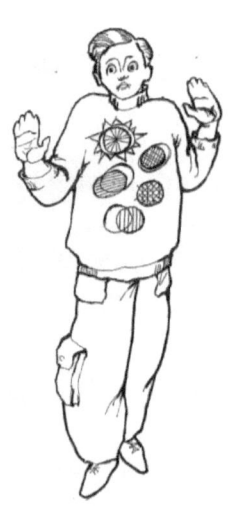

b. Acupuncture points to bring SHEN back to reality in panic

name	function	action
Ki1-GB34-GB24 lead SHEN to its root, treat anxiety that has no external cause and feeling of tragedy		
GB24 RI YUE 日月 Sun and Moon	MU of Gallbladder, nourish YIN of Gallbladder	move QI down, treat mental instability and inability to decide
GB34 YANG LING QUAN 陽陵泉 YANG Mound Spring	HE-Soil of Gallbladder, HUI-meeting of muscles and tendons	regulate and move QI of Gallbladder down
Ki1 YONG QUAN 湧泉 Gushing Spring	JING-Well-Wood of Kidney, root of SHAO YIN	move rebel QI and YANG down, open Heart orifices, awaken SHEN
BL44-GV16, BL62 stabilize SHEN		
BL44 SHEN TANG 神堂 Spirit Hall		stabilize SHEN, calm Heart, treat excess in chest, regulate QI, move QI rising in panic down
BL62 SHEN MAI 申脈 SHEN Hour Vessel	open YANG QIAO MAI	purify head and eyes, restore presence and vigilance
GV16 FENG FU 風府 Wind Mansion	meeting of DU MAI with YANG WEI MAI, one of points of bone marrow	move Source QI and JING up to brain, benefit anxiety of elderly, **tonify gently**
H7-CV14 bring SHEN back		
CV14 JU QU 巨闕 Great Tower Gate	MU of Heart, regulate Heart YIN	calm SHEN and Heart, dissolve phlegm, open chest, move turbid QI down
H7 SHEN MEN 神門 SHEN Gate	SHU-YUAN-Soil of Heart	calm SHEN, cool Heart, open Heart orifices

c. Acupuncture points to treat *contemplation without anchor* in panic

name	function	action
GB43-GB24-GB40 tonify Gallbladder QI		
GB43 XIA XI 侠谿 Pinched Ravine	RONG-Water of Gallbladder, tonify Wood	purify head, ears and eyes, return order and mental uprightness
GB40 QIU XU 丘墟 Hill Ruins	YUAN of Gallbladder, Group LUO of leg	disperse Gallbladder fire, regulate SHAO YANG
Ki20-Ki21-LU7 regulate excessive contemplation (worry)		
Ki20 FU TONG GU 腹通谷 Abdomen Communication Valley	meeting of Ki. Meridian with CHONG MAI	treat fear (with a sense of suffocation in throat)
Ki21 YOU MEN 幽門 Dark door	meeting of Ki. Meridian with CHONG MAI	calm restlessness and suffering
LU7 LIE QUE 列缺 Broken Sequence	LUO of Lung, open REN MAI	treat rebel QI and fear that closes Upper JIAO

8. Exhaustion (LAO 勞), SU WEN, Chapter 39 (Figure 48)

勞	LAO	exhaustion	外	WAI	exterior	故	GU	so
則	ZE	this	內	NEI	interior	氣	QI	
喘	CHUAN	gasp	皆	JIE	all	耗	HAO	consume
息	XI	breath	越	YUE	cross	矣	YI	period
汗	HAN	sweat						
出	CHU	exit						

Exhaustion following strenuous effort (LAO 勞) *causes gasping for breath and sweat.*

There are no boundaries between the interior and exterior (of the body).

So QI 氣 *is consumed* (HAO 耗).

Figure 48. Exhaustion (LAO 勞), SU WEN, **Chapter 39.** The numbers show the sequence in the text

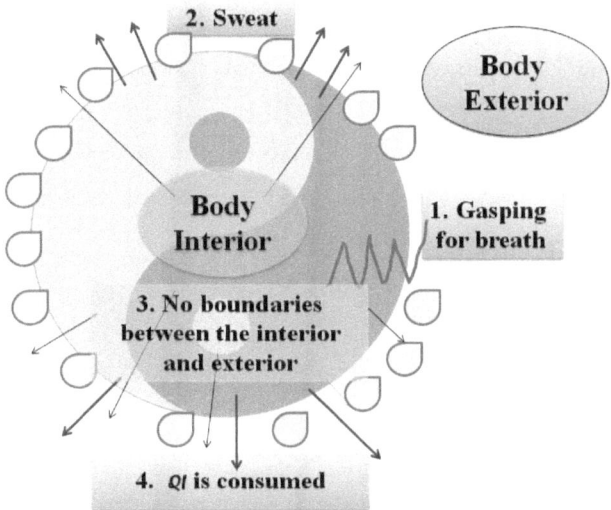

❖ SU WEN, Chapter 39: *Exhaustion following strenuous work* (LAO 勞) *causes gasping for breath and sweat. There are no boundaries between the interior and exterior* (of the body).

The character LAO 勞 is composed of the character 炏 'fire' written twice, above ⼓ 'cover', below which is 力, 'physical strength, muscle contraction'.[247] LAO 勞 describes 'burning of physical strength': exhaustion, physical fatigue after work or exercise. Lung-Metal suffers from a lack of air (DA QI 大氣), causing respiratory difficulties, and as a result QI deficiency. Exhausted Lung-Metal does not maintain the boundaries between the interior and exterior of the body. QI flow in meridians on the skin is impaired, therefore skin pores do not close and body liquids and JING QI 精氣 are lost by sweat.

SU WEN, Chapter 21, shows how inappropriate behavior exhausts and damages the five ZANG and Stomach-FU, causing perspiration (loss of body liquids and JING 精 of the damaged organ) or respiratory difficulties:

---

247 Wieger, Lesson 126

夜	YE	night	持	CHI	carry	疾	JI	quick	驚	JING	panic
行	XING	walk	重	ZHONG	heavy	走	ZOU	walk	而	ER	and
則	ZE	this	遠	YUAN	far off	恐	KONG	fear	奪	DUO	loss
喘	CHUAN	gasp	行	XING	walk	懼	JU	dread	精	JING	
出	CHU	exit	汗	HAN	sweat	汗	HAN	sweat	汗	HAN	sweat
於	YU	from	出	CHU	exit	出	CHU	exit	出	CHU	exit
腎	SHEN	kidney	於	YU	from	於	YU	from	於	YU	from
淫	YIN	excess	腎	SHEN	kidney	肝	GAN	liver	心	XIN	heart
氣	QI										
病	BING	disease									
肺	FEI	lung									

In night walking, the panting originates in Kidney; excessive QI causes Lung disease...

In walking over long distance with heavy load, sweat originates in Kidney.

In running fast and being in fear and dread (KONG JU 懼恐), *sweat originates in Liver.*

In panic (JING 驚) *which causes the loss of seed* (JING 精), *sweat originates in Heart.*

In work which requires exhausting body movements, sweat originates in Spleen. In overdrinking or overeating, sweat originates in Stomach.[248]

According to SU WEN, Chapter 21:
- Walking at night exhausts Kidney, provoking respiratory (inhalation) difficulties, since Kidney governs inhalation and Lung governs exhalation. During night sleep, Kidney directs Defensive QI (WEI QI 衛氣) flow from the surface of the body to the interior to clean the five ZANG, which creates dreaming. During night walking, Defensive QI does not enter the body but flows **in excess** on the body surface - skin (governed by Lung). The exhausted Kidney does not generate Lung properly: excessive flow of Defensive QI on the skin and inhalation difficulties lead to Lung disease.

---

248 For this sentence in Chinese characters see page 87

- Physical exhaustion damages Kidney, Liver and Spleen, causing the loss of body liquids and JING 精:
  - Walking a long distance with a heavy load exhausts bones – Kidney; therefore it is Kidney liquids that are lost in perspiration.
  - Running in fear and dread (KONG JU 懼恐) affects muscles and tendons – Liver; therefore it is Liver liquids that are lost in perspiration.
  - Hard work which requires strenuous body movements exhausts Spleen, responsible for the muscular force of limbs; therefore it is Spleen liquids that are lost in perspiration.

- Overeating and overdrinking cause food congestion (excess condition) in Stomach; therefore it is Stomach liquids that are lost in perspiration.
- Loss of seed (JING 精) in panic exhausts Kidney. Exhausted Kidney cannot cool (control) Heart. Heart is exhausted by heat and it is Heart liquids that are lost in perspiration.

❖ SU WEN, Chapter 39, Exhaustion: *QI 氣 is consumed.*
Loss of body liquids and JING 精 through perspiration and QI 氣 deficiency through respiratory difficulties cause exhaustion which develops into *Empty-Heat syndrome* and 'burns' QI 氣, therefore QI 氣 is lost, consumed. Chronic fatigue without physical exertion can be a sign of depression, common nowadays in overactive and agitated people.

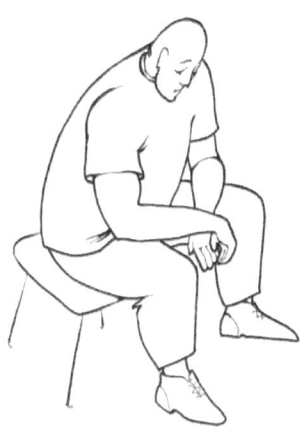

9. Obsessive thinking (SI 思), SU WEN, Chapter 39 (Figure 49)

思	SI	thinking	神	SHEN		正	ZHENG	right	故	GU	so
則	ZE	this	有	YOU	has	氣	QI		氣	QI	
心	XIN	heart	所	SUO	where	留	LIU	stay	結	JIE	tie, knot
有	YOU	has	歸	GUI	return	而	ER	and	矣	YI	period
所	SUO	where				不	BU	not			
存	CUN	stabilize				行	XING	move			

In obsessive thinking (SI 思) Heart (XIN 心) is stabilized (CUN 存),
SHEN 神 returns (to its starting point),
Upright QI (ZHENG QI 正氣) stagnates and does not flow.
So QI 氣 is knotted (JIE 結).

Thinking (SI 思)[249] is the emotion of Spleen-Soil, the center of the body. Soil Modality represents centripetal and repetitive movement, including memory and learning.

The character SI 思 is translated as 'thought, thinking, reason', but SU WEN, Chapter 39, is describing causes of disease, therefore in this text SI 思 is translated as 'repetitive thoughts' or 'obsessive thinking'.

Spleen governs absorption of Nourishing QI (RONG QI 榮氣), flavors, liquids and substances from food and beverages, and transportation in the body. Wood-Liver controls Soil-Spleen thus providing its ability to transform and transport.

❖ SU WEN, Chapter 39: *In obsessive thinking (SI 思), Heart (XIN 心) is stabilized / stored / retained in one place (CUN 存).*
Obsessive, repetitive thoughts obstruct the QI flow in Middle JIAO (Stomach, Spleen and Liver function of digestion), and 'stabilize-immobilize' (CUN 存) Heart-Consciousness.

The character CUN 存, translated as 'establish, stabilize, retain, maintain, exist, store', appears twice in LING SHU, Chapter 8, to

---

249 See page 56 for the character SI 思

emphasize the stabilization of YI 意 and of ZHI 志, and to describe the thinking process, which is a long term process:[250]

When YI 意 ***is stabilized*** *(CUN 存) this is called* ZHI 志.
When ZHI 志 ***is stabilized*** *(CUN 存) and transformed (BIAN 變), this is called thought (SI 思).*

Figure 49. Obsessive thinking (SI 思), SU WEN, **Chapter 39.**
The numbers show the sequence in the text

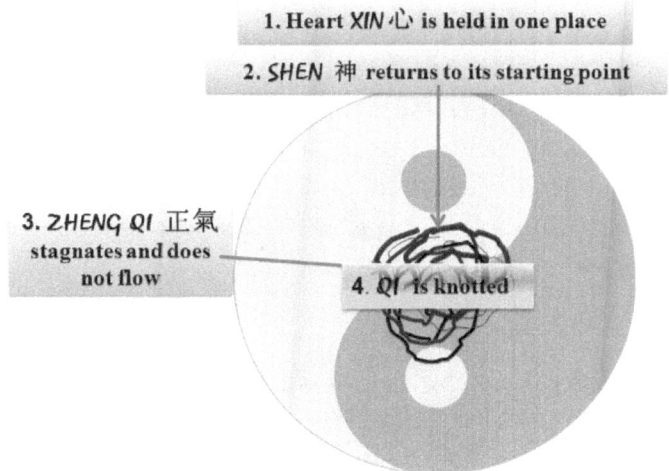

Heart determines the expansion of Consciousness in the here and now. If Heart-Consciousness is 'stabilized-immobilized' (CUN 存) it does not organize YI 意, ZHI 志 is not transformed and thoughts do not change but constantly turn around a fixed idea.

❖ SU WEN, Chapter 39, Obsessive thinking: SHEN 神 *returns*.
Heart-Consciousness, obsessed with a single idea, does not expand and communicate with the environment. SHEN 神 is 'the Spirit in motion' and has endless cycles of *'going away and coming back'*. SHEN 神 is light towards the environment - the brightness of SHEN (SHEN MING 神明). When SHEN 神 'returns to its starting point', 'closes', the brightness of SHEN 神 - communication with the environment - is lost.

---

250 See pages 104, 105 LING SHU, Chapter 8

Following SHEN 神 *as it goes away and comes back, that is called* HUN 魂 (LING SHU, Chapter 8).²⁵¹ Obsessive thinking-Soil injures (reversed control) HUN 魂 (Wood aspect of SHEN 神), which cannot follow 'closed' SHEN 神.

The first two stages of damage caused both by obsessive thinking and by panic are damage to Heart-Consciousness and SHEN 神. In obsessive thinking SHEN 神 'closes' and does not '*go away*' and in panic SHEN 神 does not '*return*'.

❖ SU WEN, Chapter 39, Obsessive thinking: Upright QI (ZHENG QI 正氣) *stagnates and does not flow. QI is knotted* (JIE 結).
ZHENG QI 正氣 - 'Upright, Rectitude QI', the regular flow of all body QI, represents wind, the Wood aspect of QI flow. Gallbladder and Liver assure the smooth flow of ZHENG QI 正氣.
ZHENG QI 正氣 *is the regular wind* (ZHENG FENG 正風). *It flows only in one direction, it is not in excess and it is not deficient* (LING SHU, Chapter 75).

The same character ZHENG 正 is used to describe Gallbladder *as Rectitude of the Center* (ZHONG ZHENG 中正) (SU WEN, Chapter 8). Usually there is a natural stimulation (control) of the thinking process (Soil) by Wood-Liver. Obsessive thinking causes an excess of Spleen-Soil which obstructs (by reversed control) ZHENG 正- QI of Liver-Wood. Spleen 'ties' obstructed (stagnant) ZHENG QI in the center of the body and forms knots (JIE 結).

Kidney generates Gallbladder - one of the six Organs of Extraordinary Longevity (QI HENG ZHI FU 奇恒之腑) which store JING 精. Obsessive thinking obstructs Gallbladder and causes it to lose connection with its roots – Water-Kidney-ZHI 志; therefore Gallbladder - *Rectitude of the Center* – does not balance Water and Fire. Repetitive thoughts, which knot QI and disturb Gallbladder's anchor to reality – ZHI 志, impair adaptation to the environment. Another Wood aspect, contemplation (LU 慮) which arranges thoughts, is injured in panic.

---

251 See page 104

YU ZHENG 鬱證 **constrained (tied) QI syndrome expressed as depression**

Spleen, either directly or indirectly, has an important role in the etiology of depression syndrome (YU ZHENG 鬱證) since obsessive thinking knots-constrains (JIE 結) QI. Spleen-Soil, the center, holds the human body together (prevents disintegration) and provides nourishment for the four other ZANG. QI of Soil - dampness - usually combines with the four other types of pernicious QI (wind, heat, cold or dryness) and obstructs Spleen and other ZANG functions. Similarly obsessive thinking combines with other emotions (pleasure, sadness, fear or anger), constrains (YU 鬱) body function and may develop into depression. SU WEN, Chapter 71, describes methods to remove constraints (YU 鬱) for each Modality:

When the Wood [QI] is oppressed, open its way DA 達 *(vomit),*
When the Fire [QI] is oppressed, effuse it FA 發 *(sweat),*
When the Soil [QI] is oppressed, take it away DUO 奪 *(purge it down),*
When the Metal [QI] is oppressed, drain it XIE 泄 *(stimulate urination),*
When the Water [QI] is oppressed, break it ZHE 折 *(regulate water passages).*[252]

During the JIN Dynasty (1115-1234) and the YUAN Dynasty (1277-1367), Chinese medicine treatments were directed to releasing YU 鬱. ZHU ZHEN HENG (1282-1358) in DAN XI XIN FA 丹溪心法 described six different types of YU 鬱:

1. YU 鬱 of Blood   4. YU 鬱 of food
2. YU 鬱 of QI   5. YU 鬱 of dampness
3. YU 鬱 of fire   6. YU 鬱 of phlegm

ZHANG JIE BIN (MING Dynasty, 1368-1644) and YE TIEN SHI (JING Dynasty 1644-1911) consider that the emotions (especially anger, sadness and obsessive thinking) cause the syndrome YU ZHENG 鬱證 which impairs the function of Spleen, Liver and Heart.

---

[252] Translation of Unschuld and Tessenow (71-501-11)

Regulating QI by acupuncture in cases of obsessive thinking

Thinking causes	points	points synergy
a. Heart to 'stabilize'	H6 CV15 PC6	H6-BL15-ST14-ST15-ST18 CV15-SI3-Ki1,CV15-CV12-SI3-ST40-BL43 PC6-SP9 (S. de Morand), PC6-BL15 CV13, BL66
b. SHEN to 'close'	BL44	BL44-PC6-K25, H7, GV20
c. ZHENG QI obstruction	SP8 LU5-LIV5	SP8-ST36-ST41/ST44, LIV13

a. Acupuncture points to treat obsessive thinking which 'closes SHEN'

name	function	action
BL44-PC6-K25, H7, GV20		
BL44 SHEN TANG 神堂 Spirit Hall	stabilize SHEN,	calm Heart, regulate QI, treat excess in chest, move QI rising in panic down (S. de Morand, p. 593)
Ki25 SHEN CANG 神藏 Spirit Storehouse	stabilize SHEN,	regulate and move Gallbladder QI down
H7 SHEN MEN 神門 SHEN Gate	SHU-YUAN-Soil of Heart	calm SHEN, cool Heart, open Heart orifices
GV20 BAI HUI 百會 Hundred Meetings	meeting of DU MAI with six YANG	move YANG QI flow down in DU MAI, purify head and brain, treat restlessness with heavy head, memory loss

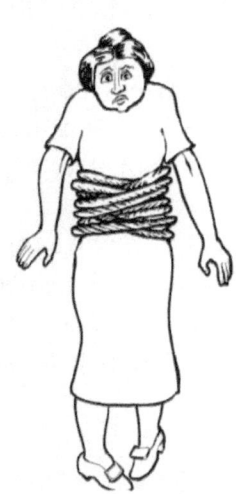

b. Acupuncture points to treat 'stabilized' Heart in obsessive thinking

name	function	action
H6-BL15-ST14-ST15-ST18 release conflict between SHAO YIN and YANG MING		
H6 YIN XI 陰郄 YIN Cleft	XI of Heart	nourish YIN, calm SHEN, consolidate exterior (BIAO)
BL15 XIN SHU 心俞 Heart SHU	SHU of Heart, regulate Heart YANG	move rebel QI down, dissolve phlegm, unbind chest: treat shock, pressure in chest
ST14 KU FANG 庫房 Storeroom		move rebel QI down, dissolve phlegm, unbind chest: treat shock, pressure in chest
ST15 WU YI 屋翳 Cover of the Room		release WEI QI and QI flow from inside chest towards exterior, treat *repression of worries, displease, melancholy* (S. de Morand. p. 446)
ST18 RU GEN 乳根 Breast Root	passage of Great LUO of Stomach	release ZONG QI and Lung, benefit QI and Blood, treat sorrow and mental pain
CV15-SI3-Ki1 treat epilepsy, **CV15**-CV12-SI3-ST40-BL43 treat schizophrenia		
CV15 JIU WEI 鳩尾 Turtledove Tail	LUO of REN MAI, YUAN of GAO - liquid fat	restore communication between inside and outside in divided consciousness
SI3 HOU XI 後谿 Back Ravine	SHU-Wood of Small Intestine, open DU MAI	calm SHEN, treat epilepsy, regulate orifices
Ki1 YONG QUAN 湧泉 Gushing Spring	JING-Well-Wood of Kidney, root of SHAO YIN	move rebel QI down, open Heart orifices, awaken SHEN, move YANG down
CV12 ZHONG WAN 中脘 Central Venter	MU of Stomach, HUI-meeting of FU, 'knot' of TAI YIN, start of Lu. Meridian	dissolve phlegm, move stagnations, regulate Stomach
ST40 FENG LONG 豐隆 Bountiful Bulge	LUO of Stomach	dissolve *phlegm-fire* (heat), calm SHEN
BL43 GAO HUANG SHU 膏肓俞 SHU of Liquid Fat	gather JING in Upper JIAO	strengthen Source QI, Kidney, Spleen, brain and bone marrow
PC6-SP9, PC6-BL15 release conflict between SHAO YIN and YANG MING		
PC6 NEI GUAN 內關 Inner Barrier	LUO of Master of Heart, open YIN WEI MAI	release three YIN, open chest, remove congestion between pelvis and chest, regulate QI, awaken SHEN
SP9 YIN LING QUAN 陰陵泉 YIN Mound Spring	HE-Water of Spleen	tonify Spleen YANG, treat dampness and cold mucus which cause palpitation, abdominal pain and stomach rumble
CV13, BL66 treat retained Heart		
BL66 TONG GU 通谷 Valley of Communication	RONG-Water of Bladder	treat agitation that constrains flow in head and eyes
CV13 SHANG WAN 上脘 Upper Venter	meeting of REN MAI, St. and S.I. Meridians	treat rebel QI, fear with palpitation, anxiety which ties QI below heart

c. Acupuncture points to treat ZHENG QI obstruction (obsessive thinking)

name	function	action
SP8-ST36-ST41/ST44, LIV13 move obstructions from Spleen-Soil		
SP8 DI JI 地機 Earth's Process	XI of Spleen, communicate with Soil	remove obstructions in Spleen Meridian, calm thoughts, treat loss of semen, vaginal discharge, anuria
ST36 ZU SAN LI 足三里 Leg Three Miles	HE-Soil of Stomach, tonify QI, Sea of Food point, potentiate other points	regulate WEI QI, regulate YANG deficiency above and YIN excess below: *lack of SHEN, prolonged melancholy, a sense of despair as if caught by ghosts* (S. de Morand. p. 438), fatigue
ST41 JIE XI 解谿 Ravine Divide	JING-River-Fire of Stomach, tonify Soil, synergy with ST36	move Stomach-*fire*, connect Upper and Middle JIAO, treat *sadness, depression, lack of appetite for life and food, troubled or loose SHEN, emotionalism* (S. de Morand. p. 442)
ST44 NEI TING 内庭 Inner Courtyard	RONG-Water of Stomach, synergy with ST36	cool and move QI of YANG MING and fire down from head, treat *hatred of the noise of men and search for silence* (S. de Morand. p. 443)
LIV13 ZHANG MEN 章門 Chapter Gate	MU of Spleen, HUI-meeting of 5 ZANG, meeting of Liv., Ki., H., Sp., Lu., G.B. Meridians	treat Upper JIAO obstruction and rebel QI which obstructs WEI QI (LING SHU, 59)
LU5-LIV5 release obstruction of QI flow through East-West axis		
LU5 CHI ZE 尺澤 Cubit Marsh	HE-Water of Lung	cool and release Lung QI and TAI YIN, diaphragm obstruction with sadness and restlessness, treat depression (sadness, crying, melancholy) (S. de Morand. p. 490), **disperse on the left**
LIV5 LI GOU 蠡溝 Woodworm Canal	LUO of Liver	calm and regulate Liver, treat melancholy, lack of joy and energy, worries with sighs, **puncture on the right**

7

Damage caused by six combinations of emotions,
LING SHU, Chapter 8

LING SHU, Chapter 8, presents two descriptions (referred to here as 8-3 and 8-4) of damage caused by six combinations of intense emotions/passions. These six combinations of emotions, in the order in which they appear in LING SHU, Chapter 8-3, are:

1. Apprehension, distress, obsessive thinking, worry (CHU TI SI LU 怵惕思慮), which cause fear and dread (KONG JU 懼恐)
2. Sorrow and grief (BEI AI 悲哀)
3. Joy and pleasure (XI LE 喜樂)
4. Melancholy and sadness (CHOU YOU 愁憂)
5. Overflowing anger (SHENG NU 盛怒)
6. Fear and dread (KONG JU 懼恐)

Damage caused by these six combinations of emotions according to LING SHU, Chapter 8-3:

A. Apprehension, distress, obsessive thinking, worry (CHU TI SI LU 怵惕思慮) damage SHEN, cause fear and dread (KONG JU 懼恐) and the anchor of life (JING 精) is lost
B. Expression of life is lost in sorrow and grief (BEI AI 悲哀)
C. Storage is lost in joy and pleasure (XI LE 喜樂)
D. Melancholy and sadness (CHOU YOU 愁憂) disrupt QI flow,
E. Organization and control are lost in overflowing anger (SHENG NU 盛怒)
F. Ability of being oneself is lost in fear and dread (KONG JU 懼恐)

LING SHU, Chapter 8-4, describes damage to ZANG 臟 functions, JING 精 storage, BEN SHEN 本神 and body tissues, caused by the same six combinations of **persistent** emotions, and forecasts the season of death:

A. Damage to Heart, SHEN and flesh in apprehension, distress obsessive thinking, worry (CHU TI SI LU 怵惕思慮), fear and dread (KONG JU 懼恐)

B. Damage to Lung, PO 魄 and mental sanity in excessive joy and pleasure (XI LE 喜樂)
C. Damage to Spleen, YI 意 and limbs in sorrow and grief (BEI AI 悲哀)
D. Damage to Liver, HUN 魂 and JING 精 in melancholy and sadness (CHOU YOU 愁憂)
E. Damage to Kidney, ZHI 志 and back in uncontrollable overflowing anger (SHENG NU 盛怒)
F. Damage to Kidney, JING 精 and bones in fear and dread (KONG JU 懼恐)

Damage caused by six combinations of emotions according to LING SHU, Chapter 8-3

A. Apprehension and distress, obsessive thinking and worry (CHU TI SI LU 怵惕思慮) **damage SHEN, cause fear and dread** (KONG JU 懼恐) **and the anchor of life** (JING 精) **is lost,** LING SHU, Chapter 8-3

是 SHI		so
故 GU		
怵 CHU		apprehension
惕 TI		distress
思 SI		thinking
慮 LU		worry, contemplation
者 ZHE		comma
則 ZE		this
傷 SHANG		injure
神 SHEN		
神 SHEN		
傷 SHANG		injure
則 ZE		this
恐 KONG		fear
懼 JU		dread
流 LIU		flow
淫 YIN		overflow
而 ER		and
不 BU		not
止 ZHI		stop, end

So apprehension, distress, obsessive thinking and worry (CHU TI SI LU 怵惕思慮) *injure* SHEN 神.
The injury to SHEN 神 *is expressed as fear and dread* (KONG JU 懼恐). (JING 精) *flows down, overflows and cannot stop* (BU ZHI 不止).

LING SHU, Chapter 8-3, introduces four emotions, arranged in two pairs, causing two additional harmful emotions:

1. Apprehension and distress (CHU TI 怵惕) injure ZHI 志 - Water of SHEN 神
2. Obsessive thinking and worry (SI LU 思慮) injure YI 意 - Soil of SHEN 神
3. Fear and dread (KONG JU 懼恐) resulting from the above four emotions cause additional injury to ZHI 志-Water, expressed as the loss of JING 精

❖ LING SHU, Chapter 8-3: *So apprehension, distress, obsessive thinking and worry* (CHU TI SI LU 怵惕思慮) *injure SHEN* 神.

The characters CHU 怵 'apprehension' and TI 惕 'distress' (Figure 50) have the same radical 心/忄 'heart'. The phonetic of the character CHU 怵 is 术 'a top heavy grain plant (millet or sorghum):'[253] CHU 怵 is the meeting of Heart-Consciousness with an object fixed in place and is translated as 'apprehension', 'fear', 'timidity'. The phonetic of TI 惕 is 易, 'movement', 'change',[254] showing 日 'the sun' and 勿 'flags moving in the wind'. TI 惕 is the meeting of Heart-Consciousness with endless change which prevents anchoring, and is translated as 'to be cautious, careful, alert, distressed'.

Figure 50. The characters CHU 怵 **'apprehension' and** TI 惕 **'distress' in ancient seal and classical script**

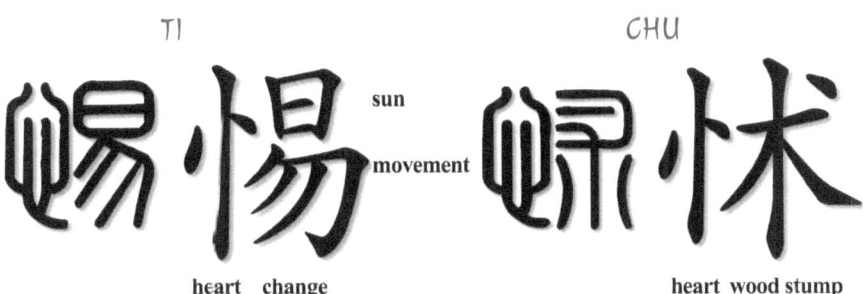

Both apprehension (CHU 怵) and distress (TI 惕) are expressions of fear, and therefore injure Kidney–Water; the injured Kidney cannot control Heart properly and damages SHEN.

---

253 http://zhongwen.com/d/165/x186.htm
254 http://zhongwen.com/d/177/x167.htm

In LING SHU, Chapter 8-3, SI LU 思慮,²⁵⁵ usually translated as thinking and contemplation, are harmful emotions and therefore translated as 'obsessive thinking and worry'.

Thought (SI 思) is the emotion of Spleen-Soil. Obsessive thinking (SI 思) knots QI (SU WEN, Chapter 39)²⁵⁶ – 'disconnects the head from the heart', obstructs Spleen, and therefore disturbs the absorption of QI from food.

Worry or obsessive contemplation (LU 慮) injures both Spleen-Soil and Liver-Wood. Liver, the Army General, does not stimulate (control) Spleen, therefore LU 慮 becomes worry, rather than 'the tiger of thoughts'²⁵⁷ (contemplation and discrimination).

Obsessive thinking and worry (SI LU 思慮) constantly revolve around a single theme without connecting to Heart-Consciousness, damaging Stomach, Spleen-YI 意 and Heart-SHEN (reversed generation). Apprehension (CHU 怵) and distress (TI 惕) injure Kidney-ZHI 志, the anchor of SHEN. Together, apprehension and distress, obsessive thinking and worry, injure SHEN by disturbing the Fire-Soil-Water (SHEN - YI - ZHI 神意志) axis - the vertical axis of the TAI JI symbol. YI 意 the Center and ZHI 志 the North-anchor-of-SHEN (on the TAI JI symbol) are closely related:
LING SHU, Chapter 8: *When YI 意 is established this is called ZHI 志*;²⁵⁸
LING SHU, Chapter 47: *ZHI 志 and YI 意 lead JING SHEN 精神 (Vital Spirits), gather HUN 魂 and PO 魄, adapt to cold and heat, harmonize joy and anger.*²⁵⁹

When YI 意 and ZHI 志 (Soil - Water) are out of balance, SHEN (Fire) does not function – it is impossible to bake bread in an oven (Fire) without flour (Soil) and water.

---

255 See pages 56, 128 for the characters SI 思, LU 慮
256 See page 166
257 See page 128
258 See page 116
259 See page 162

❖ LING SHU, Chapter 8-3, apprehension and distress, obsessive thinking and worry: *The injury to* SHEN *is expressed as fear and dread* (KONG JU 懼恐). (JING 精) *flows down, overflows and cannot stop* (BU ZHI 不止).

Apprehension and distress, obsessive thinking and worry, injure SHEN and intensify the injury to Kidney-Water, resulting in the third pair of harmful emotions – fear (KONG 恐) and dread (JU 懼).[260] *Fear* (KONG 恐) *moves* QI *downwards* (SU WEN, Chapter 39),[261] causing QI flow obstructions and swelling in Lower JIAO.

BU ZHI 不止 is translated as 'unstoppable' or 'allowing no anchor'. The two interpretations of the characters BU ZHI 不止 are related to each other. Apprehension, distress, worry, obsessive thinking, fear and dread injure YI-ZHI 意志; and provoke uncontrolled, unstoppable JING QI flow downwards to the abdomen and pelvis (bleeding or diarrhea) causing loss of JING 精 - the anchor of SHEN 神. JING 精 is essential for QI flow, Blood production and body animation. The abundance of JING SHEN 精神 (SHEN carrying JING, Vital Spirits) assures life and personal development.[262] Loss of JING 精 is a serious condition that results in many diseases.

Syndromes in Chinese medicine which describe damage to SHEN and JING 精 caused by apprehension, distress, obsessive thinking, worry

Syndrome	Acupuncture points
1. *Deficient Kidney* JING, SHEN JING BU ZU 腎精不足	Ki3-SP6-CV4-GV20-GB39-BL52
2. *Dual* QI *and Blood Deficiency*, QI XUE LIANG XU 氣血兩虛	BL15-BL17-SP6-ST36, CV10-CV12
3. *Liver and Gallbladder* QI *Deficiency*, GAN DAN QI XU 肝膽氣虛	LIV13-LIV14,GB35-GB40-GB43,CV4

---

260 See page 54 for the characters KONG 恐 (fear) and JU 懼 (dread)
261 See page 166
262 See page 163

1. *Deficient Kidney* JING, SHEN JING BU ZU 腎精不足
apprehension, distress, obsessive thinking and worry

Etiology	fear, obsessions, hereditary or chronic disease, excessive sexual activity in a man, many pregnancies, age, prolonged fatigue, weak constitution
Signs	fear, fatigue, does not respond, 'not there', tinnitus, dental diseases, impotence, knee and low back pain, memory loss
Tongue	pale or slightly pink, thin body with thin coating
Pulse	weak (RUO 弱), thin (XI 細)
Strategy	tonify Kidney, nourish JING, tonify bone marrow
Points	Ki3-SP6-CV4-GV20-GB39-BL52 (tonify)

Acupuncture points to treat *Deficient Kidney* JING
apprehension, distress, obsessive thinking and worry

name	function	action
Ki3-SP6-CV4-GV20-GB39-BL52 **tonification of all points**		
Ki3 TAI XI 太谿 Great Ravine	SHU-YUAN-Soil of Kidney	tonify Kidney YIN, release ascent of CHONG MAI and REN MAI, treat degenerative diseases
SP6 SAN YIN JIAO 三陰交 Meeting of Three YIN	meeting of Sp., Liv. and Ki. Meridians	tonify and nourish Blood, QI and YIN, move YIN up, nourish Spleen, stop diarrhea
CV4 GUAN YUAN 關元 Origin Pass	Sea of Blood, MU of Small Intestine, meeting of REN MAI with CHONG MAI and Sp., Liv. and Ki. Meridians	warm and tonify Kidney, nourish Blood and JING, assist ascent of CHONG MAI and REN MAI
GV20 BAI HUI 百會 Hundred Meetings	meeting of DU MAI with six YANG Meridians	move YANG down by moving QI flow of DU MAI down, purify head and brain, treat agitation accompanied by heavy head
GB39 XUAN ZHONG 懸鐘 Suspended Bell	HUI-meeting of bone marrow, meeting of Leg 3 YANG	move YANG QI from the upper body down, tonify bones and bone marrow, nourish JING
BL52 ZHI SHI 志室 ZHI Chamber	influence ZHI, gather JING	warm QI, tonify Kidney, ZHI and JING

2. Dual QI and Blood deficiency, QI XUE LIANG XU 氣血兩虛
apprehension, distress, obsessive thinking and worry

Etiology	fear, obsessions, QI and Blood injured by hereditary or chronic disease, bleeding
Signs	fear, fatigue, pale complexion, pale lips and nails, shortness of breath, sweating without exertion, heart murmurs, dryness (skin, hair, nose, mouth, eyes), distorted vision, spots in visual field, sensitivity to wind, dizziness
Tongue	pale with thin coating
Pulse	weak (RUO 弱), thin (XI 細), empty (XU 虛)
Strategy	tonify QI and Blood
Points	BL15-BL17-SP6-ST36, CV10-CV12 (tonify)

Acupuncture points to treat Dual QI and Blood deficiency
apprehension, distress, obsessive thinking and worry

name	function	action
BL15-BL17-SP6-ST36 tonify QI and Blood, **tonification of all points**		
BL15 XIN SHU 心俞 Heart SHU	SHU of Heart, regulate Heart YANG	calm SHEN, move congestion of Heart Blood, clear heat from Heart
BL17 GE SHU 膈俞 Diaphragm SHU	HUI-meeting of Blood, influence diaphragm	open chest, tonify and move blood
SP6 SAN YIN JIAO 三陰交 Meeting of Three YIN	meeting of Sp., Liv. and Ki. Meridians	tonify and nourish Blood, QI, Spleen and YIN, move YIN up, stop diarrhea
ST36 ZU SAN LI 足三里 Leg Three Miles	HE-Soil of Stomach, tonify QI, Sea of Food point, potentiate other points	regulate YANG deficiency above and YIN excess below, regulate WEI QI, treat long lasting melancholy and mental fatigue
CV10-CV12 tonify QI and Blood by stimulating SAN JIAO		
CV12 ZHONG WAN 中脘 Central Venter	MU of Stomach, HUI-meeting of FU, 'knot' of TAI YIN, start of Lu. Meridian	dissolve phlegm, move stagnations, regulate Stomach
CV10 XIA WAN 下脘 Lower Venter	meeting of REN MAI with Sp. Meridian	stimulate QI and Blood production in Upper JIAO

3. *Liver and Gallbladder* QI *Deficiency*, GAN DAN QI XU 肝膽氣虛 apprehension, distress, obsessive thinking and worry

Etiology	Fear injures Kidney and disturbs the upward movement of Liver and Gallbladder. Obsession injures Spleen and blood production
Signs	latent fear, no desire for confrontations, inability to decide, swelling and congestion on the sides of the upper abdomen, visual disturbances, insomnia with palpitations
Tongue	pale usually with thin coating
Pulse	weak (RUO 弱), thin (XI 細), Liver pulse is empty (XU 虛) or wiry (XUAN 弦)
Strategy	tonify Liver and Gallbladder QI
Points	LIV13-LIV14, GB35-GB40-GB43, CV4 (tonify)

Acupuncture points to treat *Liver and Gallbladder* QI *deficiency* - apprehension, distress, obsessive thinking and worry

name	function	action
LIV13-LIV14, GB35-GB40-GB43, CV4 tonify Liver and G.B., **tonify all points**		
LIV13 ZHANG MEN 章門 Chapter Gate	MU of Spleen, HUI- meeting of five ZANG, meeting of Liv., Ki., H., Sp., Lu., G.B. Meridians	treat Upper JIAO obstruction and rebel QI which obstructs WEI QI (LING SHU, 59)
LIV14 QI MEN 期門 Cycle Gate	MU of Liver, regulate Liver YIN, meeting of Liv., Sp. Meridians and YIN WEI MAI	raise QI from abdomen to chest, benefit Gallbladder, calm agitation accompanied by arrhythmia and obsession
GB35 YANG JIAO 陽交 Meeting of YANG	XI of YANG WEI MAI	regulate Gallbladder QI, treat 'trembling spirit'
GB43 XIA XI 俠谿 Pinched Ravine	RONG-Water of Gall bladder, tonify Wood	purify head, ears and eyes, return order and mental uprightness
GB40 QIU XU 丘墟 Hill Ruins	YUAN of Gallbladder, Group LUO of leg	disperse Gallbladder fire, regulate SHAO YANG
CV4 GUAN YUAN 關元 Origin Pass	Sea of Blood, MU of Small Intestine, meeting of REN MAI with CHONG MAI and Sp., Liv. and Ki. Meridians	warm and tonify Kidney, nourish Blood and JING, assist ascent of CHONG MAI and REN MAI

B. The *loss of life* in sorrow and grief (BEI AI 悲哀), LING SHU, Chapter 8-3

因	YIN	so	竭	JIE	exhaust, fatigue
悲	BEI	sorrow	絕	JUE	exhaust, interrupt, cut
哀	AI	grief	而	ER	and
動	DONG	move, agitate	失	SHI	lose
中	ZHONG	center	生	SHENG	life
者	ZHE	of			

So sorrow and grief (BEI AI 悲哀) *agitate the center* (of man),
There are fatigue and interruptions (JIE JUE 竭絕), *and life is lost* (SHI SHENG 失生).

❖ LING SHU, Chapter 8-3: *sorrow and grief* (BEI AI 悲哀) *agitate* (DONG 動) *the center* (of man)

Sorrow and grief (BEI AI 悲哀) are emotions of Lung-Metal. The character BEI 悲 is translated as 'sorrow', 'sadness', 'grief', and the character AI 哀 as 'deep grief and mourning'.[263] The characters BEI AI 悲哀, sorrow and grief, express the emotions in a final separation which is not accompanied by the severing of the relationship: the death of a loved one, the interruption of an important activity, leaving a favorite place. Sorrow and grief result from the inability to continue to realize the relationship.

The **cent**er of man is the chest which includes Heart, Lung and Master of Heart (pericardium, communication system of Heart). According to SU WEN, Chapter 39: *Sorrow* (BEI 悲) *compresses the communication system of Heart… So, QI vanishes.*[264] In sorrow and grief Master of Heart (Center of Chest) 'closes down', and therefore the rhythm of QI and Blood flow and communication with the exterior are damaged. In sorrow and grief, the chest 'closes' and all contact with the outside ceases, similarly to the closing of the door of the house following the death of the resident.

---

263 See page 52 for the characters BEI AI 悲哀
264 See page 181

Lung impaired by sorrow and grief does not cool the chest, and therefore the 'closed' chest-center of man heats up and dries. The heat in the chest (Heart, Master of Heart and Lung) is expressed outwardly as agitation and restlessness.

❖ LING SHU, Chapter 8-3, sorrow and grief: *There are fatigue and interruptions* (JIE JUE 竭絕)…

In sorrow and grief the fatigue (JIE 竭), following the interruption (JUE 絕) of communication between agitated Fire-Heart-chest and Water-Kidney-pelvis, may lead to death (loss of life).

Fatigue following the interruption of communication between chest and pelvis in sorrow and grief may result from:
1. The loss of brain liquids through tears.
2. Damage to Heart and Master of Heart preventing the ascent of Kidney JING and Liver Blood to the chest.

1. In sorrow and grief, the loss of brain liquids through tears causes fatigue

Sorrow and grief damage communication between Fire-Heart-chest and Water-Kidney-pelvis, leading to loss of brain liquids through tears and fatigue. SU WEN, Chapter 81,[265] explains how sorrow and grief cause loss of brain liquids through tears:

> Therefore, once there is sadness and grief (BEI AI 悲哀), then tears flow. When tears flow, they have originated from the water. As for the basis[266] of water, that is accumulated water. As for the accumulated water, that is the extreme YIN. As for the extreme YIN, that is the essence (JING 精) of the Kidneys. The reason why the water of basic essence (ZONG JING ZHI SHUI 宗精之水) does not come out is that the essence (JING 精) holds it. It supports it; it wraps it up. Hence, the water does not flow.
> Now, the essence (JING 精) of the water is the will (ZHI 志); the essence (JING 精) of the fire is the spirit (SHEN 神). When water

---

265 SU WEN, Chapter 28, also relates sorrow, agitation of Heart and tears
266 basis or ancestral gathering

and fire affect each other, both spirit and will (ZHI 志) are sad. Therefore, the water of the eyes is generated. Hence, a saying states: 'Heart sadness (BEI 悲) is called will (ZHI 志) sadness.' The [essence of the] will (ZHI 志) and the essence (JING 精) of the Heart, they both collect in the eyes. Therefore, when both are sad, then the spirit QI is transmitted to the essence of the Heart. [...] Above, there is no transmission to the will (ZHI 志), and the will (ZHI 志) alone is sad. Hence, tears leave [the eyes]. Tears and snivel are (substances related to) brain.[267]

According to SU WEN, Chapter 81, Kidney JING 精 stores body liquids in the brain - Sea of Marrow (SUI HAI 髓海), one of the six Organs of Extraordinary Longevity (QI HENG ZHI FU 奇恒之腑).[268]

Sorrow and grief cause conflict between Water and Fire and *interrupt* communication between the upper and lower body - between SHEN-Heart and ZHI-Kidney. Heart and brain (the upper body) lose the support of ZHI 志 and the supply of Kidney JING. The brain does not receive enough Kidney JING 精, and **insufficiency** of JING 精 in the brain prevents the storage of body liquids. Body liquids flow out as tears from the eyes (their entrance door to the brain) and as nasal liquids from the nose. The loss of brain liquids causes fatigue.

According to LING SHU, Chapter 36, sorrow damages communication between Heart and Kidney, 'contracts' the communications system of Heart (Master of Heart) and impairs the descent of body liquids from Lung (chest) to Kidney. Body liquids accumulated in the chest are lost as tears - crying without control. LING SHU, Chapter 36:
> *So the JIN YE 津液 (superficial and internal body liquids) of the 5 ZANG and 6 FU all ascend and gather at the eyes. If sorrow (BEI 悲) reaches the Heart, QI of the Heart communication system (XIN XI JI 心系急) is contracted. The Heart communication system*

---

267 Translation by Unschuld and Tessenow, pp. 722-725, characters 81-572-7 - 81-573-6

268 One of the Four Seas (SI HAI 四海)

being contracted, the Lung is distended. The distention of the Lung causes overflowing of the YE 液 *toward the upper body. The Heart communication system must not therefore be contracted, and the Lung must not therefore be distended because they ascend and descend jerkily and in disorder. This is why, it provokes cough (suffocation) and tears.*

2. In sorrow and grief, damage to Heart and Master of Heart prevents the ascent of Kidney JING and Liver Blood to the chest and causes fatigue

'Closure and agitation' of the chest in sorrow and grief interrupt communication between the chest and pelvis (Kidney and Liver) by:
   a. damaging the QI flow in Twelve Meridians (JING MAI 經脈) and/or
   b. damaging the QI flow in Six Layers (LIU JING 六經).

a. Sorrow and grief damage Master of Heart and the QI flow in Twelve Meridians (JING MAI 經脈), preventing the ascent of Kidney JING to the chest, and cause fatigue

In the sequence of flow in Twelve Meridians, Kidney Meridian transfers QI 氣 in the chest directly to Master of Heart/Pericardium Meridian (Figure 51). Sorrow and grief 'close and agitate' the chest and Master of Heart Meridian cannot receive Kidney QI carrying JING 精, causing **insufficiency** of JING QI 精氣 in the chest, and fatigue.

b. Sorrow and grief damage Master of Heart and the QI flow in Six Layers (LIU JING 六經), preventing the ascent of Liver Blood to the chest, and cause fatigue

Of the Six Layers of QI flow (LIU JING 六經), the JUE YIN 厥陰 layer is nourished by Master of Heart/Pericardium and Liver Meridians (Figure 51), therefore Master of Heart and Liver are closely related. The JUE YIN 厥陰 layer regulates Blood flow in the body. Sorrow and grief damage Master of Heart and thus impair Liver function - the ascent of Liver Blood to the chest - and cause fatigue.

Figure 51. JUE YIN 厥陰 and SHAO YIN 少陰 **layers and their meridians in Six Layers** (LIU JING 六經) **of** QI **flow**

QI flows from Kidney Meridian to Master of Heart /Pericardium Meridian. The JUE YIN layer includes Master of Heart/Pericardium and Liver Meridians. The SHAO YIN layer includes Heart and Kidney Meridians.

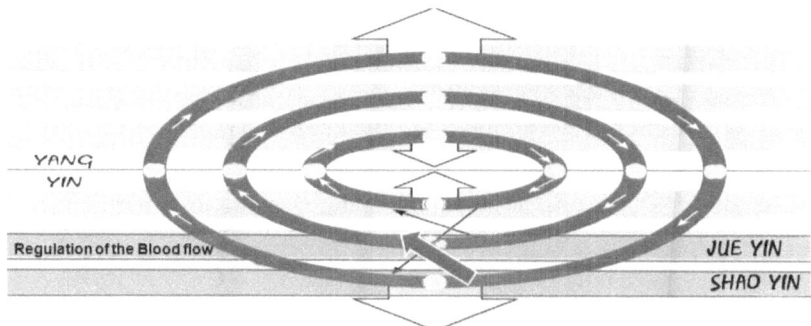

An additional explanation is that the SHAO YIN 少陰 layer, nourished by Kidney and Heart Meridians (Figure 51), maintains the balance between Water and Fire. In this way, Kidney and Heart are closely related. Sorrow and grief damage Heart by compressing its communication system, and therefore impair Kidney function – ascent of JING QI 精氣.

Liver and Kidney represent the lower body (Lower JIAO). An interruption of communication between the chest and lower body causes insufficiency of Blood and JING QI 精氣 in the chest, and provokes fatigue and exhaustion.

❖ LING SHU, Chapter 8-3, sorrow and grief: *life is lost* (SHI SHENG 失生)
In sorrow and grief, fatigue leads to death following the interruption of communication between agitated Fire-Heart-chest and Water-Kidney-pelvis. LING SHU, at the beginning of Chapter 8, explains the origin of life:
Heaven in me is DE 德, *Earth in me is* QI 氣. DE 德 *flows downwards,* QI *blooms and this is life* (SHENG 生). *Thus, life comes from what is called* JING 精.[269]

---

[269] See page 95

Life is lost - life loses its expression in a person overcome by sorrow and grief after the separation from someone or something dear (real or symbolic death). Sorrow and grief agitate the center of man interrupting communication between Heaven and Earth, between Heart and Kidney:

- DE 德 from Heaven is not received by Heart properly
- Kidney does not distribute enough JING QI 精氣 of Earth
- Body liquids are lost by tears
- Liver does not move Blood up to the chest
- Defensive QI (immune system) (WEI 衛) and Nourishing QI (RONG 榮) are depleted and assure neither defenses against pernicious QI nor proper body nourishment [270]

Sorrow and grief may lead to death if the arid desert of grief is not traversed and the mourning is not properly conducted. Separation, real or symbolic death, without an appropriate mourning process, weakens the body's defenses and may lead to serious illness resulting in loss of life.

> According to Damasio: *Sadness and anxiety can notably alter the regulation of sexual hormones, causing not only changes in sexual drive but also variations in menstrual cycle. Bereavement, again a state dependent on brainwide processing, leads to a depression of the immune system such that individuals are more prone to infection and, whether as a direct result or not, more likely to develop certain types of cancer. One can die of a broken heart.*[271]

A commonly untreated cause of grief and sorrow is a miscarriage or abortion, which causes separation and mourning expressed in the woman's body. Abortion is considered to be an event to be forgotten. However, a new life visited the woman and the fundamental, archaic relationship was brutally interrupted leaving a scar in the mother's body and soul. Abortion affects especially Master of Heart, responsible

---

270 See pages 42, 46
271 Damasio, A. R. *Descartes' Error: Emotion, Reason, and the Human Brain*, p. 120

for the distribution of blood between the mother and the embryo. Sorrow and grief may be treated through the regulation of QI flow by acupuncture to prevent *loss of life*.

Syndromes in Chinese medicine which describe the *loss of life* caused by sorrow and grief

Syndrome	Acupuncture points
1. *Heart and Lung QI Deficiency,* XIN FEI QI XU 心肺氣虛	PC5/PC7, PC4-CV18, **BL13-BL15-BL20**, BL42
2. *Liver Fire Assailing Lung,* GAN HUO FAN FEI 肝火犯肺	BL18-LIV2, **BL13**, BL42-LU7, SP15
3. *Heart Deficiency and Lung Heat,* XIN XU FEI RE 心虛肺熱	H6-Ki3, SP6, BL43, **BL15-BL23**, ST14

The major acupuncture points to treat sorrow and grief are **BL13, BL15, BL42**:

name	function	action
BL13 FEI SHU 肺俞 Lung SHU	SHU of Lung, regulate Lung YANG	release Lung
BL15 XIN SHU 心俞 Heart SHU	SHU of Heart, regulate Heart YANG	calm SHEN, move congestion of Heart blood, clear heat from Heart
BL42 PO HU 魄戶 Door of PO	regulate PO 魄	treat agitation, depression, loss of sense of reality, **tonify**

1. *Heart and Lung QI Deficiency,* XIN FEI QI XU 心肺氣虛 sorrow and grief

Etiology	Grief and separation injure Upper JIAO
Signs	mental pain, tears, difficulty in breathing, weak voice, cough when talking, nasal discharge, fatigue, sweating caused by minor effort, palpitation
Tongue	pale with thin coating
Pulse	weak (RUO 弱), thin (XI 細), floating (FU 浮)
Strategy	tonify Spleen and Lung, calm the chest pain
Points	PC5 / PC7, PC4-CV18, **BL13-BL15-BL20, BL42**

Acupuncture points to treat *Heart and Lung* QI *Deficiency*
sorrow and grief

name	function	action
PC5 or PC7 treat mental suffering		
PC5 JIAN SHI 間使 Interval Envoy	JING-River-Metal of Master of Heart - JUE YIN, Group LUO of 3 arm YIN	regulate YIN deficiency above and YIN stagnation below, open chest, calm SHEN, calm SHAO YANG, calm suffering and stop the crying
PC7 DA LING 大陵 Big Mound	SHU-YUAN-Soil of Master of Heart	calm and purify SHEN, cool Heart palpitation, cool blood, purify RONG QI
PC4-CV18 treat sudden grief		
PC4 XI MEN 郄門 XI-Cleft Gate	XI of Master of Heart	open flow in channels, cool blood, calm SHEN, purify RONG QI, calm suffering and stress in sorrow
CV18 YU TANG 堂玉 Jade palace	'knot' of JUE YIN	move QI down, open the chest, clear Lung, regulate breathing
BL13-BL15-BL20, BL42 tonify Lung, Spleen and Heart		
BL20 PI SHU 脾俞 Spleen SHU	SHU of Spleen, regulate Spleen YANG	release Spleen

2. *Liver Fire Assailing Lung,* GAN HUO FAN FEI 肝火犯肺
sorrow and grief

Etiology	Sorrow and grief cause Congested Liver QI, which is transformed into Liver Fire, injuring Lung (reversed control) and Master of Heart
Signs	sadness with tears alternates with anger, bitter taste in the mouth, swelling of the chest and hypochondria
Tongue	dark red tongue with white or yellow coating
Pulse	wiry (XUAN 弦), fast (SHU 数)
Strategy	regulate Liver fire, tonify Lung
Points	BL18-LIV2, **BL13**, **BL42**-LU7, SP15

Acupuncture points to treat *Liver Fire Assailing Lung* sorrow and grief

name	function	action
BL18-LIV2 regulate Liver fire		
LIV2 XING JIAN 行間 Moving Between	RONG-Fire of Liver	move YANG down, benefit Gallbladder, stop the wind, calm anger
BL18 GAN SHU 肝俞 Liver SHU	SHU of Liver, regulate Liver YANG	move Liver QI and blood stagnation, move stagnant blood down from head
BL13, **BL42**-LU7, SP15 tonify Lung		
LU7 LIE QUE 列缺 Broken Sequence	LUO of Lung, open REN MAI	treat rebel QI which closes Upper JIAO, move body liquids down, **tonify**
SP15 DA HENG 大横 Great Horizontal	meeting of Sp. Meridian with YIN WEI MAI	treat sorrow accompanied by cold in abdomen and problems with bowel movement, **tonify**

3. *Heart Deficiency and Lung Heat,* XIN XU FEI RE 心虛肺熱 sorrow and grief

Etiology	Sorrow injures Heart-YIN-Blood, Heart does not nourish Spleen, Spleen does not absorb RONG QI (necessary for blood production) or body liquids. Lung does not receive body liquids and becomes dry and hot
Signs	crying without reason, instability of emotions, dramatic behavior, palpitation, heat sensation in the evening, night sweat, sweating of palms and soles
Tongue	red with thin coating
Pulse	thin (XI 細), fast (SHU 數)
Strategy	tonify Heart, calm SHEN, tonify Spleen and Blood, dispel heat, regulate communication between Heart and Kidney
Points	H6-Ki3, SP6, BL43, **BL15**-BL23, ST14

Acupuncture points to treat *Heart Deficiency and Lung Heat,* sorrow and grief

name	function	action
H6-Ki3, SP6, BL43 tonify Heart, tonify Spleen and Blood, dispel heat, calm SHEN		
H6 YIN XI 陰郄 YIN Cleft	XI of Heart	nourish YIN, calm SHEN, consolidate the exterior (BIAO)
Ki3 TAI XI 太谿 Great Ravine	SHU-YUAN-Soil of Kidney	tonify Kidney YIN, release ascent of CHONG MAI and REN MAI, treat degenerative diseases, **tonify**
SP6 SAN YIN JIAO 三陰交 Meeting of Three YIN	meeting of Sp., Liv. and Ki. Meridians	tonify and nourish Blood, QI and YIN, move YIN up, nourish Spleen
BL43 GAO HUANG SHU 膏肓俞 SHU of Liquid Fat	gather JING in Upper JIAO	strengthen Source QI, Kidney, Spleen, brain and bone marrow, **moxa**
ST14 KU FANG 庫房 Storeroom		unbind the chest: treat shock, pressure in the chest, irregular breathing
BL15-BL23 regulate Heart and Kidney		
BL23 SHEN SHU 腎俞 Kidney SHU	SHU of Kidney, regulate Kidney YANG	tonify Kidney, **tonify**

C. Storage is lost in joy and pleasure (XI LE 喜樂), LING SHU, Chapter 8-3

喜	XI	joy	散	SAN	disperse
樂	LE	pleasure, joy	而	ER	and
者	ZHE	this	不	BU	not
神	SHEN		藏	CANG	store, accumulate
憚	DAN	scare away			

Joy and pleasure (XI LE 喜樂) *scare* (DAN 憚) SHEN 神, (SHEN) *is dispersed* (SAN 散) *and does not store* (CANG 藏).

❖ LING SHU, Chapter 8-3: *Joy and pleasure* (XI LE 喜樂) *scare* (DAN 憚) SHEN 神.

Joy and pleasure (XI LE 喜樂) [272] are emotions of Heart-Fire. The character XI 喜 usually means 'good', 'spontaneous', 'simple, personal,

---

272 See page 51 for the characters XI LE 喜樂

human joy and happiness'. *Joy* (XI 喜) *harmonizes* QI. *Emotions are fully expressed. Nourishing* QI *and Defensive* QI *communicate easily.* (SU WEN, Chapter 39).²⁷³ The character LE 樂 usually means joy, merriment and pleasure shared with others in festive days and celebrations. ZHUANG ZI, Chapter 31: *for those who know how to drink wine, the crucial point is the joy* (LE 樂). 樂飲酒則歡樂.

The characters XI LE 喜樂 together mean exaggerated and extroverted joy or pleasure for immediate satisfaction without control, or an addiction (alcohol, drugs, food). Any addiction gives immediate pleasure, but takes a person far away from himself, and gradually weakens SHEN. An overdose of drugs or alcohol 'scares (DAN 憚) SHEN 神' and may cause insanity. The character DAN 憚 shows the radical 心/忄 'heart' and the phonetic 單 - 口口 'a pair of mouths', above 'a pitchfork', and conveys the meaning 'to scare someone with shouting and a pitchfork'.²⁷⁴

❖ LING SHU, Chapter 8-3: joy and pleasure: SHEN *is dispersed* (SAN 散) *and does not store* (CANG 藏).

Scared and dispersed SHEN 神 is similar to a conductor leaving the orchestra in the middle of a symphony. The musicians know the melody and continue to play, but are not coordinated. SHEN 神 conducts the communication between man and his environment, and also between man and his heredity (ancestors). Joy and pleasure which cannot be controlled, or addictions, cause an excess of fire, scare, 'burn' and scatter SHEN. A person addicted to alcohol or drugs will do anything to obtain the source of his pleasure and 'burns out'. SHEN dissipates outwards, breaking the bounds of behavior, and cannot resemble itself (a person is lost to himself). Exaggerated and extroverted joy and happiness also cause SHEN 神 to lose control of its contents - secrets, and the most intimate experiences are exposed with no limits. 'Burning' the bounds of behavior 'burns' the skin (Metal-borders-Lung-skin is over-controlled by Fire-pleasures and joy) and causes skin infections, eczema and psoriasis.

---

273 See page 175
274 Wieger, Lessons 72, 104, C. Larre translated DAN 憚 as 'to scare'

Syndromes in Chinese medicine which describe damage caused by joy and pleasure with euphoria and laughter for no reason

Syndrome	Acupuncture points
1. *Heart Fire Hyperactivity and Exuberance*, XIN HUO KANG SHENG 心火亢盛	**PC7** / PC8-BL15, LI5, H3
2. *Heart and Liver Fire Effulgence*, XIN GAN HUO WANG 心肝火旺	BL18-GB20-LIV2, **PC7**-GV24
3. *No Interaction between Heart and Kidney*, XIN SHEN BU JIAO 心肾不交	**PC7**, BL43, SP6, BL52, Ki3 - Ki7
4. *Phlegm Fire Harassing Heart*, TAN HUO RAO XIN 痰火扰心	ST40-CV12, GV14-H7-GV26

The major acupuncture point to treat excessive joy and pleasure is **PC7**:

PC7 DA LING 大陵 Big Mound	SHU-YUAN-Soil of Master of Heart	calm and purify SHEN, cool Heart and palpitation, cool blood

1. *Heart Fire Hyperactivity and Exuberance* XIN HUO KANG SHENG 心火亢盛 - joy and pleasure

Etiology	Sudden emotions, combined with alcohol consumption and overeating of hot and pungent food, obstruct Heart YIN
Signs	Frequent laughter or laughing and crying alternately, agitation with nonstop - usually incoherent - speech, easily startled, palpitation, extravagant and extroverted conduct, insomnia, red complexion and eyes, dry mouth, mouth and tongue ulcers, tongue inflammation, thirst, desire for cold drinks, pain at urination, red urine
Tongue	Dry red with thin yellow coating, red tip
Pulse	slightly flooding (HONG 洪) at Heart position, fast (SHU 数)
Strategy	calm Heart, purify heat
Points	**PC7** / PC8-BL15, LI5, H3

Acupuncture points to treat *Heart Fire Hyperactivity and Exuberance* - joy and pleasure

name	function	action
PC7 / PC8-BL15, LI5, H3 tonify Heart, Spleen and Blood, dispel heat, calm SHEN		
BL15 XIN SHU 心俞 Heart SHU	SHU of Heart, regulate Heart YANG	calm SHEN, clear heat from Heart, disperse
PC8 LAO GONG 勞宮 Labor Palace	RONG-Fire of Master of Heart	clear heat from JUE YIN, purify Heart, awaken SHEN, cool blood, purify mouth
LI5 YANG XI 陽谿 YANG Ravine	JING-River-Fire of Large Intestine	purify heat from Metal, treat agitation with heat in chest and respiratory difficulties, calm SHEN and non-stop talking-with-laughter
H3 SHAO HAI 少海 Small Sea	HE-Water of Heart	tonify Heart YIN, tonify JING, treat mouth ulcers

2. *Heart and Liver Fire Effulgence* XIN GAN HUO WANG 心肝火旺 - joy and pleasure

Etiology	Frustration causes Liver QI congestion which develops into *Liver and Heart fire*, provoking agitation of HUN 魂 and SHEN
Signs	alternating laughter and anger, red eyes and face, nose and gum bleeding, feeling of distention of chest and abdomen, insomnia or dream-disturbed sleep
Tongue	red with yellow coating, red tip and sides
Pulse	wiry (XUAN 弦), fast (SHU 數) especially at Heart position
Strategy	purify *Liver fire*, calm Heart and laughter
Points	BL18-GB20-LIV2, **PC7**-GV24

Acupuncture points to treat *Heart and Liver Fire Effulgence* - joy and pleasure

name	function	action
BL18-GB20-LIV2 purify Liver fire, **PC7**-GV24 calm Heart and laughter		
LIV2 XING JIAN 行間 Moving Between	RONG-Fire of Liver	move YANG down, benefit Gallbladder, stop wind, calm anger
BL18 GAN SHU 肝俞 Liver SHU	SHU of Liver, regulate Liver YANG	move Liver QI and blood stagnation, move stagnant blood from head
GB20 FENG CHI 風池 Wind Pool	meeting of G.B., SAN JIAO Meridians, YANG WEI MAI and YANG QIAO MAI	disperse heat and *Liver wind*, regulate QI and Blood
GV24 SHEN TING 神庭 SHEN Court	meeting of DU MAI with Bl. and St. Meridians	communicate between orifices, calm SHEN, regulate mental restlessness

3. *No Interaction between Heart and Kidney* XIN SHEN BU JIAO 心腎不交 - joy and pleasure

Etiology	Emotions obstruct the interaction between SHEN and ZHI 志, or YIN *deficiency* in Kidney prevents control of Heart fire
Signs	*Kidney YIN deficiency*: low back and kidney pain or weakness, night sweats, 'five palm heat', reddish complexion, constipation, reddish or dark urine *Heart fire*: palpitation, uncontrollable laughter, 'empty' euphoria with insomnia or many dreams
Tongue	dry with peeled yellow coating
Pulse	thin (XI 細), fast (SHU 數)
Strategy	calm SHEN, tonify Kidney YIN
Points	**PC7** , BL43 , SP6, BL52 , Ki3 - Ki7

Acupuncture points to treat *No Interaction between Heart and Kidney* - joy and pleasure

name	function	action
SP6, BL52, BL43 ,Ki3 - Ki7 tonify Kidney YIN, **PC7** calm SHEN		
Ki3 TAI XI 太谿 Great Ravine	SHU-YUAN-Soil of Kidney	tonify Kidney YIN, release ascent of CHONG MAI and REN MAI, treat degenerative diseases
Ki7 FU LIU 復溜 Returning current	JING-River-Metal of Kidney, tonify Water, enhance flow in Meridians from Ki. towards M.H. (PC)	tonify Kidney YIN, tonify Heart, reduce fire, move dampness, tonify brain and bone marrow
SP6 SAN YIN JIAO 三陰交 Meeting of Three YIN	meeting of Sp., Liv. and Ki. Meridians	tonify and nourish Blood, QI and YIN, move YIN up, nourish Spleen, treat insomnia
BL52 ZHI SHI 志室 ZHI Chamber	influence ZHI, gather JING	warm QI, tonify Kidney and JING
BL43 GAO HUANG SHU 膏肓俞 SHU of liquid fat	gather JING in Upper JIAO	strengthen Source QI, Kidney, Spleen, brain and bone marrow

4. *Phlegm-fire Harassing Heart* TAN HUO RAO XIN 痰火擾心
joy and pleasure

Etiology	Fire results from overeating of hot and greasy food, intellectual strain with lack of sleep, emotional imbalance or phlegm-fire-constitution. Fire in excess obstructs Spleen function - the flow of body liquids - and produces *phlegm-fire*
Signs	*phlegm-fire* obstructs Heart, SHEN and the flow of QI: agitation, excitement with memory loss, palpitation with a feeling of heat in the chest, dizziness, tinnitus, dry mouth with bitter taste, sores around lip edges, insomnia or sleep with many dreams, wheezing, cough with yellow sputum
Tongue	red tip, yellow and greasy coating
Pulse	slippery (HUA 滑) or wiry (XUAN 弦), fast (SHU 數)
Strategy	dissolve phlegm, clear *Heart fire*
Points	ST40-CV12, GV14-H7-GV26

Acupuncture points to treat *Phlegm-fire Harrassing Heart*
joy and pleasure

name	function	action
ST40-CV12 dissolve phlegm		
CV12 ZHONG WAN 中脘 Central Venter	MU of Stomach, HUI-meeting of FU, 'knot' of TAI YIN, start of Lu. Meridian	dissolve phlegm, move stagnation, regulate Stomach
ST40 FENG LONG 豐隆 Bountiful Bulge	LUO of Stomach	dissolve *phlegm-fire* (heat), calm SHEN
GV14-H7-GV26 clear Heart fire		
GV26 SHUI GOU 水溝 Water Trough	open LUO channels in face region	calm SHEN, open Heart orifices, purify head and brain, calm uncontrollable laughter-without-reason
GV14 DA ZHUI 大椎 Big Vertebra/Wooden Mallet	meeting of DU MAI with six YANG Meridians	regulate QI and YANG flow to head and Heart, release excess heat and *damp*-heat from the upper body
H7 SHEN MEN 神門 SHEN Gate	SHU-YUAN-Soil of Heart	calm SHEN, cool Heart, open Heart orifices

D. Melancholy and sadness (CHOU YOU 愁憂) disrupt the QI flow, LING SHU, Chapter 8-3

愁	CHOU	melancholy	而	ER	and
憂	YOU	oppression by sadness, sorrow, worry	不	BU	not
者	ZHE	are	行	XING	circulate
氣	QI				
閉	BI	close			
塞	SAI	obstruct, block			

Melancholy and sadness (CHOU YOU 愁憂) close (BI 閉) and obstruct (SAI 塞) QI, and (QI) does not circulate.

Both melancholy and sadness (CHOU YOU 愁憂)[275] describe YIN-YANG aspects of the emotions of Lung-Metal:

- The character CHOU 愁 describes the passive, YIN aspect of sadness mixed with melancholy, nostalgia, a feeling of guilt and regrets
- The character YOU 憂 describes the active, YANG aspect of sadness mixed with stress, oppression, suffering, worry and soul-searching

In ZHUANG ZI, YOU 憂 means worry mixed with sadness and suffering:
ZHUANG ZI, Chapter 20: The marquis of LU answers the question as to why he looks worried (YOU 憂): *I study the way of the former kings, I do my best to carry on the achievements of the former rulers, I respect the spirits, honor worthy men, draw close to them, follow their advice, and never for an instant leave their side. And yet I can't seem to avoid disaster. That's why I'm so worried* (吾是以憂).[276]

ZHUANG ZI, Chapter 5: the marquis of LU said: *I tried to look after the regulation of the people and worried* (YOU 憂) *that they might die.* (執民之紀而憂其死).[277]

---

275 See page 52 for the characters CHOU YOU 愁憂
276 Translation by B. Watson
277 Translation by B. Watson

Melancholy and sadness close (BI 閉) *and obstruct* (SAI 塞) *the QI flow*. The character BI 閉 shows 門 'double door' locked by 才 'a bar'.²⁷⁸ The double door symbolizes Heart which opens outwards by means of the seven orifices and Lung which opens outwards by means of skin pores and points of influence (acupuncture points). The character SAI 塞 shows the radical 宀 'room, empty space', and the phonetic 基 shows 其 'two hands' and 土 'soil.'²⁷⁹ SAI 塞 conveys the meaning 'obstructing the empty space with soil', similarly to worries obstructing Spleen function.

In SU WEN, Chapter 28, the characters BI 閉 and SAI 塞, describe closing and obstruction of the diaphragm, which causes sadness (YOU 憂):

膈	GE	diaphragm	則	ZE	this causes
塞	SAI	obstruct, block	暴	BAO	sudden
閉	BI	close	憂	YOU	oppression by sadness, sorrow, worries
絕	JUE	cut, terminate	之	ZHI	of
上	SHANG	up	病	BING	disease
下	XIA	down	也	YE	period
不	BU	not			
通	TONG	communicate			

When the diaphragm is obstructed and closed (BI SAI 塞閉), *there is an interruption and no communication between the upper and lower* (body), *which causes sudden sadness* (YOU 憂) *disease*.

The diaphragm separates chest-*clear* from abdomen-*turbid*.²⁸⁰ When the diaphragm is obstructed, the communication between *clear* and *turbid* is impaired. This causes *turbid* QI congestion below the diaphragm (between the diaphragm, Spleen and Liver), and *clear* QI congestion above the diaphragm (below Center of Chest, Heart and Lung).

---

278 Wieger, Lesson 96
279 Wieger, Lesson 47
280 See page 43

The inner pathway of Lung Meridian begins in Middle JIAO and descends towards Large Intestine, then ascends through the diaphragm to the chest, and just before reaching the collarbone starts to flow on the surface of the body. Therefore, obstruction of the diaphragm prevents QI flow to Lung. Lung QI deficiency is expressed as sudden sadness (YOU 憂) with a feeling of pressure in the chest.

Melancholy and sadness (CHOU YOU 愁憂) disrupt the functioning of Heart, Spleen and Lung (Fire-Soil-Metal - the right side on the TAI JI symbol, representing downward flow), and also disturb Liver (Metal over-controls Wood):
- Melancholy and sadness impede Heart QI function - communication between the body interior and its environment - and therefore prevent adaptation to the changing environment
- Sadness mixed with worry and suffering (YOU 憂) impedes Spleen QI function - transportation and transformation
- Melancholy and sadness impede Lung QI function - breathing, QI flow inwards and downwards, flow in the meridians
- Melancholy and sadness disturb Liver QI function - smooth QI flow

Melancholy and sadness (CHOU YOU 愁憂) as well as sorrow and grief (BEI AI 悲哀) are emotions of Metal Modality, but there is a difference between injury by melancholy and sadness and injury by sorrow and grief. Sorrow and grief agitate the body center, exhausting QI and causing severe damage that can be lethal.

Melancholy and sadness accompanied by obsessive thinking obstruct QI flow slowly and constitute a chronic condition.

Syndromes in Chinese medicine which describe obstructions caused by melancholy and sadness:

Syndrome	Acupuncture points
1. *Lung and Spleen QI Deficiency* FEI PI QI XU 肺脾氣虛	BL20-**BL13**, BL43-CV4-CV6, SP8-LU6-CV12, LU1
2. *Heart and Spleen Dual Deficiency* XIN PI LIANG XU 心脾兩虛	BL20-SP6-SP4, GV20, LIV13, **BL15**-BL17
3. *No Interaction between Liver and Spleen* GAN PI BU JIAO 肝脾不交	LIV13-LIV3-LIV14, ST36-SP4
4. Lily Bulb Disease BAI HE BING 百合病[281]	
a. *Lung and Heart YIN Deficiency* XIN FEI YIN XU 心肺陰虛	LU1-**BL13**/BL42, SP6, BL15-PC8-H7
b. *Phlegm-Heat or Phlegm-Fire* TAN RE/TAN HUO 痰熱 / 痰火	ST40-ST44-GV14, PC8-LU5, **BL15**-PC7-CV12
c. *Liver YIN Deficiency* GAN YIN XU 肝陰虛	LIV14-Ki3-SP6-**BL15**, GV19-CV12
d. *Heart and Lung QI Deficiency* XIN FEI QI XU 心肺氣虛	**BL13**-**BL15**-H7-ST36 or LU1-BL44-BL42
e. *Lung and Kidney YIN Deficiency* FEI SHEN YIN XU 肺腎陰虛	**BL13**-BL20-BL23-Ki3-SP4, GV14-GV20
f. *No Interaction between Heart and Kidney* XIN SHEN BU JIAO 心腎不交[282]	BL23-**BL15**-GV4-CV4, GV20-H7, YIN TANG
g. *Loss of Interaction between YIN and YANG*, YIN YANG SHI JIAO 陰陽失交	BL23-**BL15**-GV4-CV4, GV20-H7, YIN TANG, SP6
5. YU ZHENG 鬱證, depression syndrome caused by constrained QI[283]	

---

[281] ZHANG ZHONG JING, *Essential Prescriptions of the Golden Coffer*, JIN GUI YAO LUE 金匱要略. The disease was named after the Lily Bulb, the plant used for the treatment of this disease

[282] See page 236 No Interaction between *Heart and Kidney* in joy and pleasure

[283] See page 211, SU WEN, Chapter 39, obsessive thoughts, and page 289 LING SHU, Chapter 8-4, melancholy and sadness

The major acupuncture points to treat melancholy and sadness are BL13-BL15 (similarly to sorrow and grief):

name	function	action
BL13 FEI SHU 肺俞 Lung SHU	SHU of Lung, regulate Lung YANG	release Lung
BL15 XIN SHU 心俞 Heart SHU	SHU of Heart, regulate Heart YANG	calm SHEN, move congestion of Heart Blood, clear heat from Heart

1. *Lung and Spleen QI deficiency* FEI PI QI XU 肺脾氣虛 melancholy and sadness

Etiology	melancholy and sadness injure Lung and Spleen
Signs	SHEN is 'not there': fatigue with spontaneous sweat, anxious thoughts, mental pain with crying, loose stools, cold limbs. Pressure in the chest, weak voice, shortness of breath, dry and weak cough at effort and speech
Tongue	pale and flaccid with thin coating
Pulse	weak (RUO 弱), thin (XI 細), empty (XU 虛)
Strategy	tonify Lung and Spleen, release QI flow of TAI YIN
Points	BL20-**BL13**, BL43-CV4-CV6, SP8-LU6-CV12, LU1

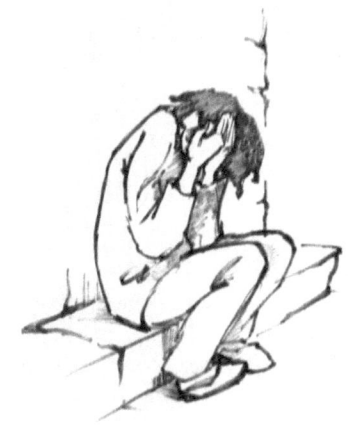

Acupuncture points to treat *Lung and Spleen QI Deficiency*
melancholy and sadness

name	function	action
BL20-BL13 tonify Spleen and Lung		
BL20 PI SHU 脾俞 Spleen SHU	SHU of Spleen, regulate Spleen YANG	tonify Spleen
BL43-CV4-CV6 tonify QI production by Spleen and Lung		
CV4 GUAN YUAN 關元 Origin Pass	Sea of Blood, MU of Small Intestine, meeting of REN MAI with CHONG MAI and Sp., Liv. and Ki. Meridians	warm and tonify Kidney, nourish Blood and JING, assist ascent of CHONG MAI and REN MAI
CV6 QI HAI 氣海 Sea of QI	MU of QI	tonify QI and especially Source QI
BL43 GAO HUANG SHU 膏肓俞 SHU of liquid fat	gather JING in Upper JIAO	strengthen Source QI, Kidney. Spleen, brain and bone marrow
SP8-LU6-CV12, LU1 release QI flow of TAI YIN		
SP8 DI JI 地機 Earth's Mechanism	XI of Spleen, restore communication with soil	remove obstructions of Spleen Meridian
CV12 ZHONG WAN 中脘 Central Venter	MU of Stomach, HUI-meeting of FU, 'knot' of TAI YIN, start of Lu. Meridian	move stagnation, regulate Stomach
LU6 KONG SUI 飛揚 Collection Hole	XI of Lung	disseminate and move Lung QI down
LU1 ZHONG FU 中府 Middle palace	MU of Lung, regulate Lung YIN, entry point, meeting with Sp. Meridian	open QI passage to Upper JIAO, disseminate and move Lung QI down

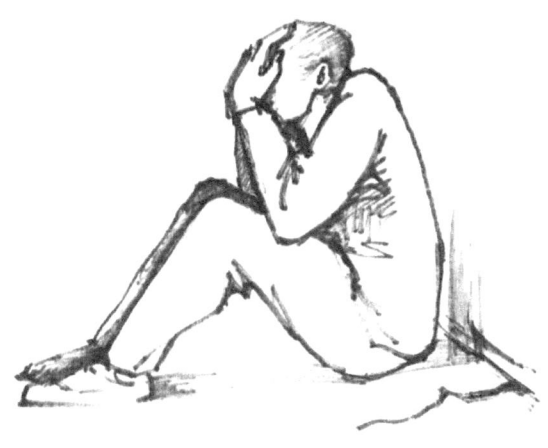

2. Heart and Spleen Dual Deficiency, XIN PI LIANG XU
心脾兩虛 - melancholy and sadness

Etiology	Melancholy and sadness with worry cause Spleen deficiency; Spleen does not nourish Blood, causing Heart deficiency.
Signs	Spleen deficiency: pressure in upper abdomen, loss of appetite, loose stools, constant thoughts, memory loss, difficulty concentrating. Heart and Blood deficiency: palpitation, shortness of breath, insomnia, recurrent dreams, pale complexion, nails and lips.
Tongue	pale and flaccid with thin coating
Pulse	weak (RUO 弱), thin (XI 細)
Strategy	tonify Heart and Spleen, calm thoughts
Points	BL20-SP6-SP4 (tonify), GV20, LIV13, **BL15**-BL17 (tonify)

Acupuncture points to treat *Heart and Spleen Dual Deficiency* - melancholy and sadness

name	function	action
BL20-SP6-SP4, GV20, LIV13 tonify Spleen and calm thoughts, **BL15**-BL17 tonify Heart and Blood		
BL20 PI SHU 脾俞 Spleen SHU	SHU of Spleen, regulate Spleen YANG	tonify Spleen, **tonify**
SP6 SAN YIN JIAO 三陰交 Meeting of Three YIN	meeting of Sp., Liv., and Ki. Meridians	tonify and nourish Blood, QI and YIN, move YIN up, nourish Spleen, stop diarrhea, **tonify**
SP4 GONG SUN 公孫 Grandfather-Grandson	opening of CHONG MAI, LUO of Spleen	move Spleen QI upwards through CHONG MAI, **tonify**
LIV13 ZHANG MEN 章門 Chapter Gate	MU of Spleen, HUI-meeting of five ZANG, meeting of Liv., Ki., H., Sp., Lu., G.B. Meridians	treat Upper JIAO obstruction and rebel QI which obstructs WEI QI (LING SHU, Chapter 59)
GV20 BAI HUI 百會 Hundred Meetings	meeting of DU MAI with six YANG Meridians	move YANG down by moving QI flow of DU MAI down, purify head and brain, treat agitation accompanied by heavy head, release obsession and wrong ideas
BL17 GE SHU 膈俞 Diaphragm SHU	HUI-meeting of Blood, influence diaphragm	open chest, tonify and move blood, **tonify**

3. *No Interaction between Liver and Spleen* GAN PI BU JIAO
肝脾不交 - melancholy and sadness

Etiology	Melancholy and sadness obstruct the QI flow, congest Liver QI. Liver over-controls Spleen
Signs	Liver: irritability, frustration, suppressed aggression, chest and hypochondriac pain and pressure, irregular periods, premenstrual syndrome, Spleen: anxiety, obsessive thinking, loss of appetite, fatigue, sensitive abdomen, soft stool alternating with constipation
Tongue	pale, large with dark coating
Pulse	thin (XI 細), wiry (XUAN 弦)
Strategy	tonify Spleen, calm Liver
Points	LIV13-LIV3-LIV14, ST36-SP4

Acupuncture points to treat *Lung and Spleen* QI *Deficiency*
melancholy and sadness

name	function	action
ST36-SP4 tonify Spleen		
ST36 ZU SAN LI 足三里 Leg Three Miles	HE-Soil of Stomach, tonify QI, Sea of Food point, potentiate other points	regulate YANG deficiency above and YIN excess below, regulate WEI QI, treat lack of SHEN, long lasting melancholy and mental fatigue
SP4 GONG SUN 公孫 Grandfather-Grandson	open CHONG MAI, LUO of Spleen	move Spleen QI upwards through CHONG MAI
LIV13-LIV3-LIV14 calm Liver		
LIV3 TAI CHONG 太沖 Great Rush	SHU-YUAN-Soil of Liver	release and harmonize Liver
LIV13 ZHANG MEN 章門 Chapter Gate	MU of Spleen, HUI-meeting of five ZANG, meeting of Liv., Ki., H., Sp., Lu., G.B. Meridians	treat Upper JIAO obstruction and rebel QI which obstructs WEI QI (LING SHU, 59)
LIV14 QI MEN 期門 Cycle Gate	MU of Liver, regulate Liver YIN, meeting of Liv., Sp. Meridians and YIN WEI MAI	benefit G.B., move QI up from abdomen to chest, calm agitation with arrhythmia and obsession

4. Lily Bulb Disease BAI HE BING 百合病 according to ZHANG ZHONG JING

Etiology	Melancholy, sadness, constant worry combined with heat dry body liquids, Heart Blood and Lung liquids, causing *phlegm-fire*. *Phlegm-fire* obstructs the orifices, dries Heart Blood, causes YIN deficiency and thus injures SHEN; disturbs the Lung function of lowering and injures PO 魄
Signs	Depression and anxiety with a subjective feeling of heat or cold. The three main signs of Lily Bulb Disease: 1. wants to walk and cannot 2. wants to sleep and cannot 3. wants to eat and cannot
Diseases	Multiple sclerosis, Parkinson's disease, Conversion Disorder: blindness, muteness, deafness, paralysis, movement difficulties

4a. Lily Bulb Disease, *Lung and Heart* YIN *Deficiency*
XIN FEI YIN XU 心肺陰虛 - melancholy and sadness

Etiology	Internal heat following external heat dries body liquids, Latent heat dries body YIN, Extreme sadness causes heat in the chest and injures Lung and Heart YIN.
Signs	Feeling cold or hot, regardless of the environment, sadness and anxiety, loneliness, craving sweet taste, dry mouth with bitter taste, red urine. The three signs of Lily Bulb Disease: cannot walk, sleep or eat (alternately anorexia and bulimia)
Tongue	red
Pulse	fast (SHU 數), minute (WEI 微)
Strategy	tonify Lung YIN and purify Heart
Points	LU1-**BL13**/BL42, SP6, **BL15**-PC8-H7 (**disperse**),

Acupuncture points to treat Lily Bulb Disease, *Lung and Heart* YIN *Deficiency* - melancholy and sadness

name	function	action
LU1-**BL13**/BL42, SP6 tonify Lung YIN		
LU1 ZHONG FU 中府 Middle palace	MU of Lung, regulate Lung YIN, entry point, QI passage to Upper JIAO, meeting of Lu. and Sp. Meridians	disseminate and move Lung QI down
BL42 PO HU 魄戶 Door of PO	regulate PO 魄	treat agitation, depression, loss of sense of reality
SP6 SAN YIN JIAO 三陰交 Meeting of Three YIN	meeting of Sp., Liv. and Ki. Meridians	tonify and nourish Blood, QI YIN and Spleen, move YIN up
BL15-PC8-H7 (**disperse**) purify Heart		
PC8 LAO GONG 勞宮 Labor Palace	RONG-Fire of Master of Heart	disperse heat from JUE YIN, purify Heart, awaken SHEN, cool blood, purify mouth
H7 SHEN MEN 神門 SHEN Gate	SHU-YUAN-Soil of Heart	calm SHEN, cool Heart, open Heart orifices

4b. Lily Bulb Disease, *Phlegm-heat or Phlegm-fire*
TAN RE 痰熱/TAN HUO 痰火 - melancholy and sadness

Etiology	*Phlegm fire/heat* resulting from the drying of body liquids by *Heart fire* or latent heat
Signs	feeling of pressure, heat, congestion and pain in the diaphragm and chest, dysfunctional orifices, sexual dysfunction, sticky phlegm, headache with pressure, unrealistic ideas, alternate laughing and crying, fever, the three signs of Lily Bulb Disease
Tongue	thick greasy coating, red tip
Pulse	slippery (HUA 滑), fast (SHU 數)
Strategy	dissolve phlegm, cool YANG MING, purify Heart
Points	ST40-ST44-GV14, PC8-LU5, **BL15**-PC7-CV12

Acupuncture points to treat Lily Bulb Disease, *Phlegm-Heat or Phlegm-Fire* - melancholy and sadness

name	function	action
ST40-ST44-GV14 dissolve phlegm, cool YANG MING		
ST40 FENG LONG 豐隆 Bountiful Bulge	LUO of Stomach	dissolve *phlegm-fire/heat*, calm SHEN
ST44 NEI TING 內庭 Inner Courtyard	RONG-Water of Stomach	cool and move QI of YANG MING and fire down from the head, dissolve phlegm
GV14 DA ZHUI 大椎 Big Vertebra/Wooden Mallet	meeting point of DU MAI with six YANG Meridians	regulate QI and YANG flow to head and Heart, release excess heat and *damp-heat* from the upper body
PC8-LU5 purify Heart		
PC8 LAO GONG 勞宮 Labor Palace	RONG-Fire of Master of Heart	disperse heat from JUE YIN, purify Heart, awaken SHEN, cool blood, purify mouth
LU5 CHI ZE 尺澤 Cubit Marsh	HE-Water of Lung	cool Lung, release Lung QI and TAI YIN, depression, sadness, melancholy, blockage of diaphragm with sadness and restlessness (S. de Morand, page 490)
BL15-PC7-CV12 calm restlessness		
CV12 ZHONG WAN 中脘 Central Venter	MU of Stomach, HUI-meeting of FU, 'knot' of TAI YIN, start of Lu. Meridian	move stagnations, regulate Stomach
PC7 DA LING 大陵 Big Mound	SHU-YUAN-Soil of Master of Heart	calm and purify SHEN, cool blood and Heart (palpitation), purify RONG QI

4c. Lily Bulb Disease, *Liver* YIN *Deficiency* GAN YIN XU
肝陰虛 - melancholy and sadness

Etiology	Melancholy and sadness obstruct the QI flow, causing *Liver QI congestion*, leading to *Liver fire* which dries body liquids and results in *Liver* YIN *deficiency*
Signs	reddish complexion, dry eyes, irritation, headache, hiccups with sour liquid, red urine; the three signs of Lily Bulb Disease: cannot walk, cannot sleep and cannot eat because of the pressure in the chest and hypochondrium
Tongue	red with yellow coating
Pulse	thin (XI 細), wiry (XUAN 弦), fast (SHU 數)
Strategy	tonify YIN, tonify Liver YIN, regulate YANG
Points	LIV14-Ki3-SP6-BL15, GV19-CV12

Acupuncture points to treat Lily Bulb Disease, *Liver* YIN *Deficiency* - melancholy and sadness

name	function	action
LIV14-Ki3-SP6-**BL15** tonify YIN, tonify Liver YIN		
LIV14 QI MEN 期門 Cycle Gate	MU of Liver, regulate Liver YIN, meeting of Liv., Sp. Meridians and YIN WEI MAI	raise QI from abdomen to chest, benefit Gallbladder, calm agitation with arrhythmia and obsession
Ki3 TAI XI 太谿 Great Ravine	SHU-YUAN-Soil of Kidney	tonify Kidney YIN, release ascent of CHONG MAI and REN MAI, treat degenerative diseases
SP6 SAN YIN JIAO 三陰交 Meeting of Three YIN	meeting of Sp., Liv. and Ki. Meridians	tonify and nourish Blood, QI and YIN, move YIN up, nourish Spleen
GV19-CV12, regulate YANG		
CV12 ZHONG WAN 中脘 Central Venter	MU of Stomach, HUI-meeting of FU, 'knot' of TAI YIN, start of Lu. Meridian	move stagnations, regulate Stomach
GV19 HOU DING 後頂 Behind the Vertex	influence HUN 魂	regulate YANG, calm Liver fire rising and HUN 魂

4d. Lily Bulb Disease, *Heart and Lung* QI *Deficiency*
XIN FEI QI XU 心肺氣虛 - melancholy and sadness

Etiology	Melancholy and sadness, failure, anxiety and obsessive thoughts gradually empty Lung and Heart
Signs	depression, anxiety, introversion; the three signs of Lily Bulb Disease develop gradually: cannot walk, sleep (insomnia with shortness of breath and cold sweat) nor eat
Tongue	pale, swollen with thin coating
Pulse	weak (RUO 弱), floating (FU 浮)
Strategy	tonify Lung and Heart QI
Points	**BL13-BL15**-H7-ST36 or LU1-BL44-BL42

Acupuncture points to treat Lily Bulb Disease, *Heart and Lung QI Deficiency* - melancholy and sadness

name	function	action
BL13-BL15-H7-ST36 tonify Lung and Heart QI		
H7 SHEN MEN 神門 SHEN Gate	SHU-YUAN-Soil of Heart	calm SHEN, cool Heart, open Heart orifices
ST36 ZU SAN LI 足三里 Leg Three Miles	HE-Soil of Stomach, tonify QI, Sea of Food point, potentiate other points	regulate YANG deficiency above and YIN excess below, regulate WEI QI, treat lack of SHEN, sighs, prolonged melancholy, mental fatigue
LU1-BL44-BL42, tonify Lung and Heart QI		
LU1 ZHONG FU 中府 Middle palace	MU of Lung, regulate Lung YIN, entry point, QI passage to Upper JIAO, meeting of Lu. and Sp. Meridians	disseminate and move Lung QI down, stop sweat, tonify Lung YIN
BL42 PO HU 魄戶 Door of PO	regulate PO 魄	treat agitation, depression, loss of sense of reality
BL44 SHEN TANG 神堂 Spirit Hall	stabilize SHEN	calm Heart, regulate QI, treat excess in chest, move QI rising in panic down (S. de Morand, page 593)

4e. Lily Bulb Disease, *Lung and Kidney YIN Deficiency*
FEI SHEN YIN XU 肺腎陰虛 - melancholy and sadness

Etiology	Melancholy and sadness heat the chest, dry body liquids and cause *Lung* and *Kidney YIN Deficiency*
Signs	red cheeks, sad and crying easily, shortness of breath, lack of strength, impotence and non-retention of urine, low back and knee pain, 'five palm heat' with sensation of heat in bones. The three signs of Lily Bulb Disease: anorexia, difficulty in walking, difficulty falling asleep
Tongue	red with cracks
Pulse	thin (XI 細), fast (SHU 數)
Strategy	tonify YIN, regulate YANG
Points	**BL13**-BL20-BL23-Ki3-SP4, GV14-GV20 **(puncture in regulation)**

Acupuncture points to treat Lily Bulb Disease, Lung and Kidney YIN *Deficiency* - melancholy and sadness

name	function	action
BL13-BL20-BL23-Ki3-SP4 tonify YIN		
BL20 PI SHU 脾俞 Spleen SHU	SHU of Spleen, regulate Spleen YANG	tonify Spleen YIN, **disperse**
BL23 SHEN SHU 腎俞 Kidney SHU	SHU of Kidney, regulate Kidney YANG	tonify Kidney YIN, **disperse**
Ki3 TAI XI 太谿 Great Ravine	SHU-YUAN-Soil of Kidney	tonify Kidney YIN, release ascent of CHONG MAI and REN MAI, treat degenerative diseases
SP4 GONG SUN 公孫 Grandfather-Grandson	opening of CHONG MAI, LUO of Spleen	move Spleen QI upwards through CHONG MAI, treat mental diseases, calm SHEN
GV14-GV20 regulate YANG		
GV14 DA ZHUI 大椎 Big Vertebra/ Wooden Mallet	meeting of DU MAI with six YANG Meridians	regulate QI and YANG flow to head and Heart, release excess heat and damp-heat from upper body, **regulate**
GV20 BAI HUI 百會 Hundred Meetings	meeting of DU MAI with six YANG Meridians	move YANG down by moving QI flow of DU MAI down, purify head and brain, treat agitation accompanied by heavy head, release obsession and wrong ideas, **regulate**

4f. Lily Bulb Disease, *No Interaction between Heart and Kidney*

XIN SHEN BU JIAO 心腎不交 - melancholy and sadness

Compare joy and pleasure (page 236).

The three signs of Lily Bulb Disease: cannot walk, eat or sleep (stretches and curls in bed, sleep interrupted by disturbing dreams) are observed here.

Acupuncture points to tonify Kidney and Heart and to calm Heart are: BL23-**BL15**-GV4-CV4 (tonify), GV20-H7, YIN TANG (disperse).

Acupuncture points to treat Lily Bulb Disease, *No Interaction between Heart and Kidney* - melancholy and sadness

name	function	action
BL23-**BL15**-GV4-CV4 tonify Kidney and Heart		
BL23 SHEN SHU 腎俞 Kidney SHU	SHU of Kidney, regulate Kidney YANG	tonify Kidney YIN, **tonify**
CV4 GUAN YUAN 關元 Origin Pass	Sea of Blood, MU of Small Intestine, meeting of REN MAI with CHONG MAI and Sp., Liv. and Ki. Meridians	warm and tonify Kidney, nourish Blood and JING, assist ascent of CHONG MAI and REN MAI, **tonify**
GV4 MING MEN 命門 Destiny Gate	reunion between DU MAI and DAI MAI	tonify Kidney and Source YANG, benefit the lumbar spine, **tonify**
GV20-H7, YIN TANG calm Heart		
GV20 BAI HUI 百會 Hundred Meetings	meeting of DU MAI with six YANG meridians	move YANG down by moving QI flow of DU MAI down, purify head and brain, treat agitation accompanied by heavy head, release obsession and wrong ideas, **disperse**
H7 SHEN MEN 神門 SHEN Gate	SHU-YUAN-Soil of Heart	calm SHEN, cool Heart, open Heart orifices, **disperse**
YIN TANG 印堂 Hall of Seal	extra meridian point	move YANG down, calm SHEN, **disperse**

4g. Lily Bulb Disease, *Loss of Interaction between* YIN *and* YANG, YIN YANG SHI JIAO 陰陽失交 - melancholy and sadness

Etiology	*No Interaction between Heart and Kidney* (see above) deteriorates to *Loss of Interaction between* YIN *and* YANG
Signs	YIN and YANG alternate: reddish and pale complexion alternately, not wanting to talk or cannot stop talking even when wanting to, joy and mental pain alternate, heart rhythm disorders, stretching and yawning, feeling miserable; the three signs of Lily Bulb Disease: cannot walk, sleep (wanting to lie down and cannot) or eat
Tongue	red
Pulse	thin (XI 細), fast (SHU 數), without force (WU LI 無力)
Strategy	tonify Kidney and Heart, calm Heart
Points	BL23-**BL15**-GV4-CV4 (tonify), GV20-H7, YIN TANG (disperse), SP6 (tonify) This treatment is similar to treatment for *No Interaction between Heart and Kidney* (see above, page 251)

E. Organization and control are lost in overflowing anger (SHENG NU 盛怒), LING SHU, Chapter 8-3

盛	SHENG	abundant
怒	NU	anger
者	ZHE	this
迷	MI	deceive, deviate
惑	HUO	lost, confused
而	ER	and
不	BU	not
治	ZHI	control, govern

Overflowing anger (SHENG NU 盛怒) *causes deviation* (MI 迷), *confusion* (HUO 惑) *and loss of control* (BU ZHI 不治).

Anger NU 怒 is emotion of Liver-Wood. The character NU 怒[284] shows violence against the feminine, recipient, YIN aspect of a person. The character 盛 with phonetic SHENG (second tone) is translated as 'flourishing', 'abundant'; the character 盛 with phonetic CHENG (fourth tone) is translated as 'hold', 'contain'.[285] SHENG NU 盛怒 conveys the meaning increasing 'overflowing anger',[286] that cannot be contained and controlled.

SHENG NU 盛怒 may be expressed in two ways:
- Aggression expressed outwardly with immediate consequences
- Introverted, accumulated anger leading to restrained aggression which obstructs QI flow (body function) and modifies behavior. Restrained aggression attracts conflict situations and causes a negative attitude to life

Inability to distance oneself from anger transfers it to other people and the environment. ZHUANG ZI, Chapter 20, talks with humor about the need for anger to be attached to something:

---

284 See page 54 for the character NU 怒
285 http://zhongwen.com/d/178/x177.htm
286 Dictionnaire Ricci, 4333

If a man is crossing a river in a boat, and another empty vessel comes into collision with it, even though he be a man of a choleric temper, he will not be angry with it. If there be a person, however, in that boat, he will bawl out to him to haul out of the way. If his shout be not heard, he will repeat it; and if the other do not then hear, he will call out a third time, following up the shout with abusive terms. Formerly he was not angry, but now he is; formerly (he thought) the boat was empty, but now there is a person in it. If a man can empty himself of himself, during his time in the world, who can harm him?[287]

MI HUO 迷惑 describe a deviation from the right direction combined with confusion. The character MI 迷 shows the radical 辶/辵 'movement' (foot moving) and the phonetic 米 'grain of rice'.[288] MI 迷 is 'losing seeds in motion', 'loss of life due to non-organized movement', 'deviation from the personal pathway' and is translated as 'confused', 'lost', 'bewitched' or 'charmed'.

Expressions in Chinese which include the character MI 迷 are related to destruction and deviation:
- MI GONG 迷宮 - Deviation Palace, the labyrinth
- MI XIN 迷心 - superstition
- MI HUN TANG 迷魂湯 - a potion causing deviation of HUN 魂, spells which cause memory loss.[289]

The character HUO 惑 shows the phonetic 或 which means 'perhaps' or 'both',[290] above the radical 心 'heart'. HUO 惑 conveys the meaning 'confusion of Heart' and is translated as 'confuse', 'mislead', 'baffle', 'doubt', 'uncertainty'.[291] HUO LUAN 惑亂 describes a problematic situation, a deviation.

---

287 Translation by Legge, J.
288 http://zhongwen.com/d/176/x103.htm
289 Dictionnaire Ricci, 3467
290 Wieger, Lesson 71
291 http://zhongwen.com/d/180/x98.htm

*Anger (NU 怒) moves QI upwards.*²⁹² Overflowing anger causes deviation, increased harmful ascent of QI and blood towards the head and chest (*Liver YANG rising*) - causing a false order of QI flow which conceals madness (QI flow disorder) - (KUANG 狂)²⁹³ like a fire that is spread by strong winds. Liver-HUN 魂 loses its virtue 'humanity, kindness, benevolence' (REN 仁). Uncontrolled ascent of QI and blood depletes Lower JIAO and causes *Kidney QI Deficiency* (loss of anchor to reality) leading to 'loss of control or inability to be cured' (BU ZHI 不治). The character ZHI 治 may be translated as 'control' or 'healing'.²⁹⁴

In Man, the harmonious flow of Earth QI towards Heaven is represented on the left, ascending phase of the TAI JI symbol, from Kidney to Heart through Liver-Gallbladder (Figure 19). Anger injures Liver and Gallbladder - the transit organ (FU 腑), the YANG aspect of Liver. Gallbladder in Man represents *Rectitude of the Center* (ZHONG ZHENG 中正) (SU WEN, Chapter 8) and oversees the rectitude of the Kidney-Heart axis and the rectitude of Man-SHEN 神 between Heaven and Earth. Overflowing anger disrupts the harmonious QI flow from Earth to Heaven. Injury to the balanced QI flow from Earth to Heaven is seen in Greek mythology in the uprising of angry Titans against the gods, and in Buddhism in the angry and jealous world of the asuras ('demigods' or 'antigods').

SU WEN, Chapter 52, and LING SHU, Chapter 9, do not recommend treating an angry person, since in anger a person is not himself (SHEN 神 is disturbed). It is impossible to regulate QI flow by acupuncture when SHEN 神 is in a disturbed state. Treatment will be effective after a person calms down and returns to himself.

Overflowing anger separates QI and Blood
Severe cases (of anger, NU 怒) *are manifested in vomiting blood and diarrhea* (SU WEN, Chapter 39).²⁹⁵ In anger, QI and blood rise suddenly

---

292 See page 166, SU WEN, Chapter 39
293 See page 252
294 http://zhongwen.com/d/180/x98.htm
295 See page 170

and overflow channels and blood vessels in head and chest, causing blood congestion and bleeding (vomiting blood). Anger also depletes QI of the abdomen and pelvis (Middle and Lower JIAO) causing Spleen and Kidney QI deficiency, expressed in the loss of body liquids through diarrhea.

SU WEN, Chapter 3, describes rage/'great anger' (DA NU 大怒) causing the ascent of YANG QI to the head and chest, separation of 'substantial forms' (Blood) and QI of upper and lower body, and damage to tendons:

陽 YANG	而 ER	and	有 YOU	has	汗 HAN	sweat
氣 QI	血 XUE	blood	傷 SHANG	injure	出 CHU	exit
者 ZHE	of	菀 YU	pull	於 YU	to	偏 PIAN	one side
大 DA	big	於 YU	to	筋 JIN	tendon	沮 JU	fade
怒 NU	anger	上 SHANG	up	縱 ZONG	relax	使 SHI	makes
則 ZE	of	使 SHI	make	其 QI	these	人 REN	man
形 XING	form	人 REN	man	若 RUO	like	偏 PIAN	hemiplegia
氣 QI		薄 BO	feeble	不 BU	not	枯 KU	
絕 JUE	separate	厥 JUE	exhaust	容 RONG	contain		

In great anger (DA NU 大怒) *YANG QI separates 'substantial forms'* (Blood) *from QI,*
So the blood rises and causes loss of force through QI exhaustion (BO JUE 薄厥) *in man.*
The tendons are injured and loosen as if they cannot contain (QI).
Sweating on only one side of the body (is a sign of) *hemiplegia* (the paralysis of one side of the body).

The overflow of blood to the head exhausts QI (BO JUE 薄厥) and impairs body function (causes *loss of force*), leading to partial loss of movement due to paresis (a neurological disorder - inability to move a muscle or group of muscles, loss of muscle mass) or cerebral bleeding. Rochat de la Vallée translates BO JUE 薄厥 as 'flexing by pressure'.[296] Following an excessive ascent of blood and QI (including

---

296 Rochat de la Vallée, E., *Les 11 Premiers Traites*, p. 75

Defensive QI - WEI QI - which provides muscle tonus) to the head and chest, Liver cannot release blood and QI to nourish tendons and muscles. Blood and WEI QI deficiency in tendons and muscles causes weakness and partial paralysis.

Sweating on only one side of the body is a sign of weakness on the other side, which may lead to hemiplegia (paralysis of one side of the body). Imbalance between the upper and lower body is expressed by imbalance between the left side of the body (which is dominated by QI) and the right side (which is dominated by Blood). Heart problems and cerebral hemorrhage in the elderly often occur following overflowing anger.

Overflowing anger and wind
Wind is QI of Wood-Liver. ZHUANG ZI, Chapter 2, associates wind and anger:

夫 FU	so	其 QI	its	是 SHI	be	作 ZUO	act
大 DA	big	名 MING	name	唯 WEI	only	則 ZE	then
塊 KUAI	clump	為 WEI	is	无 WU	not	萬 WAN	10.000
噫 YI	vomit	風 FENG	wind	作 ZUO	act	竅 QIAO	opening
氣 QI						怒 NU	anger
						呺 HAO	scream

The Great Clod belches out breath and its name is wind. So long as it doesn't come forth, nothing happens. But when it does, then ten thousand hollows begin crying wildly (in anger, NU 怒).[297]

A breeze is considered to be a source of inspiration and a metaphor for the smooth flow of Liver QI; a strong wind is a metaphor for *Liver QI rising*. A hurricane is a metaphor for *Liver fire/YANG rising* and is expressed as overflowing anger and agitation (KUANG 狂). Liver-Wood is injured by wind (of external or internal origin).

---

297 Translation by B. Watson

SU WEN, Chapter 42, describes anger caused by external wind, which has penetrated Liver or Heart and has attached to internal wind and/or fire:

心	XIN	heart	病	BING	disease	肝	GAN	liver	善	SHAN	like
風	FENG	wind	甚	SHEN	many	風	FENG	wind	怒	NU	anger
之	ZHI	of	則	ZE	then	之	ZHI	of	時	SHI	period
狀	ZHUANG	look	言	YAN	speak	狀	ZHUANG	look	憎	ZENG	hate
多	DUO	many	不	BU	not	多	DUO	many	女	NU	
汗	HAN	sweat	可	KE	possible	汗	HAN	sweat	子	ZI	woman
惡	E	hate	快	KUAI	fast	惡	E	hate	診	ZHEN	examine
風	FENG	wind	診	ZHEN	examine	風	FENG	wind	在	ZAI	locate
焦	JIAO	burn	在	ZAI	locate	善	SHAN	like	目	MU	eye
絕	JUE	cut	口	KOU	mouth	悲	BEI	sorrow	下	XIA	below
善	SHAN	like	其	QI	this	色	SE	color	其	QI	this
怒	NU	anger	色	SE	color	微	WEI	slight	色	SE	color
嚇	HE	terrify	赤	CHI	red	蒼	CANG	blue	青	QING	green
赤	CHI	red				嗌	YI	throat			
色	SE	color				乾	GAN	dry			

Wind of Heart syndrome is expressed as profuse sweating, aversion to wind, burnt and cracked lips, and a tendency to frightening anger and red complexion.
When disease progresses speech is slow and the mouth is red.
Wind of Liver syndrome is expressed as profuse sweating, aversion to wind, a tendency to sorrow (BEI 悲), bluish-green complexion, dry throat, a tendency to lasting anger (NU 怒) and avoiding sexual relations with women. Examination shows greenish color under the eyes.

Common signs of damage by external wind which has penetrated Heart and Liver are profuse sweating and aversion to wind.
External wind penetrating Heart is expressed as frightening anger (NU HE 怒嚇) accompanied by red complexion, damage to Spleen YIN (burnt and cracked lips, mouth inflammation) and speech disorders.

External wind penetrating Liver is expressed as anger (NU 怒) with sorrow (BEI 悲). Wind-Wood over-nourishes Heart-Fire and damages (reversed control) Lung-Metal. Other symptoms are: blue-green complexion, dry throat (the internal pathway of Liver Meridian passes through the throat), sexual dysfunction and greenish color under the eyes.

Loss of control in overflowing anger and QI of war
QI of war is similar to uncontrolled anger and represents an acute disease in society which has to run its course, and only then can its disastrous outcomes be treated. QI of war presents as actions that are confused and uncontrolled and inability to find a just solution to accumulating problems. No matter the source of QI of war, its outcome is always a surprise associated with multiple disasters. Explosion of collective hatred accumulated during generations or collective hypnotic hatred is similar to overflowing anger. Hatred injures the rectitude of Man between Heaven and Earth and the ability to examine the situation at a distance, which is each person's responsibility. Of course, there can be justified collective anger, but history has many examples of righteous collective rages which became collective drama.

The army general in Ancient China was supposed to have an unobstructed Liver, enabling *planning and contemplation of the situation* (MU LU 謀慮) and Gallbladder with emphasized *Rectitude of the Center* (ZHONG ZHENG 中正) (SU WEN, Chapter 8). He predicted the future and avoided extreme situations by intuition, was realistic, and by observing stars, planets and the landscape was capable of choosing the right time and place to win the battle.

Syndromes in Chinese medicine which describe the loss of organization and control caused by overflowing anger

Frustrations and inability to react or realize desires and aspirations impair proper communication of Liver with the environment. Liver YIN QI congests, disrupting a smooth QI flow, prevents (reversed generation) Kidney YIN flow upwards and bursts into uncontrollable overflowing anger (described in Chinese Medicine as *Liver fire/YANG rising* which injures Spleen, Lung, Heart and Kidney). Sometimes repressed anger bursts out as if without cause. Syndromes in Chinese medicine which describe similar situations are:

Syndrome	Acupuncture points
1. *Liver QI Congested and Knotted,* GAN QI YU JIE 肝氣鬱結	**LIV3-LIV6**, H7-PC6-GV24
2. *Congested QI Transforms into Fire,* QI YU HUA HUO 氣鬱化火	**LIV3-LIV8**-3-SP6, LIV2-GV19-GB43
3. *Liver and Gallbladder Fire Flaring Upwards,* GAN DAN HUO SHANG YAN 肝膽火上炎	GB41-**LIV2**, ST44, PC5
4. *Dual Liver Blood and Kidney YIN Deficiency,* GAN XUE SHEN YIN LIANG XU 肝血腎陰兩虛	**LIV3-LIV8**, Ki3-Ki7, CV4-SP6
5. *Loss and Deficiency of Liver YIN,* GAN YIN KUI XU 肝陰虧虛	LIV14-**LIV8**, BL17-BL18, GB34
6. *Confusion of Heart and of SHEN,* XIN SHEN HUO LUAN 心神惑亂	**LIV3-LIV6**, SP6-Ki7-BL44-BL52, PC5, GV22
7. *No Interaction between Liver and Spleen,* GAN PI BU JIAO 肝脾不交[298]	LIV13-**LIV3**-LIV14, ST36-SP4

Major acupuncture points to calm overflowing anger: **LIV3**, **LIV2**, **LIV8**, **LIV6**:

LIV3 TAI CHONG 太沖 Great Rush	SHU-YUAN-Soil of Liver	release and harmonize Liver
LIV2 XING JIAN 行間 Moving Between	RONG-Fire of Liver	move YANG down, benefit Gallbladder, stop wind, calm anger
LIV6 ZHONG DU 中都 Capital Center	XI of Liver	sedate and regulate Liver, release congested Liver QI and blood, treat gynecological disorders
LIV8 QU QUAN 曲泉 Spring at the bend	HE-Water of Liver, tonify Wood	tonify Liver YIN (specially in Ki. YIN deficiency), nourish Liver Blood, clear excess heat, move dampness, regulate Lower JIAO

---

298 See page 245 for *No Interaction between Liver and Spleen* in melancholy and sadness

1. *Liver QI Congested and Knotted,* GAN QI YU JIE 肝氣鬱結 - anger

Etiology	Errors in life, problems in human relations, unfulfilled desires
Signs	unstable, introverted, dissatisfied, sometimes depressed, sighs, feeling of fullness and pressure in the chest, abdominal bloating, especially in hypochondrium, hiccups, loss of appetite, anorexia, nausea and vomiting, irregular bowel movements.
	irregular periods, PMS with breast swelling. Sensation of a lump (plum pit) in throat
Tongue	dark or normal with thin white coating
Pulse	wiry (XUAN 弦), with force (YOU LI 有力)
Strategy	release Liver QI, calm SHEN
Points	**LIV3-LIV6**, H7-PC6-GV24

Acupuncture points to treat *Liver QI congested and knotted* - anger

name	function	action
LIV3-LIV6 release Liver QI, H7-PC6-GV24 calm SHEN		
H7 SHEN MEN 神門 SHEN Gate	SHU-YUAN-Soil of Heart	calm SHEN, cool Heart (insomnia, stress, memory loss), open Heart orifices
PC6 NEI GUAN 內關 Inner Barrier	LUO of Master of Heart, open YIN WEI MAI	release 3 YIN, regulate QI, move rebel QI down, awaken SHEN, open chest, remove blockages between pelvis and chest
GV24 SHEN TING 神庭 SHEN Court	meeting of DU MAI with Bl. and St. Meridians	communicate between orifices, calm SHEN, regulate mental restlessness

2. *Congested QI Transforms into Fire,* QI YU HUA HUO 氣鬱化火 - anger

Etiology	*Congested Liver* YIN QI transforms into *Liver* YANG/*fire* rising to the head
Signs	*Liver fire rises*: red face and eyes, headaches, tinnitus, dizziness; *fire* injures Spleen and Stomach: a burning sensation in the esophagus and stomach, gingivitis, the rise of gastric juices, pain and swelling in hypochondrium;
	fire dries body liquids: bitter taste in the mouth, dry lips, constipation
Tongue	dry red with dry yellow coating
Pulse	wiry (XUAN 弦), fast (SHU 數)
Strategy	regulate *Liver* YANG/*fire*, nourish YIN
Points	**LIV3-LIV8**-Ki3-SP6, **LIV2**-GV19-GB43

Acupuncture points to treat *Congested QI Transforms into Fire* - anger

name	function	action
LIV3-LIV8 regulate *Liver YANG/fire*, Ki3-SP6 nourish YIN		
Ki3 TAI XI 太谿 Great Ravine	SHU-YUAN-Soil of Kidney	tonify Kidney YIN, release ascent of CHONG MAI and REN MAI, treat degenerative diseases
SP6 SAN YIN JIAO 三陰交 Meeting of Three YIN	meeting of Sp., Liv. and Ki. Meridians	tonify and nourish Blood, QI and YIN, move YIN up, nourish Spleen, stop diarrhea
LIV2-GV19 disperse *Liver fire*, GB43 cool Gallbladder		
GV19 HOU DING 後頂 Behind the Vertex	influence HUN 魂	regulate YANG, calm Liver fire rising and HUN 魂
GB43 XIA XI 俠谿 Pinched Ravine	RONG-Water of Gallbladder, tonify Wood	purify head, ears and eyes, return order and mental uprightness, **tonify**

3. *Liver and Gallbladder Fire Flaring Upwards*
GAN DAN HUO SHANG YAN 肝膽火上炎 - anger

Etiology	Hot and spicy food (meats, chili, alcohol), agitation, chronic lack of sleep
Signs	agitation, anger, irritability, rage, insomnia with nightmares, red face and eyes; severe headache, dizziness; dry mouth with bitter taste, hypochondriac pain, constipation, dark urine.
Tongue	red with yellow coating
Pulse	wiry (XUAN 弦), fast (SHU 數)
Strategy	disperse and purify *Liver and Gallbladder fire*, release fire from the head through cooling of YANG MING,
Points	GB41-**LIV2**, ST44, PC5

Acupuncture points to treat *Liver and Gallbladder Fire Flaring Upwards* - anger

name	function	action
GB41- **LIV2**, ST44, PC5 disperse and purify *Liver and Gallbladder fire*		
GB41 ZÚ LÍN QÌ 足臨泣 Bend to Cry of Foot	SHJ-Wood of G.B., open DAI MAI	regulate G.B. QI, open communication between upper and lower body
PC5 JIAN SHI 間使 Interval Envoy	JING-River-Metal of Master of Heart - JUE YIN, Group LUO of 3 arm YIN	regulate YIN deficiency above and YIN stagnation below, open chest, calm SHEN, calm SHAO YANG, calm suffering and stop the crying
ST44 NEI TING 內庭 Inner Courtyard	RONG-Water of Stomach	cool and move QI of YANG MING and fire down from head

4. *Dual Liver Blood and Kidney* YIN *Deficiency*
GAN XUE SHEN YIN LIANG XU 肝血腎陰兩虛 - anger

Etiology	Age, weak constitution, chronic disease
Signs	*Liver Blood deficiency*: irritability, anger in the elderly, tinnitus, dry inflamed eyes, decreased vision, pain in the lower back and knees, chest and hypochondriac pain; *Kidney* YIN *deficiency*: dry throat, night sweats, 'five palm heat'
Tongue	pale with red edges, almost without coating
Pulse	thin (XI 細), floating (FU 浮), fast (SHU 數)
Strategy	release Liver, nourish Liver Blood, tonify Blood and Kidney YIN
Points	LIV3-LIV8, Ki3-Ki7, CV4-SP6

Acupuncture points to treat *Dual Liver Blood and Kidney* YIN *Deficiency* - anger

name	function	action
LIV3-LIV8 release Liver and nourish Liver Blood, Ki3-Ki7 tonify Kidney YIN		
Ki3 TAI XI 太谿 Great Ravine	SHU-YUAN-Soil of Kidney	tonify Kidney YIN, release ascent of CHONG MAI and REN MAI, treat degenerative diseases, **tonify**
Ki7 FU LIU 復溜 Returning Current	JING-River-Metal of Kidney, tonify Water, enhance QI flow in meridians from Ki. towards M.H. (PC)	tonify Kidney YIN, tonify Heart, reduce fire, move dampness, tonify brain and bone marrow
CV4-SP6 tonify Blood		
SP6 SAN YIN JIAO 三陰交 Meeting of Three YIN	meeting of Sp., Liv. and Ki. Meridians	tonify and nourish Blood, QI and YIN, move YIN up, nourish Spleen
CV4 GUAN YUAN 關元 Origin Pass	Sea of Blood, MU of S.I., meeting of REN MAI with CHONG MAI, Sp., Liv. and Ki. Meridians	warm and tonify Kidney, nourish Blood and JING, assist ascent of CHONG MAI and REN MAI

5. *Loss and Deficiency of Liver* YIN, GAN YIN KUI XU 肝陰虧虛 - anger

Etiology	Long lasting anger with tendency to YIN deficiency causes loss of body liquids and JING in the upper part of the body (head)
Signs	YIN *deficiency* with *empty* YANG *rising* to the head: headache, dry eyes, intolerance to light, red face and eyes, tinnitus, vertigo; hot flushes, 'five palm heat', insomnia or restless dreams, night sweats;
	Liver YIN does not nourish muscles: loss of muscle strength, loss of sensation in the muscles
Tongue	red and dry with little coating
Pulse	thin (XI 細), wiry (XUAN 弦), fast (SHU 數)
Strategy	tonify Liver YIN, nourish Liver Blood, muscles and tendons
Points	LIV14-**LIV8**, BL17-BL18, GB34

Acupuncture points to treat *Loss and Deficiency of Liver* YIN
anger

name	function	action
LIV14-LIV8 tonify Liver YIN		
LIV14 QI MEN 期門 Cycle Gate	MU of Liver, regulate Liver YIN, meeting of Liv., Sp. Meridians and YIN WEI MAI	raise QI from abdomen to chest, benefit G.B., calm agitation with arrhythmia and obsession
BL17-BL18, GB34 nourish Liver Blood, muscles and tendons		
BL17 GE SHU 膈俞 Diaphragm SHU	HUI-meeting of Blood, influence diaphragm	open the chest, tonify and move blood, **disperse**
BL18 GAN SHU 肝俞 Liver SHU	SHU of Liver, regulate Liver YANG	tonify Liver YIN, move Liver QI and blood stagnation, move stagnant blood from head
GB34 YANG LING QUAN 陽陵泉 YANG Mound Spring	HE-Soil of Gallbladder, HUI-meeting of muscles and tendons	regulate and move G.B. QI down

6. *Confusion of Heart and of* SHEN, XIN SHEN HUO LUAN
心神惑亂 - anger

Etiology	Long-lasting *Liver QI congestion* causes *Heart QI* and *Blood deficiency* and injures SHEN and JING
Signs	dementia/Alzheimer, alternating sadness and anger, aggression, yawning and stretching
Tongue	pale
Pulse	wiry (XUAN 弦)
Strategy	release *Liver QI congestion*, tonify JING, regulate YIN of the upper body, regulate SHEN
Points	**LIV3-LIV6**, SP6-Ki7-BL44-BL52, PC5, GV22

Acupuncture points to treat *Confusion of Heart and of SHEN* - anger

name	function	action
LIV3-LIV6 release Liver QI		
SP6-Ki7-BL44-BL52, PC5, GV22 tonify JING, regulate YIN of the upper body, regulate SHEN		
Ki7 FU LIU 復溜 Returning current	JING-River-Metal of Kidney, tonify Water, enhance QI flow in Meridians from Ki. towards M.H. (PC)	tonify Kidney YIN, tonify Heart, reduce fire, move dampness, tonify brain and bone marrow
SP6 SAN YIN JIAO 三陰交 Meeting of Three YIN	meeting of Sp., Liv. and Ki. Meridians	tonify and nourish Blood, QI and YIN, move YIN up, nourish Spleen
BL44 SHEN TANG 神堂 Spirit Hall	stabilize SHEN	calm Heart, regulate QI, treat excess in chest
BL52 ZHI SHI 志室 ZHI Chamber	influence ZHI, gather JING	warm QI, tonify Kidney and JING
PC5 JIAN SHI 間使 Interval Envoy	JING-River-Metal of Master of Heart - JUE YIN, Group LUO of three arm YIN	regulate YIN deficiency above and YIN stagnation below, open chest, calm SHEN, calm SHAO YANG, calm suffering and stop the crying
GV22 XIN HUI 囟會 Fontanelle Meeting		strengthen JING, create new ideas

F. Ability of being oneself is lost in fear and dread
(KONG JU 懼恐), LING SHU, Chapter 8-3

恐 KONG fear
懼 JU dread
者 ZHE this
神 SHEN
蕩 DANG agitate
憚 DAN scare away

而 ER and
不 BU no
收 SHOU gathering

In fear and dread (KONG JU 懼恐) SHEN is restless (DANG 蕩) and scared away (DAN 憚),
and (the person) cannot gather himself (SHOU 收) (cannot be himself).

❖ LING SHU, Chapter 8-3: *In fear and dread* (KONG JU 懼恐) SHEN 神 *is restless* (DANG 荡) *and scared away* (DAN 憚)…

Fear and dread (KONG JU 懼恐)²⁹⁹ are expressed as restless agitation (DANG 荡). The character DANG 荡 describes movement and is translated as 'vagrant', 'licentious', 'to sway', 'to shake'.³⁰⁰ The agitation in the chest (Heart-SHEN) caused by sorrow and grief (BEI AI 悲哀), is written with another character, DONG 動 ('action', 'movement').³⁰¹ Sorrow of Heart is transmitted to Kidney-ZHI 志: *Heart sorrow* (BEI 悲) *is called ZHI* 志 *sorrow* (BEI 悲) 心悲名曰志悲 (SU WEN, Chapter 81). Both sorrow and fear cause agitation of Center of Chest (Heart-SHEN).

In fear and dread SHEN 神 is scared away (DAN 憚).³⁰² Joy and pleasure also scare SHEN away (DAN 憚), and therefore SHEN is dispersed and does not store.³⁰³ 'SHEN scared away (DAN 憚)' is a process similar to 'SHEN *has nowhere to return to*' in panic (JING 驚) causing *disorder of QI* flow.³⁰⁴ When SHEN is *scared away*, QI flows in disorder causing *Heart fire*, which disperses QI from the body and damages JING 精 storage in Kidney. Fear (KONG 恐) *makes* JING 精 retreat (SU WEN, Chapter 39),³⁰⁵ and therefore disturbs QI flow.

LING SHU, Chapter 8-3, starts: *The injury to* SHEN (caused by apprehension, distress, obsessive thinking and worry) *is expressed as fear and dread* (KONG JU 懼恐). (JING 精) *flows down, overflows and cannot stop*. Obsessive thinking and worry may continuously create fear and dread (Soil controls Water). Fear and dread injure the lower body, especially Kidney JING 精.³⁰⁶

---

299 See page 54 for the characters KONG 恐 JU 懼
300 http://zhongwen.com/d/191/x186.htm
301 See page 233
302 See page 232 for the character DAN 憚 in joy and pleasure
303 See page 233
304 See page 197
305 See page 187
306 See page 219

The final topic of this chapter, deals with injury to the upper body, especially Heart/SHEN, caused by fear and dread.

Kidney-Water, weakened by fear and dread, do not control Heart-Fire: the flow of JING QI 精氣 and body liquids upwards from Kidney to Heart is impaired. The first and last topics in chapter 8-3 combined together describe the damage caused by fear and dread to the upper and lower body, the central axis Fire-Water (as on the TAI JI symbol).

❖ LING SHU, Chapter 8-3, fear and dread: the person *cannot gather himself* (SHOU 收) (cannot be himself).

Fear and dread scare SHEN and 'separate' Kidney and Heart (YIN and YANG): Heart fire damages Kidney (reversed control). Therefore a man loses his anchor at all levels of existence and stops being himself.

Types of fear

The nature and expression of fear varies depending on its cause and intensity. Fear can damage either or both YIN and YANG aspects of Kidney:
- The YANG aspect of fear (KONG 恐) is expressed outwardly and causes an active reaction (flight).
- The YIN aspect of fear - dread (JU 懼) is not expressed outwardly and contracts (freezes) inside.

ZHUANG ZI, Chapter 2, describes little 'agitating' fears and big 'freezing' fears:

少	XIAO	small	大	DA	great
恐	KONG	fear	恐	KONG	fear
惴	ZHUI	agitated	縵	MAN	stunned
惴	ZHUI	anxious	縵	MAN	unsettled

Their little fears (XIAO KONG 少恐) *are mean and trembly*;
Their great fears (DA KONG 大恐) *are stunned and overwhelming*.[307]

---

307 Translation by B. Watson

The expression *as if someone were about to arrest them* (KONG RU REN JIANG BU ZHI 恐如人將捕之) is used to describe fear:
- in autumn (SU WEN, Chapter 49)
- in Gallbladder diseases (LING SHU, Chapter 4)
- in injury to Kidney Meridian (LING SHU, Chapter 10)

SU WEN, Chapter 49:

所	SUO what which	秋	QIU autumn	陰	YIN	陰	YIN
謂	WEI called	氣	QI	氣	QI	陽	YANG
恐	KONG fear	萬	WANG 10,000	少	XIAO little	相	XIANG together
如	RU are	物	WU being	陽	YANG	薄	BO abundance
人	REN man	未	WEI not	氣	QI	故	GU therefore
將	JIANG soon	有	YOU has	入	RU enter	恐	KONG fear
捕	BU capture	畢	BI finish	陰	YIN	也	YE period
之	ZHI him	去	QU leave				

As for the so-called 'they are in fear as if someone were about to arrest them (KONG RU REN JIANG BU ZHI 恐如人將捕之),' [that is to say:] [Under the dominance of] the autumn QI the myriad beings have not completely vanished yet.
The YIN QI is present in small quantities and the YANG QI enters [the interior]. YIN and YANG [QI] strike at each other. Hence, [people suffer from] 'fear.'[308]

SU WEN, Chapter 49, describes fear in autumn, caused by an imbalance of YIN and YANG. Autumn is the period when YANG QI retreats towards the interior, and YIN QI is still weak. YANG QI enters the body, like myriad beings entering the ground to hibernate, through the skin surface, and there confronts exiting YIN QI. The agitation of YANG QI entering into the body combines with the anxiety of YIN QI exiting.

The imbalance of YIN and YANG causes the instability of the axis Water-Fire (Kidney-Heart). A person feels as if not in his right place, a lack of stability and support causing *fear as if someone were about to arrest (capture)* him.

---

308 Translation by Unschuld and Tessenow, pp. 730, characters 49-272-4

LING SHU, Chapter 4:

膽	DAN gallbladder	口	KOU mouth	心	XIN heart	恐	KONG fear
病	BING disease	苦	KU bitter	下	XIA below	人	REN man
者	ZHE are	嘔	OU vomit	澹	DAN agitation	將	JIANG soon
善	SHAN often	宿	XIU bile	澹	DAN palpitation	捕	BU capture
太	TAI extreme	汁	ZHI			之	ZHI him
息	XI breath						

In Gallbladder disease there are often sighs.
There is a bitter taste in the mouth and vomiting of bile.
There are palpitation and agitation below the heart,
The man fears as if someone were about to arrest him (KONG REN JIANG BU ZHI 恐人將捕之).

LING SHU, Chapter 4, describes the situation of instability and fear *as if someone were about to arrest him* in Gallbladder diseases. Gallbladder - *Rectitude of the Center* (ZHONG ZHENG 中正) - stores JING 精 and oversees the rectitude of the Kidney-Heart axis in Man and the rectitude of Man-SHEN 神 between Heaven and Earth.

SU WEN, Chapter 10, describes fear-distress (TI 惕)[309] caused by damage to Kidney Meridian: *Heart* (of a man) *is distressed* (*anxious*, TI 惕) *as if someone were about to arrest him* (XIN TI TI RUO REN JIANG BU ZHI 心惕惕若人將捕之)

It is important to strengthen Kidney and Gallbladder to prevent fear and dread.

---

309 See page 217 for the character TI 惕

Action without action as a treatment for fear according to ZHUANG ZI

ZHUANG ZI, Chapter 19, proposes a treatment for fear by non-action, calm and keeping SHEN 神 gathered, giving an example of the drunken man who has no knowledge and fear of what is going on and therefore does not get injured:

夫	FU so	骨	GU bone	其	QI his	死	SI death
醉	ZHUI drunken	節	JIE joint	神	SHEN	生	SHENG life
者	ZHE comma	與	YU with	全	QUAN entire	驚	JING panic
之	ZHI of	人	REN man	也	YE period	懼	JU dread
墜	ZHUI fall	同	TONG similar	乘	CHENG carriage	不	BU not
車	CHE carriage	而	ER but	亦	YI also	入	RU man
雖	SUI even	犯	FAN injury	不	BU not	乎	HU !
疾	JI bruise	害	HAI injure	知	ZHI know	其	QI his
不	BU not	與	YU with	也	YE period	胷	XIONG chest
死	SI die	人	REN man	墜	ZHUI fall	中	ZHONG center
		異	YI different	亦	YI also	故	GU cause
				不	BU not	遻	E meet
				知	ZHI know	物	WU things
				也	YE period	而	ER and
						不	BU not
						慴	SHE fear

Take the case of a drunken man falling from his carriage - though he may suffer injury, he will not die. His bones and joints are the same as those of other men, but the injury which he receives is different: His spirit is entire. He knew nothing about his getting into the carriage, and knew nothing about his falling from it. The thought of death or life, or of any alarm or affright, does not enter his breast; and therefore he encounters danger without any shrinking from it.[310]

---

310 Translation by Legge, J.

ZHUANG ZI, Chapter 23, calls this place of calm without fear, which holds SHEN 神 gathered, Terrace of the Spirit (LING TAI 靈臺). Terrace of the Spirit cannot be defined and cannot be fortified by knowledge:

靈	LING	soul, spirit	而	ER	and	而	ER	and
臺	TAI	terrace	不	BU	not	不	BU	not
有	YOU	has	知	ZHI	know	其	QI	its
持	CHI	support	其	QI	its	可	KE	possible
			所	SUO	by which	持	CHI	support
			持	CHI	support	者	ZHE	of
						也	YE	period

The Terrace of Spirit (LING TAI 靈臺) *has* (its) *support,*
But (we) *do not know what supports it,*
And (we) *cannot support it.*

The Art of Nourishing Life (YANG SHENG 養生) **as the treatment against fear according to** LAO ZI

The Art of Nourishing Life (YANG SHENG 養生),[311] which had an important role in ancient Chinese tradition, is based on techniques of the gathering and preservation of JING 精 by Kidney-QI-ZHI 志, in order to prevent disease and assure long life. JING 精 reserves are called 'Cinnabar Field' (DAN TIAN 丹田), the symbol of life, support and source for refining QI and preventing fear.

Today, especially among city dwellers, constant mental activity moves body QI upward to the chest and head, creating QI deficiency in the lower body (hips and legs) and causing deficiency of JING 精 reserves in DAN TIAN 丹田, resulting in emotional instability and fear. Daily exercise and a proper diet are necessary for the Art of Nourishing Life which treats DAN TIAN deficiency.

---

311 See page 145, LING SHU, Chapter 8-1

According to LAO ZI, Chapter 3, in order to govern human society, as well as the human body, it is essential to empty Heart of desires, passions and wills, and to fill the belly (DAN TIAN) with JING QI 精氣:

是	SHI		虛	XU	empty	弱	RUO	weaken
以	YI	therefore	其	QI	their	其	QI	their
聖	SHENG	sage	心	XIN	heart	志	ZHI	emotions, will
人	REN	man	實	SHI	fill	強	QIANG	strengthen
之	ZHI	of	其	QI	their	其	QI	their
治	ZHI	govern	腹	FU	abdomen	骨	GU	bones

Therefore the sage, in the exercise of his government,
Empties their minds, fills their bellies,
Weakens their wills, and strengthens their bones.[312]

LAO ZI, Chapter 59, emphasizes the importance of deep rootedness and a firm foundation for the prolongation of life: *To be deeply rooted in a firm foundation* is to be rooted in DAN TIAN 丹田; that means in Kidney YIN (gathering and storage of JING 精) and in Kidney YANG (overflowing JING QI 精氣), which provide a support for the axis Kidney-Heart.

是	SHI	be	長	CHANG	long
謂	WEI	say	生	SHENG	life
深	SHEN	deep	久	JIU	enduring
根	GEN	root	視	SHI	sight, vision
固	GU	firm	之	ZHI	of
柢	DI	basis, foundation	道	DAO	way

This is to be deeply rooted (GEN 根) *in a firm foundation* (DI 柢), *the way of long life* (CHANG SHENG 長生) *and eternal vision.*[313]

---

312 Translation by Legge, J.
313 Translation by Beck, S.

Syndromes in Chinese medicine which describe the loss of ability to be oneself caused by fear and dread

Syndrome	Acupuncture points
1. *Blood* YIN *Deficiency*, XUE YIN XU 血陰虛	SP6-BL17, H6-Ki3-BL15-BL18
2. *Heart and Gallbladder* QI *Deficiency*, XIN DAN QI XU 心膽氣虛	BL19-GB35-LIV14 or GB24, H7-GV24, BL15-CV6
3. *Phlegm Fire Harassing Heart* TAN HUO RAO XIN 痰火擾心	PC7-LI11-GB41, ST40-CV12
4. *Heart Fire Hyperactivity and Exuberance* XIN HUO KANG SHENG 心火亢盛[314]	SI7-H7, PC8, Ki4, Ki27
5. *Blood Deficiency and Liver* QI *Congested and knotted* XUE XU GAN QI YU JIE 血虛肝氣鬱結	LIV3-LIV6-LIV14, BL17-SP6-BL20, PC7/PC6, BL47

1. *Blood* YIN *Deficiency*, XUE YIN XU 血陰虛
fear and dread

Etiology	Prolonged illness, bleeding and anorexia cause *Blood* YIN *deficiency*, preventing Heart-SHEN nourishment and provoking *Empty* YANG *rising*
Signs	instability, palpitation, night sweats, insomnia with erotic dreams and ejaculation, tinnitus, 'five palm heat', low back pain, fear, pale complexion,
Tongue	red and dry
Pulse	thin (XI 細), wiry (XUAN 弦), fast (SHU 數)
Strategy	tonify Blood YIN, regulate YANG, calm SHEN
Points	SP6-BL17, H6-Ki3-BL15-BL18

---

314 See page 234, joy and pleasure

Acupuncture points to treat *Blood* YIN *Deficiency*
fear and dread

name	function	action
SP6-BL17 tonify Blood YIN		
SP6 SAN YIN JIAO 三陰交 Meeting of Three YIN	meeting of Sp., Ki. and Liv. Meridians	tonify and nourish Blood, QI, YIN and Spleen, move YIN up
BL17 GE SHU 膈俞 Diaphragm SHU	HUI-meeting of Blood, influence diaphragm	open chest, tonify and move blood, **tonify**
H6-Ki3-BL15-BL18 regulate YANG, calm SHEN		
Ki3 TAI XI 太谿 Great Ravine	SHU-YUAN-Soil of Kidney	tonify Kidney YIN, release ascent of CHONG MAI and REN MAI, treat degenerative diseases, tonify
H6 YIN XI 陰郄 YIN Cleft	XI of Heart	nourish YIN, calm SHEN, consolidate exterior (BIAO), **disperse**
BL15 XIN SHU 心俞 Heart SHU	SHU of Heart, regulate Heart YANG	calm SHEN, clear heat from Heart, move Heart blood congestion, tonify YIN
BL18 GAN SHU 肝俞 Liver SHU	SHU of Liver, regulate Liver YANG	move Liver QI and Blood

2. Heart and Gallbladder QI *Deficiency*, XIN DAN QI XU
心膽氣虛 - fear and dread

Etiology	*Gallbladder* QI *deficiency* and *Liver* YANG *deficiency* prevent proper Heart nourishment
Signs	Inability to decide, shyness, inability to control fear, fear causes shortness of breath and weak voice, sensation of a foreign body or phlegm stuck in the throat (plum pit); confusion of Heart and of SHEN: palpitation with sweat, insomnia or many dreams, pale complexion
Tongue	pale with thin coating
Pulse	weak (RUO 弱), wiry (XUAN 弦) or sometimes slippery (HUA 滑)
Strategy	tonify and calm Gallbladder, calm SHEN, nourish Heart and Heart Blood
Points	BL19-GB35-LIV14 or GB24, H7-GV24, BL15-CV6

Acupuncture points to treat *Heart and Gallbladder* QI *Deficiency* - fear and dread

name	function	action
BL19-GB35-LIV14 or GB24 tonify and calm Gallbladder		
BL19 DAN SHU 膽俞 Gall bladder SHU	SHU of Gallbladder, regulate G.B. YANG	tonify and regulate G.B. QI, tonify deficiency, **needle in direction of QI flow**
GB35 YANG JIAO 陽交 Meeting of YANG	XI of YANG WEI MAI	regulate Gallbladder QI, treat 'trembling spirit', **tonify**
LIV14 QI MEN 期門 Cycle Gate	MU of Liver, regulate Liver YIN, meeting of Liv., Sp. Meridians and YIN WEI MAI	raise QI from abdomen to chest, benefit Gallbladder, calm agitation with arrhythmia, **tonify**
GB24 RI YUE 日月 Sun and Moon	MU of Gallbladder, nourish YIN of G.B.	move QI down, treat mental instability and inability to decide
H7-GV24, BL15-CV6 calm SHEN, nourish Heart and Heart Blood		
H7 SHEN MEN 神門 SHEN Gate	SHU-YUAN-Soil of Heart	calm SHEN, cool Heart, open Heart orifices
GV24 SHEN TING 神庭 SHEN Court	meeting of DU MAI with Bl. and St. Meridians	communicate between orifices, calm SHEN, regulate mental restlessness
BL15 XIN SHU 心俞 Heart SHU	SHU of Heart, regulate Heart YANG	calm SHEN, clear heat from Heart, tonify Heart YIN
CV6 QI HAI 氣海 Sea of QI	MU of QI	move QI and Blood

3. *Phlegm-Fire Harassing Heart* TAN HUO RAO XIN 痰火擾心 fear and dread

Compare joy and pleasure (page 237). When fear is a prominent sign, the treatment is: PC7-LI11-GB41, ST40-CV12

Acupuncture points to treat *Phlegm-Fire Harassing Heart*
fear and dread

name	function	action
ST40-CV12 dissolve phlegm		
CV12 ZHONG WAN 中脘 Central Venter	MU of Stomach, HUI-meeting of FU, 'knot' of TAI YIN, start of Lu. Meridian	dissolve phlegm, move stagnation, regulate Stomach
ST40 FENG LONG 豐隆 Bountiful Bulge	LUO of Stomach	dissolve *phlegm-fire* (heat), calm SHEN
PC7-LI11-GB41 clear Heart fire		
PC7 DA LING 大陵 Big Mound	SHU-YUAN-Soil of Master of Heart	calm and purify SHEN, cool Blood and Heart (palpitation), purify RONG QI
LI11 QU CHI 曲池 Pool at the Bend	HE-Soil of Large Intestine	regulate QI and Blood, dissipate heat from upper body, treat fear with memory loss
GB41 ZÚ LÍN QÌ 足臨泣 Bend to Cry of Foot	SHU-Wood of Gallbladder, regulate QI of G.B., open DAI MAI	open communication between upper and lower body

4. *Heart Fire Hyperactivity and Exuberance* XIN HUO KANG SHENG 心火亢盛 - fear and dread

Compare joy and pleasure. When fear is a prominent sign, the treatment is: SI7-H7 (LUO-YUAN), PC8, Ki4, K27

Acupuncture points to treat *Heart Fire Hyperactivity and Exuberance* - fear and dread

name	function	action
SI7-H7 regulate Heart fire, PC8 disperse Heart fire, Ki4, Ki27 disperse fire		
H7 SHEN MEN 神門 SHEN Gate	SHU-YUAN-Soil of Heart	calm SHEN, cool Heart, open Heart orifices
SI7 ZHI ZHENG 支正 Upright Branch	LUO of Small Intestine	clear heat, calm SHEN, release exterior
PC8 LAO GONG 勞宮 Labor Palace	RONG-Fire of Master of Heart	clear heat from JUE YIN, purify Heart, awaken SHEN, cool Blood, purify mouth
Ki4 DA ZHONG 大鍾 Big Bell	LUO of Kidney, enhance QI flow in meridians from Ki. towards M.H.(PC)	open Upper JIAO, treat fear
Ki27 SHU FU 俞府 SHU Mansion	meeting point of all SHU	unbind chest, treat insomnia, mouth inflammation/sores

5. *Blood deficiency and Liver* QI *Congested and Knotted* XUE
XU GAN QI YU JIE 血虛肝氣鬱結 - fear and dread

Etiology	*Congested Liver* QI causes *Liver Blood deficiency* preventing Heart nourishment. SHEN and HUN become agitated
Signs	easily startled, fear, restless, irritation, fullness in chest and hypochondrium especially during menstruation, irregular periods, headache, pale complexion, lips, nails
Tongue	pale with thin coating
Pulse	weak (RUO 弱), thin (XI 細)
Strategy	release and regulate Liver QI, nourish Blood, calm SHEN and HUN
Points	LIV3-LIV6-LIV14, BL17 - SP6 - BL20, PC7 / PC6, BL47

Acupuncture points to treat *Blood Deficiency and Liver* QI *Congested and Knotted* - fear and dread

name	function	action
LIV3-LIV6-LIV14 release and regulate Liver QI		
LIV3 TAI CHONG 太冲 Great Rush	SHU-YUAN-Soil of Liver	release and harmonize Liver
LIV6 ZHONG DU 中都 Capital Center	XI of Liver	sedate and regulate Liver, treat gynecological disorders
LIV14 QI MEN 期門 Cycle Gate	MU of Liver, regulate Liver YIN, meeting of Liv., Sp. Meridians and YIN WEI MAI	raise QI from abdomen to chest, benefit G.B., calm agitation with arrhythmia
BL17 – SP6 - BL20 nourish Blood		
BL17 GE SHU 膈俞 Diaphragm SHU	HUI-meeting of Blood, influence diaphragm	open chest, tonify and move blood
SP6 SAN YIN JIAO 三陰交 Meeting of Three YIN	meeting of Sp., Liv. and Ki. Meridians	tonify and nourish Blood, QI and YIN, move YIN up, nourish Spleen, stop diarrhea
BL20 PI SHU 脾俞 Spleen SHU	SHU of Spleen, regulate Spleen YANG	release Spleen
PC7 / PC6, BL47 calm SHEN and HUN		
PC7 DA LING 大陵 Big Mound	SHU-YUAN-Soil of Master of Heart	calm and purify SHEN, cool blood and Heart (palpitation), purify RONG QI
PC6 NEI GUAN 內關 Inner Barrier	LUO of Master of Heart, open YIN WEI MAI	release three YIN, open the chest, remove congestion between pelvis and chest, regulate QI, awaken SHEN
BL47 HUN MEN 魂門 HUN Gate	regulate HUN 魂, gather Liver JING	spread Liver QI, regulate Middle JIAO

8

Damage caused by six combinations of persistent emotions, LING SHU, Chapter 8-4

LING SHU, Chapter 8, presents two descriptions (referred to here as 8-3 and 8-4) of damage caused by six combinations of emotions/passions. LING SHU, Chapter 8-4, describes the following types of damage caused by persistent emotions:

A. Damage to Heart, SHEN 神 and flesh caused by apprehension, distress, obsessive thinking, worry (CHU TI SI LU 怵惕思慮), fear and dread (KONG JU 懼恐)
B. Damage to Spleen, YI 意 and limbs caused by sorrow and grief (BEI AI 悲哀)
C. Damage to Liver, HUN 魂 and JING 精 caused by melancholy and sadness (CHOU YOU 愁憂)
D. Damage to Lung, PO 魄 and sanity caused by excessive joy and pleasure (XI LE 喜樂)
E. Damage to Kidney, ZHI 志 and back caused by uncontrollable overflowing anger (SHENG NU 盛怒)
F. Damage to Kidney, JING 精 and bones caused by fear and dread (KONG JU 懼恐)

LING SHU, Chapter 8-4, presents for each of these six combinations of persistent emotions:
1. Damage caused to:
   - ZANG 臟 functions
   - BEN SHEN 本神 or JING 精 storage
   - Body tissues or body functions

2. Signs of premature death seen in QI and Blood deficiency:
   - since body hair is 'flowering'[315] of Lung QI, body hair falling out is a sign that Lung does not grasp QI from the air and JING QI 精氣 is deficient

---

315 Sign of good ZANG function

- since complexion is 'flowering' of Heart QI and Blood, a change in complexion is a sign that Heart-SHEN function is impaired
3. Forecast of the season of death. Body hair falling out and change of complexion are the signs of serious damage to Lung and Heart, to QI and Blood, and therefore to SHEN 神. Thus the patient cannot be treated and will die during the season which brings the QI that worsens the situation.

SU WEN, Chapter 26, emphasizes the importance of the abundance of Blood and QI for nourishing SHEN 神, which is essential for a cure and the preservation of life:

> *For nourishing SHEN 神, one must know whether the physical appearance is fat or lean, whether Nourishing QI (RONG 榮), Defensive QI (WEI 衛), Blood and QI abound or are weak. Blood and QI are SHEN 神 of man; it is impossible to nourish (SHEN) without paying attention (to Blood and QI).*
>
> 故養神者, 必知形之肥瘦, 榮衛血氣之盛衰, 血氣者人之神, 不可不謹養

A. Damage to Heart, SHEN 神 and flesh caused by apprehension, distress, obsessive thinking and worry
(CHU TI SI LU 怵惕思慮), LING SHU, Chapter 8-4

心	XIN heart	神	SHEN	破	PO ruin	毛	MAO hair
怵	CHU apprehension	傷	SHANG injure	䐃	JUN fat	悴	CUI fall
惕	TI distress	則	ZE this	脫	TOU remove	色	SE color
思	SI thinking	恐	KONG fear	肉	ROU flesh	夭	YAO death
慮	LU worry	懼	JU dread			死	SI death
則	ZE this	自	ZI oneself			於	YU in
傷	SHANG injure	失	SHI loss			冬	DONG winter
神	SHEN						

When apprehension, distress, obsessive thinking and worry (CHU TI SI LU 怵惕思慮) invade Heart, SHEN 神 is injured.
The injury to SHEN 神 is expressed as fear and dread (KONG JU 懼恐) and loss of self (ZI SHI 自失).
The flesh is diminished and the body grows thinner. Body hair breaks off; the complexion shows signs of premature death. Death will come in winter.

❖ LING SHU, Chapter 8-4: *apprehension, distress, obsessive thinking, worry* (CHU TI SI LU 怵惕思慮) *injure* SHEN 神. *The injury to* SHEN 神 *is expressed as fear and dread* (KONG JU 懼恐) *and loss of self* (ZI SHI 自失).

LING SHU, 8-4 (as well as 8-3)[316] describes damage caused to SHEN 神 by four emotions (arranged in two pairs) causing two additional harmful emotions:

1. Apprehension and distress (CHU TI 怵惕) injure ZHI 志 (Water of SHEN 神), Kidney and JING 精 storage
2. Obsessive thinking and worry (SI LU 思慮) injure YI 意 (Soil of SHEN 神), Spleen, ability to absorb Nourishing QI, flavors and liquids and build muscle and fat tissues
3. Fear and dread (KONG JU 懼恐) resulting from the above four emotions cause additional injury to ZHI 志 (Water of SHEN 神) and Kidney, causing the loss of self.

Apprehension, distress, obsessive thinking and worry disturb the central axis of the TAI JI symbol - Fire-Soil-Water (SHEN-YI-ZHI). Heart-SHEN is injured following damage to ZHI 志 (Water does not control Fire), and also obstructed following damage to YI 意 (reversed generation). *Loss of self* (ZI SHI 自失) is the loss of this central axis, and may be described as a loss of the subtle process of SHEN (SHEN JI 神機). SU WEN, Chapter 15, describes the loss of the subtle process of SHEN (SHEN JI 神機):

道	DAO		回	HUI	return
在	ZAI	hold	則	ZE	this
於	YU	in	不	BU	not
一	YI	one	轉	ZHUAN	circulate
神	SHEN		乃	NAI	then
轉	ZHUAN	circulate	失	SHI	lost
不	BU	not	其	QI	its
回	HUI	return	機	JI	subtle process

DAO 道 *is One* (oneness). SHEN 神 *flows and does not return. If* (SHEN 神) *returns there is no flow and* (SHEN 神) *loses its subtle process* (JI 機).

---

316 See page 216

❖ LING SHU, Chapter 8-4, apprehension, distress, obsessive thinking and worry: *The flesh is diminished and the body grows thinner. Body hair breaks off; the complexion shows signs of premature death. Death will come in winter.*

Loss of the subtle process of SHEN 神 is also loss of the body - the palace of SHEN. Spleen is injured by obsessive thinking and worry, and therefore does not build muscle and fat tissue, causing weight loss. Injured Spleen does not nourish Lung-body hair. Body hair loss is a sign of severe damage to QI absorption from the air. Change of complexion is another sign of serious injury to SHEN and of premature death.

The patient dies in the winter, when Water is in excess and Fire-Heart deficient. Heart, injured by apprehension, distress, obsessive thinking and worry, fear and dread, cannot function in the winter and the patient dies.

Syndromes in Chinese medicine which describe the damage to Heart, SHEN and flesh caused by apprehension, distress, obsessive thinking and worry

1. *Heart and Spleen Dual Deficiency* XIN PI LIANG XU 心脾兩虛[317]	BL20-SP6-BL15, H7-GV24-SP8
2. *Phlegm-dampness and QI Deficiency* TAN SHI QI XU 痰濕氣虛	BL20-BL21, SP9-CV12, ST36-ST40, SI19, GB37, PC7-H5-GV20
3. *No Interaction between Heart and Kidney* XIN SHEN BU JIAO 心腎不交[318]	BL23-Ki3-Ki10, BL15-Ki1, PC7-H6

1. *Heart and Spleen Dual Deficiency*, XIN PI LIANG XU 心脾兩虛 - apprehension, distress, obsessive thinking and worry

Compare melancholy and sadness (LING SHU, Chapter 8-3). When apprehension, distress, obsessive thinking and worry cause the syndrome, acupuncture points to tonify Spleen and Heart and to calm thoughts are: BL20-SP6-BL15, H7-GV24-SP8

---

317 See page 244 in melancholy and sadness, LING SHU, 8-3
318 See pages 236, 251 in joy and pleasure and in melancholy and sadness, LING SHU, 8-3

Acupuncture points to treat *Heart and Spleen Dual Deficiency* - apprehension, distress, obsessive thinking and worry

name	function	action
BL20-SP6-BL15, H7-GV24-SP8 tonify Spleen and Heart and calm thoughts		
BL20 PI SHU 脾俞 Spleen SHU	SHU of Spleen, regulate Spleen YANG	tonify Spleen, **tonify**
SP6 SAN YIN JIAO 三陰交 Meeting of Three YIN	meeting of Sp., Liv., and Ki. Meridians	tonify and nourish Blood, QI and YIN, move YIN up, nourish Spleen, stop diarrhea, **tonify**
BL15 XIN SHU 心俞 Heart SHU	SHU of Heart, regulate Heart YANG, release LUO of Heart	calm SHEN, tonify Heart YIN, **tonify**
H7 SHEN MEN 神門 SHEN Gate	SHU-YUAN-Soil of Heart	calm SHEN, cool Heart, open Heart orifices
SP8 DI JI 地機 Earth's Process	XI of Spleen, restore communication with Soil	remove obstructions in Spleen Meridian, calm thoughts
GV24 SHEN TING 神庭 SHEN Court	meeting of DU MAI with Bl. and St. Meridians	communicate between orifices, calm SHEN, regulate mental agitation and obsessions

2. *Phlegm-dampness and QI Deficiency,* TAN SHI QI XU 痰濕氣虛 - apprehension, distress, obsessive thinking and worry

Etiology	obsessive thinking and worry injure Spleen QI, apprehension and distress injure Kidney QI. Spleen and Kidney injury disturbs body liquids causing phlegm-dampness obstructing Heart orifices.
Signs	apathy, lack of concentration, sadness, fatigue, feeling of failure, unfocused eyes, recluse, insomnia, lack of appetite, depression with visual and auditory hallucinations, incoherent speech, anger, fear and laughter
Tongue	thick, swollen with teeth marks
Pulse	thin (XI 細), slippery (HUA 滑), slow (CHI 遲)
Strategy	tonify Spleen and Stomach, move dampness, disperse phlegm, open Heart orifices, treat hallucinations
Points	BL20-BL21, SP9-CV12, ST36-ST40, SI19, GB37, PC7-H5-GV20

Acupuncture points to treat *Phlegm-dampness and Qi Deficiency* - apprehension, distress, obsessive thinking and worry

name	function	action
BL20-BL21, SP9-CV12, ST36-ST40 tonify Spleen and Stomach, move dampness, disperse phlegm		
BL21 WEI SHU 胃俞 Stomach SHU	SHU of Stomach, regulate Stomach YANG	tonify Stomach, move dampness, disperse phlegm
BL20 PI SHU 脾俞 Spleen SHU	SHU of Spleen, regulate Spleen YANG	tonify Spleen, move dampness, disperse phlegm
CV12 ZHONG WAN 中脘 Central Venter	MU of Stomach, HUI-meeting of FU, 'knot' of TAI YIN, start of Lu. Meridian	move stagnations, regulate Stomach
SP9 YIN LING QUAN 陰陵泉 YIN Mound Spring	HE-Water of Spleen	tonify Spleen YANG, treat constrained dampness and cold mucus (TAN YIN) which cause palpitation, abdominal pain and stomach rumble
ST40 FENG LONG 豐隆 Bountiful Bulge	LUO of Stomach	dissolve *phlegm-fire*/heat, calm SHEN, treat hallucinations
ST36 ZU SAN LI 足三里 Leg Three Miles	HE-Soil of Stomach, tonify QI, Sea of Food point, potentiate other points	regulate YANG deficiency above and YIN excess below: treat long lasting melancholy, mental fatigue, hallucinations
PC7-H5-GV20 open Heart orifices, SI19 treat visual hallucinations, GB37 treat auditory hallucinations		
PC7 DA LING 大陵 Big Mound	SHU-YUAN-Soil of Master of Heart	calm and purify SHEN, cool Heart palpitation, cool blood
H5 TONG LI 通里 Penetrating the Interior	LUO of Heart	purify Heart, calm SHEN, release QI congestion in throat
GV20 BAI HUI 百會 Hundred Meetings	meeting of DU MAI with six YANG Meridians	move YANG down through QI flow of DU MAI, purify head and brain, treat restlessness with heavy head, release obsessions and wrong ideas
GB37 GUANG MING 光明 Bright Light	LUO of Gallbladder	treat visual hallucinations
SI19 TING GONG 聽宮 Auditory Palace	exit point, meeting of S.I., SAN JIAO and G.B. Meridians	treat auditory hallucinations

3. *No Interaction between Heart and Kidney* XIN SHEN BU JIAO

心肾不交 - apprehension, distress, obsessive thinking and worry
Compare joy and pleasure and Lily Bulb Disease in melancholy and sadness (LING SHU, 8-3), but here acupuncture points to tonify Kidney and Heart are: BL23-Ki3-Ki10, BL15-Ki1, PC7-H6

Acupuncture points to treat *No Interaction between Heart and Kidney* - apprehension, distress, obsessive thinking and worry

name	function	action
BL23-Ki3-Ki10 tonify Kidney and Heart		
BL23 SHEN SHU 肾俞 Kidney SHU	SHU of Kidney, regulate Ki. YANG	tonify Kidney YIN, **tonify**
Ki3 TAI XI 太谿 Great Ravine	SHU-YUAN-Soil of Kidney	tonify Kidney YIN, release ascent of CHONG MAI and REN MAI, treat degenerative diseases, **tonify**
Ki10 YIN GU 陰谷 YIN Valley	HE-Water of Kidney	tonify Kidney YIN, **tonify**
BL15-Ki1, PC7-H6 regulate SHAO YIN (Kidney-Heart)		
BL15 XIN SHU 心俞 Heart SHU	SHU of Heart, regulate Heart YANG, release Heart LUO	calm SHEN, move congestion of Heart Blood, clear Heart heat, tonify Heart YIN
Ki1 YONG QUAN 湧泉 Gushing Spring	JING-Well-Wood of Kidney, root of SHAO YIN	move rebel QI and YANG down, open Heart orifices, awaken SHEN, **massage**
PC7 DA LING 大陵 Big Mound	SHU-YUAN-Soil of Master of Heart	calm and purify SHEN, cool blood and Heart palpitation, purify RONG QI
H6 YIN XI 陰郄 YIN Cleft	XI of Heart	nourish YIN, calm SHEN

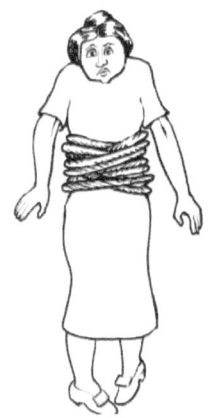

B. Damage to Spleen, YI 意 and limbs caused by melancholy and sadness (CHOU YOU 愁憂), LING SHU, Chapter 8-4

脾	PI	spleen	意	YI		四	SI	4	毛	MAO	hair
愁	CHOU	melancholy	傷	SHANG	injure	肢	ZHI	limbs	悴	CUI	fall
憂	YOU	sadness	則	ZE	this	不	BU	not	色	SE	color
而	ER	and	悗	MEN	oppression	舉	JU	lift	夭	YAO	death
不	BU	not	亂	LUAN	disorder				死	SI	death
解	JIE	release							於	YU	in
則	ZE	this							春	CHUN	spring
傷	SHANG	injure									
意	YI										

When melancholy and sadness (CHOU YOU 愁憂) without release invade Spleen, YI 意 is injured.
Injury to YI 意 causes stress and confusion (MEN LUAN 悗亂).
The four limbs do not rise.
Body hair breaks off; the complexion shows signs of premature death.
Death will come in spring.

❖ LING SHU, Chapter 8-4: *When melancholy and sadness (CHOU YOU 愁憂) without release invade Spleen, YI 憂 is injured.*

Melancholy and sadness close and obstruct QI and QI does not circulate (LING SHU, Chapter 8-3).[319] The character CHOU 愁 conveys the meaning 'autumn Heart' expressed as chronic, obsessive (*without release*) or frequent melancholy - an emotion of Lung. The character YOU 憂 conveys the meaning 'pressure on Heart'; sadness. YOU 憂 is an emotion of Lung and also of Spleen. Melancholy and sadness influence Heart and Liver,[320] impair QI circulation and damage the functioning of both Spleen and Lung. Chronic melancholy and sadness invade Spleen, become obsessive and block and knot (JIE 結) the Spleen function of transporting and transforming Nourishing QI, flavors and body liquids. Spleen dysfunction causes injury to YI 憂 (BEN SHEN of Spleen).

---

319 See page 238
320 See page 52 for the characters CHOU YOU 愁憂

❖ LING SHU, Chapter 8-4: melancholy and sadness: *Injury to YI* 意 *causes stress and confusion* (MEN LUAN 悗亂).

On the vertical central axis of the TAI JI symbol, Soil-Spleen is an intermediary between the opposites Water and Fire. Injury to Spleen-YI 意 causes confusion (LUAN 亂) in the communication between Water-Kidney-ZHI 志 and Fire-Heart-SHEN 神. Injury to Spleen-YI 意 causes confusion (LUAN 亂) in the thoughts and intent of SHEN 神 that results in changes in the mind: self-image and the image of the environment, memories, verbal expression and knowledge. The character LUAN 亂 is also used in SU WEN, Chapter 39, to describe the injury caused by panic.[321] Injury to Y' 意 also results in stress (MEN 悗). The character MEN 悗 shows the radical 心/忄 'heart' and the phonetic 免 'rabbit' and conveys the meaning 'the heart that beats like a running rabbit'. MEN 悗 is translated as 'stress' or 'a feeling of oppression', which causes contraction of the diaphragm and discomfort in the chest.

❖ LING SHU, Chapter 8-4, melancholy and sadness: *Four limbs do not rise.*

Spleen is responsible for the nourishment of the four limbs. Melancholy and sadness disturb Spleen function (transformation and transportation of Nourishing QI, flavors and body liquids) and therefore the limbs are not properly nourished and body movement is impaired. Injury to YI 意 provokes a change in body image and there is no desire, coordination or strength to move the body.

❖ LING SHU, Chapter 8-4: *Body hair breaks off; the complexion shows signs of premature death. Death will come in spring.*

Melancholy and sadness injure both Spleen and Lung. In addition, a weak Spleen cannot nourish Lung. Lung exhaustion causes body hair to fall out. Weak Spleen cannot absorb Nourishing QI, causing Blood deficiency. Heart is not properly nourished by Blood and the complexion changes. In spring, nature renews itself and strong Wood-Liver over-controls weak Spleen. Spleen stops functioning, and the patient dies.

---

321 See page 200

Syndromes in Chinese medicine which describe the injury to Spleen and YI 憂 caused by melancholy and sadness

Spleen absorbs Nourishing QI and body liquids from food and beverages which enter Stomach. Nourishing QI raises body liquids (nourishing moisture) from Middle JIAO to Upper JIAO. The weakness of Spleen in melancholy and sadness interferes with the absorption and/or flow of Nourishing QI and body liquids. Lung, injured by melancholy and sadness, does not move body liquids down to Kidney and Bladder. The flow of body liquids is disturbed and they stagnate.

Figure 52. Development of melancholy and sadness (CHOU YOU 愁憂) **into depression** (DIAN 癲)

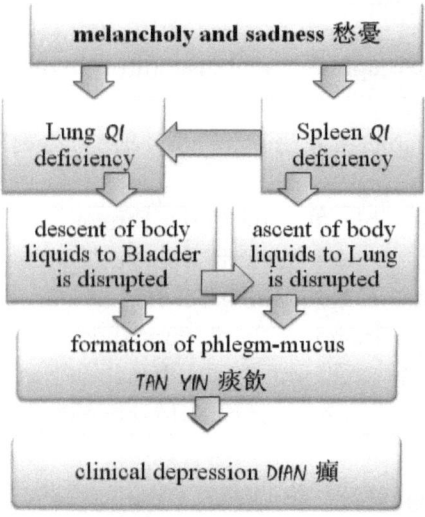

- Stagnant body liquids form TAN YIN 痰飲 (*phlegm-mucus* of cold origin, white mucus discharge) (see Figure 52). The character TAN 痰, shows the radical 疒 'disease' with 炎 'double fire' inside.[322] The character YIN 飲 is translated as 'beverage' or in Chinese medicine as 'watery discharge'. TAN YIN obstructs and slows down body functions, causing 'cold-deficiency' of Spleen-YI 憂 and Heart-SHEN 神. Stress and confusion may result from phlegm-mucus accumulation.

---

[322] http://zhongwen.com/d/183/x240.htm

- Melancholy and sadness impair Spleen function (transportation and transformation) and also Liver function (smooth flow of QI). Liver QI congests and transforms into *Liver fire* (excess heat):

  - *Liver fire* combined with the overeating of spicy and 'hot' food causes stagnant body liquids to form phlegm-fire (TAN HUO 痰火)
  - *Liver fire* which dries stagnant body liquids causes YIN *deficiency of Heart, Liver and Spleen.*

Injury to Spleen and YI 憂 by melancholy and sadness may be classified in Chinese medicine as:

1. Constrained QI syndrome (YU ZHENG 鬱證)[323] expressed as depression.

Of the six types of YU 鬱,[324] four (QI, Blood, phlegm and fire) describe situations of damage to Spleen and YI 憂 from melancholy and sadness. Melancholy and sadness disturb the function of Spleen, Heart and Liver, constrain QI (YU 鬱) and may provoke depression. YU ZHENG 鬱證 has different clinical expressions but usually includes: sadness, anxiety, emotional instability, feeling of pressure and congestion in the chest and stomach, mood swings and insomnia.

2. Clinical depression (DIAN 癲)[325]

DIAN 癲 is 'quiet' introverted YIN 'madness' which may develop into clinical depression (Figure 52). Melancholy and sadness cause Spleen and Lung QI deficiency, and phlegm-mucus of cold origin. TAN YIN 痰飲 disturb the function of the central nervous system, causing clinical depression (DIAN 癲).

According to NAN JING, difficulty 59: *At the onset of* DIAN 癲 *disease, intent is joyless* (YI BU LE 意不樂). *(The patient) is lying on his back gazing straight.*[326] Being unhappy and *gazing straight* corresponds to melancholy and sadness. *Lying on the back* may correspond to the inability to move the four limbs.

---

323 See page 211 YU ZHENG in SU WEN, 39, and page 241 LING SHU, 8-3
324 See page 211
325 See Chapter 9, page 252, for DIAN 癲 in LING SHU, Chapter 22, DIAN KUANG
326 See Chapter 9, page 361

Constrained QI syndrome (YU ZHENG 鬱證) expressed as depression, which describes injury to Spleen and YI 意 caused by melancholy and sadness

Four out of six types of YU 鬱 (QI, Blood, phlegm and fire) correspond to damage to Spleen and YI 意 by melancholy and sadness. The syndromes in Chinese medicine which describe each YU ZHENG 鬱證 are:

YU 鬱, constrained QI[327]	
a. *Liver QI Congested and Knotted* GAN QI YU JIE 肝氣鬱結[328]	LIV3-LIV6, H7-PC5, LIV14, LIV2-GV20
b. *Congested QI Transforms into Fire* QI YU HUA HUO 氣鬱化火[329]	LIV3-LIV2-GB43-LIV14, PC7-H5, GV14
YU 鬱 caused by constrained QI and phlegm	
c. *Phlegm and QI Congested and Knotted* TAN QI YU JIE 痰氣鬱結	LIV3-PC5, ST36-ST40-CV12, H6-CV23
YU 鬱 - heat causes Liver, Heart and Spleen YIN deficiency	
d. *Loss and Deficiency of Heart YIN* XIN YIN KUI XU 心陰虧虛	H3-CV14, BL15-H7, SI8, GV24
e. *Loss and Deficiency of Liver YIN* GAN YIN KUI XU 肝陰虧虛[330]	LIV3-LIV8-BL47-GB34
YU 鬱 of Blood	
f. *Blood Flow Congested and Obstructed* XUE XING YU ZHI 血行鬱滯	SP10-CV4-SP6-BL17, LI4-LIV13-CV12
g. *Heart and Spleen Dual Deficiency* XIN PI LIANG XU 心脾兩虛[331]	BL15-BL20,SP3-SP8-CV12,CV14-H5,GB13-GV24
h. *Confusion of Heart and of SHEN* XIN PI LIANG XU 心神惑亂[332]	SP6-Ki7-BL44-BL52,PC5, GV22

---

327 See page 211 SU WEN, 39
328 See page 261, LING SHU, 8-3 and pages 261,311,315,316,331. LING SHU, 8-4
329 See page 261, LING SHU, 8-3
330 See page 264 overflowing anger, and LING SHU, 8-3
331 See pages 244, 296, 313, 334 in LING SHU, 8-3 and in LING SHU, 8-4
332 See page 265, melancholy and sadness, LING SHU, 8-3

a. *Liver QI Congested and Knotted*, GAN QI YU JIE 肝氣鬱結
YU ZHENG 鬱證, melancholy and sadness

Compare overflowing anger (LING SHU, Chapter 8-3).
When chronic melancholy and sadness and YU ZHENG are expressed by this syndrome, the patient has no desire to live and in severe cases has suicidal thoughts and a tendency to self-mutilation.

Acupuncture points to release Liver QI and blood flow are LIV3-LIV6, H7-PC5, LIV14, LIV2-GV20.

Acupuncture points to treat *Liver QI Congested and Knotted*
YU ZHENG, melancholy and sadness

name	function	action
LIV3-LIV6, H7-PC5, LIV14 release Liver QI, release QI and blood flow		
LIV3 TAI CHONG 太沖 Great Rush	SHU-YUAN-Soil of Liver	release and harmonize Liver
LIV6 ZHONG DU 中都 Capital Center	XI of Liver	sedate and regulate Liver, treat gynecological disorders
H7 SHEN MEN 神門 SHEN Gate	SHU-YUAN-Soil of Heart	calm SHEN, cool Heart (insomnia, stress, memory loss), open Heart orifices
PC5 JIAN SHI 間使 Interval Envoy	JING-River-Metal of Master of Heart (JUE YIN), Group LUO of three arm YIN	regulate YIN deficiency above and YIN stagnation below, open chest, calm SHEN, calm SHAO YANG, calm suffering and stop the crying
LIV14 QI MEN 期門 Cycle Gate	MU of Liver, regulate Liver YIN, meeting of Liv., Sp. Meridians and YIN WEI MAI	raise QI from abdomen to chest, invigorate blood, benefit Gall-bladder, regulate QI, dissolve masses
LIV2-GV20 treat suicidal tendency		
LIV2 XING JIAN 行間 Moving Between	RONG-Fire of Liver	move YANG down, benefit Gall-bladder, calm anger
GV20 BAI HUI 百會 Hundred Meetings	meeting of DU MAI with six YANG Meridians	move YANG down through DU MAI, purify head and brain, treat restlessness with heavy head

b. *Congested QI Transforms into Fire,* QI YU HUA HUO 氣鬱化火 - YU ZHENG 鬱證, melancholy and sadness

Compare overflowing anger (LING SHU, Chapter 8-3).
When chronic melancholy and sadness develop into YU ZHENG, and cause this syndrome, acupuncture points to release *Liver fire/*YANG and to tonify YIN of chest and head are LIV3-LIV2-GB43-LIV14, PC7-H5, GV1

Acupuncture points to treat *Congested* QI *Transforms into Fire* - YU ZHENG, melancholy and sadness

name	function	action
LIV3-LIV2-GB43-LIV14 release *Liver fire/*YANG		
LIV3 TAI CHONG 太冲 Great Rush	SHU-YUAN-Soil of Liver	release and harmonize Liver, treat suicidal thoughts
LIV2 XING JIAN 行間 Moving Between	RONG-Fire of Liver	move YANG down, benefit Gall-bladder, calm anger
GB43 XIA XI 俠谿 Pinched Ravine	RONG-Water of Gall-bladder, tonify Wood	purify head, ears and eyes, return order and mental uprightness
LIV14 QI MEN 期門 Cycle Gate	MU of Liver, regulate Liver YIN, meeting of Liv., Sp. Meridians and YIN WEI MAI	raise QI from abdomen to chest, invigorate Blood, benefit Gall-bladder, regulate QI
PC7-H5, tonify YIN of chest and head, GV14 release heat from head		
PC7 DA LING 大陵 Big Mound	SHU-YUAN-Soil of Master of Heart	calm and purify SHEN, cool Heart palpitation, cool blood, purify RONG QI
H5 TONG LI 通里 Penetrating the Interior	LUO of Heart	purify Heart, calm SHEN, release Heart from mourning, *despair crisis* (S. de Morand)
GV14 DA ZHUI 大椎 Big Mallet	meeting of the DU MAI with the six YANG Meridians	regulate QI and YANG flow to head and Heart, release excess heat and damp-heat from upper body

c. *Phlegm and QI Congested and Knotted,* TAN QI YU JIE, 痰氣鬱結 - YU ZHENG 鬱證, melancholy and sadness

Etiology	*Congested Liver* YIN QI causes a release of *Liver* YANG, which obstructs Spleen, body liquids and causes *phlegm-heat* injuring SHEN
Signs	depression, a sense of failure, sighs, feeling of fullness and pressure in chest, abdominal bloating, especially in hypochondria, sensation of a foreign body (plum pit) in throat
Tongue	thick white greasy coating
Pulse	wiry (XUAN 弦), slippery (HUA 滑)
Strategy	regulate Liver and JUE YIN, regulate Spleen, dissolve phlegm, calm SHEN, release QI obstruction in throat
Points	LIV3-PC5, ST36-ST40-CV12, H6-CV23

Acupuncture points to treat *Phlegm and QI Congested and Knotted* - YU ZHENG, melancholy and sadness

name	function	action
LIV3-PC5 regulate Liver and JUE YIN		
LIV3 TAI CHONG 太冲 Great Rush	SHU-YUAN-Soil of Liver	release and harmonize Liver
PC5 JIAN SHI 間使 Interval Envoy	JING-River-Metal of Master of Heart (JUE YIN), Group LUO of 3 arm YIN	regulate YIN deficiency above and YIN stagnation below, calm SHAO YANG, open chest, calm SHEN
ST36-ST40-CV12 dissolve phlegm		
CV12 ZHONG WAN 中脘 Central Venter	MU of Stomach, HUI-meeting of FU, 'knot' of TAI YIN, start of Lu. Meridian	dissolve phlegm, move stagnations, regulate Stomach
ST40 FENG LONG 豐隆 Bountiful Bulge	LUO of Stomach	dissolve phlegm-fire (heat), calm SHEN
ST36 ZU SAN LI 足三里 Leg Three Miles	HE-Soil of Stomach, tonify QI, Sea of Food point	regulate YANG deficiency above and YIN excess below, long lasting melancholy, mental fatigue
H6-CV23 release QI obstruction in throat		
H6 YIN XI 陰郄 YIN Cleft	XI of Heart	nourish YIN, calm SHEN, release QI obstruction in throat
CV23 LIAN QUAN 廉泉 Ridge Spring	'knot' of SHAO YIN, meeting of REN MAI with YIN WEI MAI	dissolve phlegm, obstructions and swellings in throat, release ascent of body liquids

d. *Loss and Deficiency of Heart* YIN, XIN YIN KUI XU 心陰虧虛 YU ZHENG, melancholy and sadness

Etiology	melancholy, sadness, frustrations injure Heart QI. *Heart QI deficiency* combined with fatigue, chronic illness, weak constitution or old age causes *Heart Blood deficiency* which develops into *Heart YIN Deficiency* and *Empty Fire Rising*
Signs	anxiety and suffering, unstable personality, quick and irrelevant speech, palpitation, loss of memory and concentration, hot flashes with night sweat, dry mouth and throat, sore tongue, insomnia or light sleep with restless dream, heat in 'five palms', small quantity of reddish urine
Tongue	red, dry, especially at the tip
Pulse	fast (SHU 數), thin (XI 細)
Strategy	tonify Heart YIN
Points	H3-CV14, BL15-H7, SI8, GV24

Acupuncture points to treat *Loss and Deficiency of Heart* YIN YU ZHENG, melancholy and sadness

name	function	action
H3-CV14, BL15-H7, SI8, GV24 tonify Heart YIN		
H3 SHAO HAI 少海 Small Sea	HE-Water of Heart	tonify Heart YIN, tonify JING, treat mouth ulcers
CV14 JU QUE 巨闕 Great Tower Gate	MU of Heart, regulate Heart YIN	calm SHEN and Heart, open chest, move *turbid QI* down
BL15 XIN SHU 心俞 Heart SHU	SHU of Heart, regulate Heart YANG, release LUO of Heart	calm SHEN, tonify Heart YIN
H7 SHEN MEN 神門 SHEN Gate	SHU-YUAN-Soil of Heart	calm SHEN, cool Heart, open Heart orifices
GV24 SHEN TING 神庭 SHEN Court	meeting of DU MAI with Bl. and St. Meridians	communicate between orifices, calm SHEN, regulate mental restlessness
SI8 XIAO HAI 小海 Small Sea	HE-Soil of Small Intestine, sedate Fire	clear Heart heat, treat mouth ulcers

e. *Loss and Deficiency of Liver* YIN, GAN YIN KUI XU 肝陰虧虛 YU ZHENG, melancholy and sadness

Compare overflowing anger (LING SHU, Chapter 8-3). When chronic melancholy and sadness heat the center, dry the body liquids and cause *Liver YIN deficiency*, acupuncture points to tonify Liver YIN are LIV3-LIV8-BL47-GB34.

Acupuncture points to treat *Loss and Deficiency of Liver* YIN
melancholy and sadness

name	function	action
LIV3-LIV8-BL47-GB34 tonify Liver YIN		
LIV3 TAI CHONG 太冲 Great Rush	SHU-YUAN-Soil of Liver	release and harmonize Liver
LIV8 QU QUAN 曲泉 Spring at the bend	HE-Water of Liver, tonify Wood	tonify Liver YIN (especially in Kidney YIN deficiency), nourish Liver Blood, clear excess heat, regulate Lower JIAO
BL47 HUN MEN 魂門 HUN Gate	regulate HUN 魂, gather Liver JING	spread Liver QI, regulate Middle JIAO
GB34 YANG LING QUAN 陽陵泉 YANG Mound Spring	HE-Soil of Gallbladder, HUI-meeting of muscles-tendons	tonify muscles and tendons

f. *Blood Flow Congested and Obstructed* XUE XING YU ZHI
血行鬱滯 - YU ZHENG 鬱證, melancholy and sadness

Etiology	*Congested Liver QI* provokes the release of heat obstructing the blood flow, and causes blood congestion
Signs	emotional instability, irritability, feeling of failure, confusion, talking to oneself, confused speech, reluctance to talk or non-stop talking, continuous cursing, visual or auditory hallucinations, pulsating headache, insomnia, memory loss, pressure or pain in chest, abdomen and pelvis worse when pressure applied, dark complexion with prominent blood vessels, red spots, beauty spots, benign tumors of blood vessels
Tongue	dark purple or dark red with purple spots, white coating
Pulse	sinking (CHEN 沉), full (SHI 實) with force (YOU LI 有力), or choppy (SE 澀) or wiry (XUAN 弦)
Strategy	tonify Blood flow and QI
Points	SP10-CV4-SP6-BL17, LI4-LIV13-CV12

Acupuncture points to treat *Blood Flow Congested and Obstructed* - YU ZHENG, melancholy and sadness

name	function	action
SP10-CV4-SP6-BL17 tonify Blood flow		
SP6 SAN YIN JIAO 三陰交 Meeting of Three YIN	meeting of Sp., Liv., and Ki. Meridians	tonify and nourish Blood, QI and YIN, move YIN up, nourish Spleen
BL17 GE SHU 膈俞 Diaphragm SHU	HUI-meeting of Blood, influence diaphragm	open the chest, tonify and move blood
CV4 GUAN YUAN 關元 Origin Pass	Sea of Blood, MU of Small Intestine, meeting of REN MAI with CHONG MAI and Sp., Liv. and Ki. Meridians	warm and tonify Kidney, nourish Blood and JING, assist ascent of CHONG MAI and REN MAI
SP10 XUE HAI 血海 Sea of Blood		invigorate and cool blood
LI4-LIV13-CV12 tonify Blood flow and QI		
LI4 HE GU 合谷 Union Valley	YUAN of Large Intestine, entry point, command of face and mouth	regulate QI, release excess YANG from head
LIV13 ZHANG MEN 章門 Chapter Gate	MU of Spleen, HUI- meeting of five ZANG, meeting of Liv., Ki., H., Sp., Lu., G.B. Meridians	treat Upper JIAO obstruction and rebel QI obstructing WEI QI (LING SHU, 59)
CV12 ZHONG WAN 中脘 Central Venter	MU of Stomach, HUI-meeting of FU, 'knot' of TAI YIN, start of Lu. Meridian	dissolve phlegm, move stagnation, regulate Stomach

g. *Heart and Spleen Dual Deficiency* XIN PI LIANG XU 心脾兩虛 YU ZHENG, melancholy and sadness

Compare melancholy and sadness (LING SHU, 8-3), apprehension, distress, obsessive thinking and worry (LING SHU, 8-4).

When melancholy and sadness cause this syndrome, injury to YI 意 is expressed as obsessive-compulsive disorder: obsessive thoughts on the subject of suffering, compulsive habits, lack of imagination, memory loss, difficulty in concentration, impulsive and sometimes aggressive behavior. Acupuncture points to tonify Spleen and Heart and to calm thoughts are: BL15-BL20, SP3-SP8-CV12, CV14-H5, GB13-GV24.

Acupuncture points to treat *Heart and Spleen Dual Deficiency* - melancholy and sadness

name	function	action
BL15-BL20, SP3-SP8-CV12 ,CV14-H5 tonify Spleen and Heart and calm thoughts		
BL20 PI SHU 脾俞 Spleen SHU	SHU of Spleen, regulate Spleen YANG	tonify Spleen
BL15 XIN SHU 心俞 Heart SHU	SHU of Heart, regulate Heart YANG, release LUO of Heart	calm SHEN, tonify Heart YIN
H7 SHEN MEN 神門 SHEN Gate	SHU-YUAN-Soil of Heart	calm SHEN, cool Heart, open Heart orifices
SP8 DI JI 地機 Earth's Mechanism	XI of Spleen, communicate with Soil	remove obstructions in Sp. Meridian, calm thoughts
SP3 TAI BAI 太白 Supreme White	SHU-YUAN-Soil of Spleen	regulate Spleen and Stomach
CV12 ZHONG WAN 中脘 Central Venter	MU of Stomach, HUI-meeting of FU, 'knot' of TAI YIN, start of Lu. Meridian	dissolve phlegm, move stagnations, regulate Stomach
H5 TONG LI 通里 Penetrating the Interior	LUO of Heart	purify Heart, calm SHEN
CV14 JU QUE 巨闕 Great Tower Gate	MU of Heart, regulate Heart YIN	calm SHEN and Heart, dissolve phlegm, open chest, move *turbid* QI down
GB13-GV24 treat obsession		
GB13 BEN SHEN 本神 Root of SHEN	meeting of G.B. Meridian with YANG WEI MAI	treat obsession
GV24 SHEN TING 神庭 SHEN Court	meeting of DU MAI with Bl. and St. Meridians	calm SHEN, communicate between orifices, regulate mental agitation and obsession

h. *Confusion of Heart and of* SHEN, XIN SHEN HUO LUAN 心神惑亂 - YU ZHENG, melancholy and sadness

In melancholy and sadness, *Liver QI congestion* causes *Heart QI and Blood deficiency*, and injures SHEN 神 and JING 精. Compare overflowing anger (LING SHU, Chapter 8-3) for description and acupuncture points (which are the same): SP6-Ki7-BL44-BL52, PC5, GV22.

C. Damage to Liver, HUN 魂 and JING 精 caused by sorrow and grief (BEI AI 悲哀), LING SHU, Chapter 8-4

肝	GAN liver	魂	HUN	當	DANG at time	毛	MAO hair
悲	BEI sorrow	傷	SHANG injure	人	REN man	悴	CUI fall
哀	AI grief	則	ZE this	陰	YIN	色	SE color
動	DONG move	狂	KUANG insanity	縮	SUO contract	夭	YAO death
中	ZHONG center	忘	WANG forget	而	ER and	死	SI death
則	ZE this	不	BU no	攣	LUAN spasm	於	YU in
傷	SHANG injure	精	JING	筋	JIN tendon	秋	QIU autumn
魂	HUN	不	BU no	兩	LIANG both		
		精	JING	脅	XIE rib		
		則	ZE this	骨	GU bone		
		不	BU no	不	BU not		
		正	ZHENG rectitude	舉	JU rise		

When sorrow and grief (BEI AI 悲哀) invade Liver, there is restlessness (DONG 動) in the center and this injures HUN 魂.
Injury to HUN 魂 results in KUANG 狂 (agitated insanity), memory loss and lack of JING 精. Lack of JING 精 is the loss of rectitude (BU ZHENG 不正).
So in man, genital organs (YIN 陰) contract and there are spasms in tendons. On both sides of the body, the ribs do not rise.
Body hair breaks off; the complexion shows signs of premature death. Death will come in autumn.

❖ LING SHU, Chapter 8-4: *When sorrow and grief (BEI AI 悲哀) invade Liver, there is restlessness (DONG 動) in the center and this injures HUN 魂.*

Intense sorrow and grief (emotions of Lung) interrupt communication with the environment, and cut off all life's pleasures. This type of sorrow and grief follows a separation from someone or something very important to the person, and may be compared to phantom pain after limb amputation, in which there is a feeling of pain as if in the limb which is actually not there.

Sorrow and grief agitate the center (of man) (LING SHU, Chapter 8-3)[333] - Master of Heart (the source of pleasure). Sorrow and grief obstruct (heat and agitate) the chest and Lung.

Figure 53. Injury to Master of Heart, Lung and Liver caused by sorrow and grief (BEI AI 悲哀)

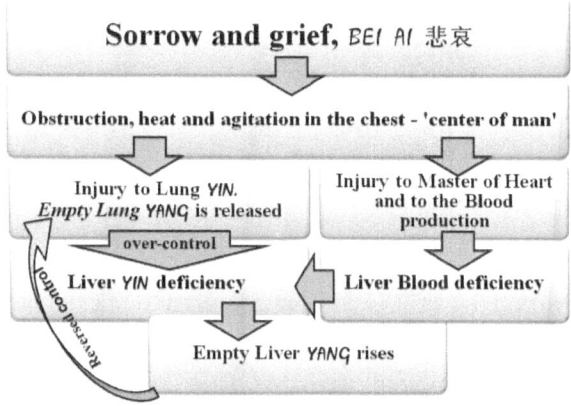

The restlessness spreads from the center to Liver (Figure 53). Both Liver and Master of Heart belong to the JUE YIN 厥陰 layer of QI flow. The obstruction of Master of Heart disturbs blood production, and develops into *Liver Blood deficiency*, which may lead to Liver YIN deficiency. Nourishing QI absorbed from food continues to ascend to the chest from Middle JIAO and contributes to further QI congestion in the chest. Congested QI in the chest heats and damages Lung YIN, therefore *empty Lung YANG* is released and 'over-controls' Liver. Liver is injured by both Master of Heart and Lung disorder, and the smooth flow of QI in the body is disrupted. *Empty Liver YANG* rises and provides an additional injury to Lung (reversed control).

❖ LING SHU, Chapter 8-4, sorrow and grief: *Injury to* HUN 魂 *results in* KUANG 狂 (agitated insanity), *memory loss ...*

Sorrow and grief injure Liver and HUN 魂, thereby interfering with humanity and the drive to communicate with the environment (birth,

---

333 See page 223

awakening, walking, talking). *Following SHEN as it goes away and comes back, that is called HUN 魂 (LING SHU, Chapter 8-1).*[334] In sorrow and grief, HUN does not follow SHEN and gets lost: loss of oneself and loss of communication with the environment. As a result, the person becomes insane (KUANG 狂).[335] KUANG 狂 describes agitated, extroverted and violent YANG psychoses. In sorrow and grief, a man cries inside, but laughs and sings outwardly.

In sorrow and grief, *injury to HUN 魂 results in... memory loss*. Liver *fire* and HUN without direction over-control and damage Spleen and YI 意. Injury to YI 意 is expressed as inability to collect and store information/memories, so a person forgets everything, and loses his self-identity.

NAN JING, difficulty 59, describes KUANG 狂:
> *At the onset of KUANG 狂 a person does not sleep or eat, glorifies himself, his abilities and his height, laughs and sings inappropriately, is happy without reason, restless without order and without end.*[336]

LING SHU, Chapter 22, relates KUANG 狂 to sorrow (BEI 悲) and memory loss:
> *KUANG manifests at the beginning as sudden sorrow (ZI BEI 自悲). There is memory loss, suffering (KU 苦), anger (NU 怒) and a tendency to fear (KONG 恐), all of which come from sadness together with worry (YOU 憂) and hunger.*[337]

Anger, fear, sadness mixed with worry (YOU 憂, pressure on Heart) and a feeling of hunger are signs of disordered mental and bodily functioning. The desire to eat compensates for flaring emotions.

---

334 See page 104
335 See page 352
336 See Chapter 9, page 378
337 See Chapter 9, page 379

❖ LING SHU, Chapter 8-4, sorrow and grief: *Injury to HUN 魂 results in… lack of JING 精. Lack of JING 精 is the loss of rectitude* (BU ZHENG 不正).

In sorrow and grief, absorption of JING 精 from food or air by Spleen and Lung is impaired, causing JING 精 deficiency. Kidney and Organs of Extraordinary Longevity (QI HENG ZHI FU 奇恒之腑) suffer from JING 精 deficiency, provoking a loss of the vertical axis between Heart-Fire and Kidney-Water (which signifies the rectitude between Heaven and Earth). Gallbladder (YANG of Liver), one of the six Organs of Extraordinary Longevity, is also called *Rectitude of the Center* (ZHONG ZHENG 中正) in Man (SU WEN, Chapter 8). *Rectitude of the Center* in Man is the balanced flow of QI from Earth to Heaven, from Kidney to Heart, passing through Liver-Gallbladder (the ascending phase of the TAI JI symbol).

In sorrow and grief, JING 精 deficiency of Gallbladder and Kidney disturbs *Rectitude of the Center*: there is no regulation of Water and Fire. The body liquids (Water) do not flow but stagnate as a result of the dysfunction of Lung, Kidney and Spleen. Fire-heat transforms the stagnant liquids into *phlegm-fire* (TAN HUO 痰火), which obstructs QI flow and the 'Heart orifices' (sense organs – communication with the environment), disrupting brain activity and the mind.

❖ LING SHU, Chapter 8-4, sorrow and grief: *So in man, genital organs* (YIN 陰) *contract and there are spasms in tendons. On both sides of the body, the ribs do not rise.*

The expression of sexuality is related to:
- Liver, since Liver Meridian (Leg JUE YIN 厥陰) passes through the genitals
- Muscle of Ancestors (ZONG JIN 宗筋), which 'gathers' the muscles of abdomen, pelvis, and genitals
- Extraordinary Meridian CHONG MAI 衝脉
- YANG MING 陽明, one of the Six Layers (LIU JING 六經) of QI flow, which includes Stomach and Large Intestine Meridians

Liver nourishes muscles and tendons. Liver QI and JING 精 deficiency cause the insufficient nourishment of the genitals and tendons (muscles), provoking contractions and spasms.

According to NAN JING, difficulty 24:

> QI *deficiency in* JUE YIN 厥陰 *causes spasms in tendons, contractions of genitals and rolling of tongue.* JUE YIN 厥陰 *is Liver Meridian. Liver is the meeting of tendons* (muscles). *Tendons gather at the genitals and branch at the root of the tongue.*

Liver nourishes muscles and tendons. Liver Meridian passes through the anterior perineum and the Muscle of Ancestors (ZONG JIN 宗筋), which 'gathers' the muscles of abdomen, pelvis, and genitals. When Liver QI is deficient, Liver Meridian does not nourish ZONG JIN 宗筋 and therefore genitals, muscles and tendons contract and do not function. An internal branch of Liver Meridian passes through the throat; therefore when Liver QI is deficient, the tongue rolls. Liver Meridian also flows through rib muscles, essential to the process of breathing. Liver QI deficiency provokes contractions of muscles between the ribs, resulting in respiratory difficulties.

❖ LING SHU, Chapter 8-4, sorrow and grief: *Body hair breaks off; the complexion shows signs of premature death. Death will come in autumn.*

Lung injured by sorrow and grief does not nourish body hair. Sorrow and grief cause deficiency of JING, QI and Blood, injuring Heart, as seen in the change of complexion. Autumn is a period in which Metal QI controls and directs the inward gathering of QI and over-controls deficient Liver. Liver ceases functioning and the patient dies.

Syndromes in Chinese medicine which describe the damage to Liver, HUN 魂 and JING 精 caused by sorrow and grief

1. Injury to JUE YIN 厥陰 (Liver and Master of Heart),
2. *Agitated insanity* (KUANG 狂)[338]
3. *Restless* ZANG (ZANG ZAO 臟躁)
4. *Plum pit* QI (MEI HE QI 梅核氣)

---

338 See page 338

1. *Injury* to JUE YIN 厥陰		LIV3/LIV2-LIV6-CV18, PC5-LIV5-GB40-GB34, PC3-BL47-BL40, PC7-ST40-GV26
2. Agitated insanity, KUANG 狂 (Figure 54)		
	2a. *Congested QI Transforms into Fire* QI YU HUA HUO, 氣鬱化火[339]	LIV2-GB43-PC7-PC8, GV14-PC5
	2b. *Phlegm-Fire Harasses the Upper Body* TAN HUO SHANG RAO 痰火上擾, (aggravation of *Congested QI Transforms into Fire*)	GV14-GV26, GV24-PC6-H7, ST40-LIV3
	2c. *Excess Fire in YANG MING*, YANG MING HUO SHENG 陽明火盛	LI11-LI4-ST44-GV14-TW6,PC6-PC8
	2d. *Blood flow Congested and Obstructed* XUE XING YU ZHI 血行鬱滯[340]	SP6-SP10,ST25-LI4-LI11, GV14
	2e. YIN *Deficiency and Fire Effulgence* YIN XU HUO WANG 陰虛火旺	SP6-Ki3-Ki1-H7-H6-ST27
3. Restless ZANG, ZANG ZAO 臟躁 (Figure 54)		
	3a. *Liver QI Congested and Knotted* GAN QI YU JIE 肝氣鬱結[341]	PC5-H7-BL15-BL18-LIV3-GV19
	3b. *Phlegm-fire* TAN HUO 痰火[342] (aggravation of *Liver QI Congestion*)	LIV2-PC5, ST40-ST44-CV12-GB17
	3c. *Loss and Deficiency of Heart* YIN, XIN YIN KUI XU 心陰虧虛 (*Blood and Heart* YIN *Deficiency*)[343]	H7-ST44, GV26-PC8, PC5-BL15-PC3-Ki6
	3d. *Heart and Spleen Dual Deficiency* XIN PI LIANG XU 心脾兩虛[344]	SP6-CV14-CV12, BL15-BL20-PC6
	3f. *Heart and Liver Fire Effulgence* XIN GAN HUO WANG 心肝火旺[345]	BL18-GB20-LIV2, **PC7**-GV24
May also be expressed as *Liver and Kidney* YIN *Deficiency* GAN SHEN YIN SHU 肝腎陰虛		
4. *Plum pit QI syndrome* MEI HE QI 梅核氣		
	4a. YIN *deficiency and Liver QI Congested and Knotted* YIN XU GAN QI YU JIE, 陰虛肝氣鬱結	LIV3-LIV14-CV22-ST40, Ki6-LU7
	4b. *Liver QI Congested and Knotted*, GAN QI YU JIE 肝氣鬱結[346]	LIV3-PC5-BL18, **Ki6-LU7**, H5-**CV23**
	4c. *Lung and Kidney* YIN *Deficiency and Phlegm-Fire Harasses the Upper Body* FEI SHEN YIN XU TAN HUO SHANG RAO 肺腎陰虛痰火上擾	Ki6-LU7, SP6-**CV22**-H5-ST40-ST44
	4d. *Phlegm and QI Congested and Knotted* TAN QI YU JIE, 痰氣鬱結[347]	LIV3-PC5, ST36-ST40-CV12, H6-**CV23**, Ki6-LU7

---

339 See pages 261, 292, LING SHU, 8-3 and LING SHU, 8-4
340 See pages 295, 332, 343, LING SHU, 8-4
341 See pages 261, 291, 331, LING SHU, 8-3, and LING SHU, 8-4
342 See pages 247, 267, 307, 312, 317, 332
343 See page 294 melancholy and sadness, LING SHU, 8-4
344 See pages 244, 296, 313, 334, LING SHU, 8-3 and in LING SHU, 8-4

Figure 54. Sorrow and grief cause injury to JUE YIN 厥陰, **Restless** ZANG (ZANG ZAO 臟躁), KUANG 狂 **and** *Plum pit* QI (MEI HE QI 梅核氣)

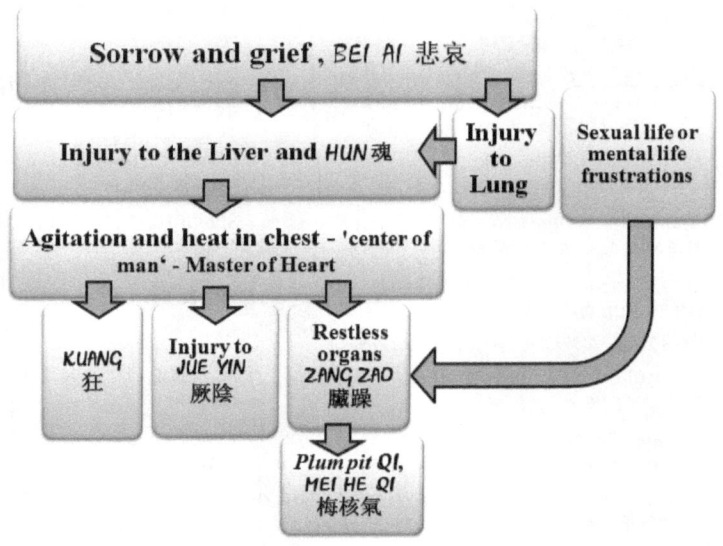

1. Injury to JUE YIN 厥陰 (Liver and Master of Heart) - sorrow and grief

Etiology	Sorrow and grief injure Liver and Master of Heart and therefore JUE YIN is unbalanced
Signs	contractions of genitals, tendons and muscles, respiratory distress, communication problems
Pulse	wiry (XUAN 弦)
Strategy	disperse *Liver fire*, JUE YIN *fire* and *phlegm-fire*, release muscles and genitals, release pressure in the chest
Points	LIV3/LIV2-LIV6-CV18, PC5-LIV5-GB40-GB34, PC3-BL47-BL40, PC7-ST40-GV26

---

345 See page 235, joy and pleasure, LING SHU, 8-3
346 See footnote 341, page 303
347 See page 293, melancholy and sadness, LING SHU, 8-4

Acupuncture points to treat injury to JUE YIN - sorrow and grief

name	function	action
LIV3/LIV2-LIV6-CV18 disperse Liver fire, nourish Liver		
LIV2 XING JIAN 行間 Moving Between	RONG-Fire of Liver	move YANG down, benefit Gall-bladder, stop wind, calm anger
LIV3 TAI CHONG 太冲 Great Rush	SHU-YUAN-Soil of Liver	release and harmonize Liver
LIV6 ZHONG DU 中都 Capital Center	XI of Liver	sedate and regulate Liver, treat gynecological disorders
CV18 YU TANG 堂玉 Jade palace	'knot' of JUE YIN	move QI down, open chest, clear Lung, regulate breathing
PC5-LIV5-GB40-GB34 release muscles and genitals		
PC5 JIAN SHI 間使 Interval Envoy	JING-River-Metal of Master of Heart - JUE YIN, Group LUO of 3 arm YIN	regulate YIN deficiency above and YIN stagnation below, open chest, calm SHEN, calm SHAO YANG, calm suffering and stop the crying
LIV5 LI GOU 蠡溝 Woodworm Canal	LUO of Liver	calm and regulate Liver, treat melancholy, lack of joy and energy, worries with sighs
GB40 QIU XU 丘墟 Hill Ruins	YUAN of Gallbladder, Group LUO of leg	disperse *Gallbladder fire*, regulate SHAO YANG
GB34 YANG LING QUAN 陽陵泉 YANG Mound Spring	HE-Soil of G.B., HUI-meeting of muscles and tendons	regulate and move QI of Gallbladder down
PC3-BL47-BL40 release heat from JUE YIN		
PC3 QU ZE 曲澤 Marsh at the Crook	HE-Water of Master of Heart	dissipate heat from Upper JIAO, cool blood and Heart, disperse toxins caused by stagnation
BL47 HUN MEN 魂門 HUN Gate	regulate HUN 魂, gather *Liver* JING	spread *Liver* QI, regulate Middle JIAO
BL40 WEI ZHONG 委中 Bend Middle	HE-Soil of Bladder, command point for the back	irrigate muscle and tendon, release phlegm obstructing SHEN
PC7-ST40-GV26 release pressure in chest		
PC7 DA LING 大陵 Big Mound	SHU-YUAN-Soil of Master of Heart	calm and purify SHEN, cool Heart (palpitation)
ST40 FENG LONG 豐隆 Bountiful Bulge	LUO of Stomach	dissolve *phlegm-fire*, calm SHEN
GV26 SHUI GOU 水溝 Water Trough	open LUO channels in face region	calm SHEN, open Heart orifices, purify head and brain, calm uncontrollable and groundless laughter

2. 'Agitated personality disorder', KUANG 狂 - sorrow and grief (Figure 54)

2a. *Congested QI Transforms into Fire*, QI YU HUA HUO 氣鬱化火 - KUANG, sorrow and grief

Compare overflowing anger (LING SHU, Chapter 8-3) and melancholy and sadness - YU 鬱 of QI (LING SHU, Chapter 8-4). Acupuncture points for KUANG in sorrow and grief to release *Liver fire/YANG* are: LIV2-GB43-PC7-PC8, GV14-PC5.

Acupuncture points to treat *Congested QI Transforms into Fire* - KUANG - sorrow and grief

name	function	action
LIV2-GB43-PC7-PC8 release *Liver fire/YANG*		
LIV2 XING JIAN 行間 Moving Between	RONG-Fire of Liver	move YANG down, benefit Gall-bladder, calm anger
GB43 XIA XI 俠谿 Pinched Ravine	RONG-Water of Gall-bladder, tonify Wood	purify head, ears and eyes, return order and mental uprightness
PC7 DA LING 大陵 Big Mound	SHU-YUAN-Soil of Master of Heart	calm and purify SHEN, cool Heart palpitation, cool blood,
PC8 LAO GONG 勞宮 Labor Palace	RONG-Fire of Master of Heart	disperse heat from JUE YIN, purify Heart, awaken SHEN, cool blood, purify mouth, treat anger
GV14-PC5 calm SHEN		
PC5 JIAN SHI 間使 Interval Envoy	JING-River-Metal of Master of Heart - JUE YIN, Group LUO of 3 arm YIN	regulate YIN deficiency above and YIN stagnation below, open chest, calm SHEN, calm SHAO YANG, calm suffering and stop crying
GV14 DA ZHUI 大椎 Big Mallet	meeting of DU MAI with six YANG Meridians	regulate QI and YANG flow to head and heart, release excess heat and damp-heat in upper body

2b. *Phlegm-fire Harasses the Upper Body*, TAN HUO SHANG RAO 痰火上擾 - KUANG, sorrow and grief

Etiology	Sorrow and grief cause *Liver QI congestion* which transforms into fire. Body liquids obstructed by sorrow, grief and fire produce *phlegm-fire*, which obstructs the Heart orifices and causes KUANG
Signs	anger, impatience, lack of manners, loss of control, madness with physical violence, shows remarkable strength, breaks things, curses, incoherent speech, alternately laughing and crying, sexual dysfunction, feeling of pressure, heat and obstruction of the diaphragm and chest, dysfunction of orifices; feeling of phlegm stuck in throat; headache with feeling of pressure, bitter taste in mouth, reddish urine, constipation
Tongue	dark red, yellow and greasy coating
Pulse	slippery (HUA 滑) or wiry (XUAN 弦), fast (SHU 數)
Strategy	purify phlegm, open Heart orifices, dissipate fire and YANG from head, calm SHEN
Points	GV14-GV26, GV24-PC6-H7, ST40-LIV3

Acupuncture points to treat *Phlegm-fire Harasses the Upper Body* - KUANG, sorrow and grief

name	function	action
GV14-GV26, GV24-PC6-H7 open Heart orifices, dissipate fire and YANG from head, calm SHEN		
GV26 SHUI GOU Water Trough 水溝	open LUO channels in face region	calm SHEN, open Heart orifices, purify head and brain, calm uncontrollable laughter without reason
GV14 DA ZHUI 大椎 Big Mallet	meeting of DU MAI with six YANG Meridians	regulate QI and YANG flow to head and Heart, release excess heat and damp-heat from upper body
H7 SHEN MEN 神門 SHEN Gate	SHU-YUAN-Soil of Heart	calm SHEN, cool Heart, open Heart orifices
PC6 NEI GUAN 內關 Inner Barrier	LUO of Master of Heart, open YIN WEI MAI	release three YIN, open chest, remove congestion between pelvis and chest, regulate QI, awaken SHEN
GV24 SHEN TING 神庭 SHEN Court	meeting of DU MAI with Bl. and St. Meridians	communicate between orifices, calm SHEN, regulate mental restlessness
ST40-LIV3 purify phlegm		
ST40 FENG LONG 豐隆 Bountiful Bulge	LUO of Stomach	dissolve *phlegm-fire*, calm SHEN
LIV3 TAI CHONG 太冲 Great Rush	SHU-YUAN-Soil of Liver	release and harmonize Liver

2c. Excess Fire in YANG MING, YANG MING HUO SHENG
陽明火盛 - KUANG, sorrow and grief

Etiology	Sorrow and grief cause *Liver fire* to invade Stomach (YANG MING), provoking KUANG (SU WEN, Chapter 30)
Signs	*Fire in YANG MING*: agitation, incoherent speech, anorexia, a tendency to undress and climb high places, red eyes. *Heat in Large Intestine*: dry, hard stools, constipation with abdominal bloating, dark red urine
Tongue	red with yellow dry coating
Pulse	sinking (CHEN 沉), full (SHI 實) with force (YOU LI 有力), fast (SHU 數)
Strategy	release heat from YANG MING, treat constipation, calm SHEN
Points	LI11-LI4-ST44-GV14-TW6, PC6-PC8

Acupuncture points to treat *Excess fire in* YANG MING - KUANG, sorrow and grief

name	function	action
LI11-LI4-ST44-GV14-TW6 release heat from YANG MING, treat constipation		
LI11 QU CHI 曲池 Pool at the Bend	HE-Soil of Large Intestine	balance QI and Blood, dissipate heat from upper body
LI4 HE GU 合谷 Union Valley	YUAN of Large Intestine, entry point, command of face and mouth.	regulate QI, release excess YANG from head
ST44 NEI TING 內庭 Inner Courtyard	RONG-Water of Stomach	cool and move QI of YANG MING down, dissolve phlegm, move fire down from head
GV14 DA ZHUI 大椎 Big Mallet	meeting of DU MAI with six YANG Meridians	regulate QI and YANG flow to head and heart, release excess heat and damp-heat from upper body
TW6 ZHI GOU 支溝 Branch Ditch	JING-River-Fire of SAN JIAO	regulate QI of SAN JIAO, treat constipation, clear heat from skin, **disperse**
PC6-PC8 calm SHEN		
PC8 LAO GONG 勞宮 Labor Palace	RONG-Fire of Master of Heart	clear heat from JUE YIN, purify Heart, awaken SHEN, cool blood, purify mouth
PC6 NEI GUAN 內關 Inner Barrier	LUO of Master of Heart, open YIN WEI MAI	release three YIN, open chest, remove congestion between pelvis and chest, regulate QI, awaken SHEN

2d. *Blood Flow Congested and Obstructed,* XUE XING YU ZHI 血行鬱滯 - KUANG, sorrow and grief

Compare melancholy and sadness, YU 鬱 of Blood (LING SHU, Chapter 8-4).

Blood stagnation may be caused by:
- brain hemorrhage due to external head injury
- chronic disease that causes brain hemorrhage
- external heat causing blood clotting in the brain

Sorrow and grief injure Liver and HUN 魂, combine with blood stagnation, and cause *empty heat*/YANG *rising* to head, expressed as KUANG. Acupuncture points to tonify QI and Blood, and to regulate *empty heat*/YANG *rising* to head are: SP6-SP10, ST25-LI4-LI11, GV14.

Acupuncture points to treat *Blood Flow Congested and Obstructed* - KUANG, sorrow and grief

name	function	action
SP10-SP6 tonify blood flow		
SP6 SAN YIN JIAO 三陰交 Meeting of Three YIN	meeting of Sp., Liv., and Ki. Meridians	tonify and nourish Blood, QI and YIN, move YIN up, nourish Spleen
SP10 XUE HAI 血海 Sea of Blood		invigorate and cool blood
ST25-LI4-LI11 tonify QI, GV14 regulate YANG rising to head		
LI4 HE GU 合谷 Union Valley	YUAN of Large Intestine, entry point, command of face and mouth	regulate QI, release excess YANG from head
LI11 QU CHI 曲池 Pool at the Bend	HE-Soil of Large Intestine, tonify Metal	balance QI and Blood, dissipate heat from upper body, **disperse**
ST25 TIAN SHU 天樞 Celestial Axis	MU of Large Intestine	dissolve phlegm, calm SHEN and talkaholism, regulate HUN and PO
GV14 DA ZHUI 大椎 Big Mallet	meeting of DU MAI with six YANG Meridians	regulate QI and YANG flow to head and heart, release excess heat from upper body

2e. YIN *Deficiency and Fire Effulgence*, YIN XU HUO WANG
陰虛火旺 - KUANG, sorrow and grief

Etiology	Long lasting sorrow and grief cause heat which dries body liquids, causes YIN *deficiency* and *empty fire* and then KUANG
Signs	KUANG: restlessness, anxiety, suspicion, irritability, fear, startled at noise, talkaholism with anger, decreased intellectual and emotional ability. YIN *deficiency*: insomnia, tinnitus, hot flashes and night sweats, feeling of heat in 'five palms' and bones, night spermatorrhea, erotic dreams
Tongue	red with peeled yellow coating
Pulse	fast (SHU 數) and wiry (XUAN 弦) or thin (XI 細)
Strategy	tonify YIN and calm SHEN
Points	SP6-Ki3-Ki1-H7-H6-ST27

Acupuncture points to treat YIN *Deficiency and Fire Effulgence* - KUANG, sorrow and grief

name	function	action
SP6-Ki3-Ki1-H7-H6-ST27 tonify YIN and calm SHEN		
SP6 SAN YIN JIAO 三陰交 Meeting of Three YIN	meeting of Sp., Liv., and Ki. Meridians	tonify and nourish Blood, QI and YIN, move YIN up, nourish Spleen
Ki3 TAI XI 太谿 Great Ravine	SHU-YUAN-Soil of Kidney	tonify Kidney YIN, release ascent of CHONG MAI and REN MAI, treat degenerative diseases
Ki1 YONG QUAN 湧泉 Gushing Spring	JING-Well-Wood of Kidney, root of SHAO YIN	move rebel QI and YANG down, open Heart orifices, improve memory, awaken SHEN
H7 SHEN MEN 神門 SHEN Gate	SHU-YUAN-Soil of Heart	calm SHEN, cool Heart, open Heart orifices
H6 YIN XI 陰郄 YIN Cleft	XI of Heart	nourish YIN, calm SHEN, stop night sweat
ST27 DA JU 大巨 Great Gigantic	passage of YANG from chest to abdomen	tonify Kidney and JING, calm SHEN, disperse QI in Middle JIAO (separate *clear* and *turbid* of Small Intestine)

3. Restless ZANG, ZANG ZAO 臟躁 - sorrow and grief (Figure 54)

Etiology	Sorrow and grief caused by frustrations in love or sex life damage HUN 魂, SHEN 神, JING 精, Blood. ZANG are not nourished properly, provoking mental disorders. Common in women with tendency to anemia.
Signs	depression, instability: tears, anger, laughter; exaggeration and theatrical expression of frustrations, loss of control, easily influenced, anemia; false paralysis or false seizures
Diseases	Inflammation of the digestive tract, especially in stomach and intestines. Respiratory system disorders: asthma

3a. *Liver QI Congested and Knotted,* GAN QI YU JIE 肝氣鬱結 - ZANG ZAO - sorrow and grief

Compare overflowing anger (LING SHU, Chapter 8-3) and melancholy and sadness which develop into YU ZHENG (LING SHU, Chapter 8-4). In sorrow and grief and ZANG ZAO, the personality is unstable. Acupuncture points to release Liver QI and to calm SHEN are PC5-H7-BL15-BL18-LIV3-GV19

Acupuncture points to treat *Liver QI Congested and Knotted*
ZANG ZAO - sorrow and grief

name	function	action
PC5-H7-BL15-BL18-LIV3-GV19 release Liver QI, calm SHEN		
PC5 JIAN SHI 間使 Interval Envoy	JING-River-Metal of Master of Heart - JUE YIN, Group LUO of 3 arm YIN	regulate YIN deficiency above and YIN stagnation below, calm SHAO YANG, open chest, calm SHEN
H7 SHEN MEN 神門 SHEN Gate	SHU-YUAN-Soil of Heart	calm SHEN, cool Heart, open Heart orifices
BL15 XIN SHU 心俞 Heart SHU	SHU of Heart, regulate Heart YANG, release LUO of Heart	calm SHEN, clear heat from Heart
BL18 GAN SHU 肝俞 Liver SHU	SHU of Liver, regulate Liver YANG	move Liver QI and Blood
LIV3 TAI CHONG 太沖 Great Rush	SHU-YUAN-Soil of Liver	release and harmonize Liver
GV19 HOU DING 後頂 Behind Vertex	influence HUN 魂	regulate YANG, calm *Liver fire rising* and HUN 魂

3b. *Phlegm-fire,* TAN HUO 痰火, **development of Liver** QI *Congestion* - ZANG ZAO - sorrow and grief

Compare Lily Bulb Disease in melancholy and sadness (LING SHU, Chapter 8-3) and sorrow and grief (LING SHU, Chapter 8-4).

Sorrow and grief cause Liver YIN QI *congestion* which develops into *Liver fire,* and injure Spleen and Lung – circulation of body liquids. *Liver fire* and stagnant body liquids form *phlegm-fire.*

Repressed anger and frustrations in sex life (real or imagined rape, traumatic separation, feelings of rejection) cause ZANG ZAO: unstable personality, loss of control, theatrical behavior, despair, shouting with tears, laughter, groundless anger, confusion. When *Phlegm-fire* develops into ZANG ZAO, acupuncture points to dissolve *phlegm-fire* and to disperse and cool Liver are LIV2-PC5, ST40-ST44-CV12-GB17.

Acupuncture points to treat *Phlegm-Fire* - ZANG ZAO sorrow and grief

name	function	action
ST40-ST44-CV12-GB17 dissolve *phlegm-fire*		
ST40 FENG LONG 豐隆 Bountiful Bulge	LUO of Stomach	dissolve *phlegm-fire*, calm SHEN
ST44 NEI TING 內庭 Inner Courtyard	RONG-Water of Stomach	cool and move QI of YANG MING and fire down from head, dissolve phlegm
CV12 ZHONG WAN 中脘 Central Venter	MU of Stomach, HUI-meeting of FU, 'knot' of TAI YIN, start of Lu. Meridian	move stagnation, regulate Stomach
GB17 ZHENG YING 正營 Nourish Rectitude	meeting of G.B, Meridian with YANG WEI MAI	dissolve *phlegm-fire* from head
LIV2-PC5 disperse and cool *Liver fire*		
PC5 JIAN SHI 間使 Interval Envoy	JING-River-Metal of Master of Heart - JUE YIN, Group LUO of 3 arm YIN	regulate YIN deficiency above and YIN stagnation below, open chest, calm SHEN, calm SHAO YANG, calm suffering and stop the crying
LIV2 XING JIAN 行間 Moving Between	RONG-Fire of Liver	move YANG down, benefit G.B., stop wind, calm anger

3c. *Loss and Deficiency of Heart* YIN, XIN YIN KUI XU 心陰虧虛
(*Blood and Heart* YIN *deficiency*) - ZANG ZAO - sorrow and grief
Compare melancholy and sadness (LING SHU, Chapter 8-4).
When this syndrome develops in sorrow and grief and ZANG ZAO, the personality is unstable. Acupuncture points to tonify Heart YIN, to calm ZANG ZAO and dreams are: H7-ST44, GV26-PC8, PC5-BL15-PC3-Ki6.

Acupuncture points to treat *Loss and Deficiency of Heart* YIN - ZANG ZAO - sorrow and grief

name	function	action
PC5-BL15-PC3-Ki6 tonify Heart YIN		
PC5 JIAN SHI 間使 Interval Envoy	JING-River-Metal of Master of Heart - JUE YIN, Group LUO of 3 arm YIN	regulate YIN deficiency above and YIN stagnation below, open chest, calm SHEN, calm SHAO YANG, calm suffering and stop the crying
BL15 XIN SHU 心俞 Heart SHU	SHU of Heart, regulate Heart YANG, release LUO of Heart	calm SHEN, tonify Heart YIN
PC3 QU ZE 曲澤 Marsh at the Crook	HE-Water of Master of Heart	dissipate heat from Upper JIAO, cool blood and Heart
Ki6 ZHAO HAI 照海 Shining Sea	open YIN QIAO MAI, raise YIN of SHAO YIN	calm SHEN, treat insomnia and sad and frightening dreams
GV26-PC8 calm ZANG ZAO attack, H7-ST44 calm dreams		
PC8 LAO GONG 勞宮 Labor Palace	RONG-Fire of Master of Heart	clear heat from JUE YIN, purify Heart, awaken SHEN, cool blood, purify mouth
GV26 SHUI GOU Water Trough 水溝	open LUO channels in face region	calm SHEN, open Heart orifices, purify head and brain, calm uncontrollable and groundless laughter
ST44 NEI TING 內庭 Inner Courtyard	RONG-Water of Stomach	cool and move QI of YANG MING and fire down from head, dissolve phlegm
H7 SHEN MEN 神門 SHEN Gate	SHU-YUAN-Soil of Heart	calm SHEN, cool Heart, open Heart orifices

3d. *Heart and Spleen Dual Deficiency,* XIN PI LIANG XU
心脾兩虛 - ZANG ZAO - sorrow and grief
Compare melancholy and sadness (LING SHU, Chapter 8-3); apprehension, distress, obsessive thinking and worry, YU ZHENG, melancholy and sadness (LING SHU, Chapter 8-4).

Unstable personality is the main sign of *Heart and Spleen Dual Deficiency* in sorrow and grief and ZANG ZAO. Acupuncture points are: SP6-CV14-CV12, BL15-BL20-PC6.

Acupuncture points to treat *Heart and Spleen Dual Deficiency,* ZANG ZAO - sorrow and grief

name	function	action
BL15-BL20-PC6 tonify Spleen and Heart		
BL20 PI SHU 脾俞 Spleen SHU	SHU of Spleen, regulate Spleen YANG	tonify Spleen, **tonify**
BL15 XIN SHU 心俞 Heart SHU	SHU of Heart, regulate Heart YANG, release LUO of Heart	calm SHEN, tonify Heart YIN, **tonify**
PC6 NEI GUAN 內關 Inner Barrier	LUO of Master of Heart, open YIN WEI MAI	release three YIN, open chest, remove congestion between pelvis and chest, regulate QI, move rebel QI down, awaken SHEN, **tonify**
SP6-CV14-CV12 treat insomnia, palpitation, memory problems		
SP6 SAN YIN JIAO 三陰交 Meeting of Three YIN	meeting of Sp., Liv. and Ki. Meridians	tonify and nourish Blood, QI and YIN, move YIN up, nourish Spleen , **tonify**
CV12 ZHONG WAN 中脘 Central Venter	MU of Stomach, HUI-meeting of FU, 'knot' of TAI YIN, start of Lu. Meridian	dissolve phlegm, move stagnations, regulate Stomach, **tonify**
CV14 JU QUE 巨闕 Great Tower Gate	MU of Heart, regulate Heart YIN	calm SHEN and Heart, dissolve phlegm, open chest, move *turbid* QI down, **tonify gently**

4. *Plum pit* QI **syndrome,** MEI HE QI 梅核氣 - sorrow and grief (Figure 54)

Plum pit QI syndrome is obstruction of the QI flow in the throat accompanied by a feeling of a lump that cannot be swallowed or spat out. In sorrow and grief, *Plum pit* QI develops from Restless ZANG (ZANG ZAO 臟躁) and is expressed as hysterical outbursts, 'loss of rectitude' with a sense of suffocation, obstruction in the throat. Plum pit QI may be treated by REN MAI, which enhances Liver QI flow in the throat: **Ki6-LU7, CV22/CV23**, and **ST40**.

Acupuncture points to treat *Plum pit* QI syndrome, MEI HE QI 梅核氣 - sorrow and grief

LU7 LIE QUE 列缺 Broken Sequence	LUO of Lung, open REN MAI	treat rebel QI and fear that closes Upper JIAO
Ki6 ZHAO HAI 照海 Shining Sea	open YIN QIAO MAI, move YIN of SHAO YIN up	calm SHEN, treat insomnia and dreams with fear and sadness
CV22 TIAN TU 天突 Celestial Chimney	Minor Celestial Window, meeting of REN MAI with YIN WEI MAI	dissolve mucus from throat, benefit throat
CV23 LIAN QUAN 廉泉 Ridge Spring	'knot' of SHAO YIN, meeting of REN MAI with YIN WEI MAI	dissolve phlegm, obstruction and swelling, release ascent of body liquids
ST40 FENG LONG 豐隆 Bountiful Bulge	LUO of Stomach	dissolve *phlegm-fire/heat*, calm SHEN

4a. YIN *deficiency and Liver* QI *Congested and Knotted*, YIN XU GAN QI YU JIE 陰虛肝氣鬱結 - *Plum pit* QI - sorrow and grief

Etiology	Frustration, sorrow and grief congest Liver QI and damage Spleen and Lung - flow of body liquids. Chronic fatigue, age, chronic disease, weak constitution cause *Kidney* YIN *deficiency*, *Liver* YIN *(Blood) deficiency*. *Empty heat* ascends and forms phlegm from obstructed liquids in chest and throat.
Signs	restlessness, anxiety, anger, feeling a lump (plum pit) in throat, menstrual irregularities, amenorrhea, YIN *deficiency*: insomnia, tinnitus, hot flashes and night sweats, impaired vision, visual disturbances, dizziness, numb pain in hypochondrium.
Tongue	red with peeled yellow coating
Pulse	fast (SHU 數), thin (XI 細)
Strategy	tonify YIN, dissolve phlegm
Points	LIV3-LIV14-**CV22-ST40, Ki6-LU7**

Acupuncture points to treat YIN *Deficiency and Liver* QI *Congested and Knotted* - *Plum pit* QI - sorrow and grief

name	function	action
LIV3-LIV14-**CV22**-ST40 tonify Liver YIN, release Liver and dissolve phlegm		
LIV3 TAI CHONG 太冲 Great Rush	SHU-YUAN-Soil of Liver	release and harmonize Liver
LIV14 QI MEN 期門 Cycle Gate	MU of Liver, regulate Liver YIN, meeting of Liv., Sp. Meridians and YIN WEI MAI	raise QI from abdomen to chest, benefit Gallbladder, calm restlessness with arrhythmia and obsession

4b. *Liver* QI *Congested and Knotted,* GAN QI YU JIE, 肝氣鬱結 - *Plum pit* QI - sorrow and grief

Compare overflowing anger (LING SHU, Chapter 8-3), melancholy and sadness - YU ZHENG and ZANG ZAO - sorrow and grief (LING SHU, Chapter 8-4).

When a sensation of lump (*plum pit*) in the throat is the main complaint, acupuncture points are LIV3-PC5-BL18, **Ki6-LU7** ,H5-**CV23**

Acupuncture points to treat *Liver* QI *Congested and Knotted* *Plum pit* QI - sorrow and grief

name	function	action
H5-**CV23** release *plum pit* in throat		
H5 TONG LI 通里 Penetrating the Interior	LUO of Heart	purify Heart, calm SHEN, release QI congestion in throat
LIV3-PC5-BL18 release Liver QI, calm SHEN.		
LIV3 TAI CHONG 太冲 Great Rush	SHU-YUAN-Soil of Liver	release and harmonize Liver
PC5 JIAN SHI 間使 Interval Envoy	JING-River-Metal of Master of Heart - JUE YIN, Group LUO of 3 arm YIN	regulate YIN deficiency above and YIN stagnation below, calm SHAO YANG, open chest, calm SHEN
BL18 GAN SHU 肝俞 Liver SHU	SHU of Liver, regulate Liver YANG	tonify Liver YIN, move Liver QI and blood stagnation, move stagnant blood down from head

4c. Lung and Kidney YIN Deficiency, and Phlegm-Fire Harasses the Upper Body, FEI SHEN YIN XU TAN HUO SHANG RAO 肺腎陰虛痰火上擾 - *Plum pit* QI - sorrow and grief

Etiology	Chronic fatigue, age, chronic disease, weak constitution cause *Kidney* YIN *deficiency*, and combined with sorrow and grief cause *Lung* YIN *deficiency*. Lung does not move body liquids down. *Empty heat* ascends and forms phlegm from obstructed liquids in chest and throat.
Signs	feeling a lump (*plum pit*) in throat YIN *deficiency*: insomnia, tinnitus, hot flashes and night sweats, tinnitus with dizziness, dry mouth and throat, thirsty but cannot drink
Tongue	red with peeled yellow coating
Pulse	fast (SHU 數), thin (XI 細)
Strategy	tonify YIN and dissolve phlegm
Points	**Ki6-LU7**, SP6-**CV22**-H5-**ST40**-ST44

Acupuncture points to treat *Lung and Kidney* YIN *Deficiency and Phlegm-Fire Harasses the Upper Body* - *Plum pit* QI sorrow and grief

name	function	action
SP6-**CV22**-H5-**ST40**-ST44 tonify YIN, dissolve phlegm		
SP6 SAN YIN JIAO 三陰交 Meeting of Three YIN	meeting of Sp., Liv. and Ki. Meridians	tonify and nourish Blood, QI and YIN, move YIN up, nourish Spleen
H5 TONG LI 通里 Penetrating the Interior	LUO of Heart	purify Heart, calm SHEN, release QI congestion in throat
ST44 NEI TING 內庭 Inner Courtyard	RONG-Water of Stomach	cool and move QI of YANG MING and fire down from head, dissolve phlegm

D. Damage to Lung, PO 魄 and sanity caused by excessive joy and pleasure (XI LE 喜樂), LING SHU, Chapter 8-4

肺 FEI	lung	魄 PO		狂 KUANG	insanity	皮 PI	skin
喜 XI	joy	傷 SHANG	injure	者 ZHE	comma	革 GE	harden
樂 LE	pleasure	則 ZE	this	意 YI		焦 JIAO	burn
無 WU	no	狂 KUANG	insanity	不 BU	not	毛 MAO	hair
極 JI	limit			存 CUN	establish	悴 CUI	fall
則 ZE	this			人 REN	man	色 SE	color
傷 SHANG	injure					夭 YAO	death
魄 PO						死 SI	death
						於 YU	in
						夏 XIA	summer

When joy and pleasure without limit (XI LE WU JI 喜樂無極) invade Lung, this injures PO 魄,

Injury to PO 魄 results in KUANG 狂 (agitated insanity). In KUANG, YI 意 loses its ability to acknowledge the existence of others.

Skin hardens and seems to be 'burned'. Body hair breaks off; the complexion shows signs of premature death. Death will come in summer.

❖ LING SHU, Chapter 8-4: *When joy and pleasure without limit (XI LE WU JI 喜樂無極) invade Lung, this injures PO 魄.*

Joy and pleasure (XI LE 喜樂),[348] the emotions of Heart, harmonize communication with the self and with the environment. *Joy (XI 喜) harmonizes QI. Emotions are fully expressed* (SU WEN, Chapter 39).[349] Joy and pleasure without limit (XI LE WU JI 喜樂無極) manifest as extreme exteriorization or a compulsive search for pleasure (addictions). *Joy and pleasure (XI LE 喜樂) scare SHEN. SHEN is dispersed and does not store* (LING SHU, Chapter 8-3).[350] Joy and pleasure (Fire) over-control Metal-PO 魄, and injure internalization, density, rest, cooling, body boundaries (skin) and the descent of body liquids. *Together with JING 精 as it exits and enters, that is called*

---

348 See page 51 for the characters XI LE 喜樂
349 See page 175
350 See page 232

PO 魄 (LING SHU, Chapter 8-1).³⁵¹ Metal-PO 魄 nourishes Water-Kidney-JING 精 storage. Endless joy and pleasure prevent PO 魄 and JING 精 from entering the body, and therefore personal integrity and the storage of JING 精 in ZANG are injured.

- LING SHU, Chapter 8-4, joy and pleasure: *Injury to PO 魄 results in KUANG 狂. In KUANG, YI 意 loses its ability to acknowledge the existence of others.*

Joy causes KUANG 狂³⁵² also according to LING SHU, Chapter 22:
> In KUANG disease the patient is bulimic; he sees ghosts and spirits, is joyful and laughs without external reason. The condition comes from great joy (DA XI 大喜).³⁵³

In SU WEN, Chapter 46, the Yellow Emperor asks QI BO about the origin of KUANG 狂. QI BO answers that KUANG emerges from YANG (exteriorization) and offers a treatment:
> Deprive the [patient] of his food and [the disease] will end. Now, food enters the YIN, and supports the growth of QI in the YANG. Hence, if one deprives the [patient] of his food, [the disease] will end. Let the [patient] consume a drink of fresh iron flakes. Now, fresh iron flakes cause QI to move down quickly.³⁵⁴

Joy and pleasure injure Lung-PO 魄 impairing communication with the inner self, and therefore provoke extreme externalization, agitated insanity (KUANG 狂), which injures Heart-SHEN. Spleen-YI 意 is not nourished properly by 'externalized' Heart and is also damaged (reversed generation) by the weakened Lung. YI 意 governs the storage and recording of the ideas and intent that enable identity and communication. In KUANG 狂, Spleen-YI 意 is damaged, and this impairs self-identity and the ability to recognize others. ZHUANG ZI, Chapter 23, shows the importance of storage of information in order to communicate:

---

351 See page 107
352 See page 302 KUANG 狂 in injury to Liver and HUN 魂 by sorrow and grief
353 See page 390
354 Translated by Unschuld, P. U. and Tessenow, H

備	BEI	encompass	藏	CANG	store	敬	JING	respect
物	WU	being	不	BU	not	中	ZHONG	center
以	YI	in order to	虞	YU	speculate	以	YI	in order to
將	JIANG	support	以	YI	in order to	達	DA	reach
形	XING	substantial forms	生	SHENG	life	彼	BI	others
			心	XIN	heart			

Contain all the beings in order to complete your reality,
Store inside yourself without getting lost in speculation in order to give life to Heart-Consciousness (XIN 心),
Be vigilant of the center in order to communicate with others.

❖ LING SHU, Chapter 8-4, joy and pleasure: *Skin hardens and seems to be 'burned'. Body hair breaks off; the complexion shows signs of premature death. Death will come in summer.*

Excessive joy and pleasure dry body liquids causing internal fire which 'burns' mind and body, especially Lung tissue – skin and body hair. Skin is dry and inflamed, '*burned*' (eczema or psoriasis). The patient's condition deteriorates, as can be seen by the change in complexion. In summer, Fire Modality dominates: heat and fire caused by excessive joy and pleasure overheat Lung (excessive control). Therefore Lung stops functioning in summer and the patient dies.

Syndromes in Chinese medicine which describe the damage to Lung and PO 魄 caused by excessive joy and pleasure

Agitated insanity, KUANG 狂	
a. *Congested QI Transforms into Fire*, QI YU HUA HUO, 氣鬱化火	LIV2-GB43-PC7-PC8, GV14-PC5
b. *Phlegm-Fire Harasses the Upper Body*, TAN HUO SHANG RAO 痰火上擾, (aggravation of *Congested QI Transforms into Fire*)	GV14-GV26, GV24-PC6-H7, ST40-LIV3
c. *Excess Fire in YANG MING*, YANG MING HUO SHENG 陽明火盛	LI11-LI4-ST44-GV14-TW6, PC6-PC8
d. *Blood Flow Congested and Obstructed*, XUE XING YU ZHI 血行鬱滯	SP6-SP10,ST25-LI4-LI11, GV14
e. *YIN Deficiency and Fire Effulgence*, YIN XU HUO WANG 陰虛火旺	SP6-Ki3-Ki1-H7-H6-ST27

See page 303 for description of syndromes corresponding to KUANG 狂 - injury to Liver and HUN 魂 by sorrow and grief, LING SHU, 8-4, which are similar to KUANG 狂 in joy and pleasure

Acupuncture points for skin diseases in excessive joy and pleasure

name	function	action
ST40-SP10-SI7-LI11-SP6-ST25 treatment of skin diseases		
ST40 FENG LONG 豐隆 Bountiful Bulge	LUO of Stomach	dissolve *phlegm-fire*, calm SHEN
SP10 XUE HAI 血海 Sea of Blood.		invigorate and cool blood, treat inflammations and infections
SI7 ZHI ZHENG 支正 *Upright Branch*	LUO of Small Intestine	clear heat, calm SHEN, release exterior
LI11 QU CHI 曲池 Pool at the Bend	HE-Soil of Large Intestine	balance QI and Blood, dissipate heat from the upper body
SP6 SAN YIN JIAO 三陰交 Meeting of Three YIN	meeting of Sp., Liv. and Ki. Meridians	tonify and nourish Blood, QI and YIN, move YIN up, nourish Spleen
ST25 TIAN SHU 天樞 Celestial Axis	MU of Large Intestine	dissolve phlegm, calm SHEN

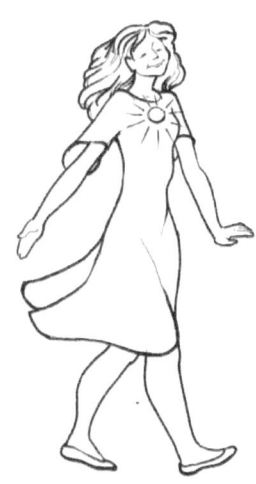

E. Damage to Kidney, ZHI 志 and back caused by uncontrollable overflowing anger (SHENG NU 盛怒), LING SHU, Chapter 8-4

腎 SHEN	kidney	志 ZHI		腰 YAO	waist	毛 MAO	hair
盛 SHENG	abundant	傷 SHANG	injure	脊 JI	spine	悴 CUI	fall
怒 NU	anger	則 ZE	this	不 BU	not	色 SE	color
而 ER	and	喜 XI	like	可 KE	capable	夭 YAO	death
不 BU	no	忘 WANG	forget	以 YI		死 SI	death
止 ZHI	stop	其 QI	his	俛 FU	bend	於 YU	in
則 ZE	this	前 QIAN	before	仰 YANG	extend	季 JI	last month of summer
傷 SHANG	injure	言 YIN	word	屈 QU	curl	夏 XIA	
志 ZHI				伸 SHEN	stretch		

When uncontrollable overflowing anger (SHENG NU BU ZHI 盛怒不止) invades Kidney, ZHI 志 is injured.
When ZHI 志 is injured, a person forgets the words spoken before.
Lower back and spine (back) are not able to bend, straighten, curl up or stretch.
Body hair breaks off; the complexion shows signs of premature death. Death will come in the last month of summer (end of July and beginning of August).

❖ LING SHU, Chapter 8-4: *When uncontrollable overflowing anger (SHENG NU BU ZHI 盛怒不止) invades Kidney, ZHI 志 is injured.*

Uncontrollable overflowing anger (SHENG NU BU ZHI 盛怒不止) [355] bursts out following:
- Significant external events,
- Unexpressed, repressed, long-lasting emotional frustration emanating from moral reasons or fear. Repressed frustration and anger require extensive use of willpower (ZHI 志). Frustrations are restrained till the 'cup is full to overflowing' or till ZHI 志 weakens, and then, like a storm, anger bursts out in the wake of an external cause of no apparent significance.

---

355 See pages 54, 253 for the characters SHENG NU 盛怒

Overflowing anger (SHENG NU 盛怒) is the emotion of Liver-Wood. Overflowing anger injures Kidney-ZHI 志 (reversed generation) and disturbs Water-Wood-Fire (Kidney-Liver-Heart), the ascending phase on the TAI JI symbol. *Anger* (NU 怒) *moves QI upwards* (SU WEN, Chapter 39).[356] Anger-Wood suddenly moves *Liver fire* and/or *Liver Blood* upwards to the chest and head,[357] and depletes the lower body – Kidney-Water (JING 精, YIN and ZHI 志).

Gallbladder, the transit organ (FU 腑), the YANG aspect of Liver, is related to anger: *Gallbladder causes anger*, DAN WEI NU 膽為怒 (SU WEN, Chapter 23).

Uncontrollable overflowing anger damages the functions of Gallbladder:
- Gallbladder does not function as *Rectitude of the Center* (ZHONG ZHENG 中正) - does not regulate the Water-Fire axis in man. In overflowing anger, the brutal ascent of *Liver QI/fire* injures the diaphragm (a muscle especially related to Gallbladder), which separates the chest (*clear*) and the abdomen (*turbid*), causing confusion of *clear* and *turbid*.
- Gallbladder loses its decisiveness and execution (JUE DUAN 決斷) (SU WEN, Chapter 8).
- Gallbladder does not regulate ZANG-FU 臟腑 (body function). *Each of the eleven organs take decisions from Gallbladder*, FAN SHI YI ZANG QU JUE YU DAN YE 凡十一藏取決於膽也 (SU WEN, Chapter 9).
- Gallbladder, one of the six Organs of Extraordinary Longevity (QI HENG ZHI FU 奇恒之腑) loses its 'roots' in Kidney-ZHI 志 and JING 精 storage is injured.

Gallbladder and ZHI 志 regulate the expression of anger, and therefore dysfunction in either or both may result in uncontrollable overflowing anger with no possibility of reasoning or stopping. Repressed frustrations and anger may injure first Liver-Gallbladder and then

---

356 See page 166
357 See page 169, SU WEN, Chapter 62

Kidney-ZHI 志. A man is lost to himself - unable to regulate, control or stop his anger. *Overflowing anger (SHENG NU 盛怒) causes deviation, confusion and loss of control* (LING SHU, Chapter 8-3).[358]

❖ LING SHU, Chapter 8-4: *When ZHI 志 is injured, the person forgets the words spoken before.*

Figure 55. Factors related to the ability to speak, according to Chinese medicine

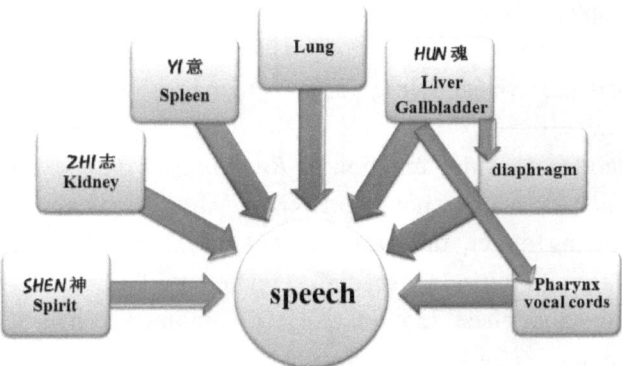

The person forgets the words spoken before may indicate memory loss, but also a disturbance in the use of language or the ability to speak. Factors which influence speech are (see Figure 55):
1. Liver-Gallbladder function:
   - Liver causes speech, GAN WEI YU 肝為語 (SU WEN, Chapter 23).
   - Throat (larynx) is the messenger of Liver and Gallbladder: *Liver is the general in the center. It receives its decisions from Gallbladder. The **throat** serves as its messenger* (SU WEN, Chapter 47).
     FU GAN ZHE ZHONG ZHI JIANG YE QU JUE YU DAN YAN WEI SHI
     夫肝者中之將也取決於膽咽為使.
   - Liver and Gallbladder rule all muscles, including the diaphragm which enables breathing and speech.

---

358 See page 253

- Choice of words comes from Gallbladder, which rules decisiveness and execution (JUE DUAN 决断) (SU WEN, Chapter 8).[359]
  The character Gallbladder-DAN 膽 shows the radical 月 'flesh', and the phonetic 詹, which has 厂 'a man standing in front of a precipice', 'danger', above 几 'separation' and 言 'word' or 'speech', conveying the meaning 'a warning of danger'.[360] The meaning of the character DAN 膽 is 'shouting to avoid danger (avoid falling from the precipice)'.
- Liver and Gallbladder (Wood) control Spleen-YI 意 (Soil). Bile secreted by Gallbladder helps Spleen to absorb flavors and QI from food. Similarly, Gallbladder (Liver YANG) organizes and regulates the registering of experiences, ideas and memories by means of Spleen-YI 意.
- Gallbladder affects brain activity, since Gallbladder Meridian flows on the head, where it has 20 points.

2. Lung, which rules breath and is therefore related to voice production.

3. The proper functioning of BEN SHEN 本神:
   - SHEN 神 rules all communication with the environment, including speech;
   - ZHI 志 contains memories of the ancestors,[361] and actualizes speech;
   - HUN 魂 provides the drive to communicate with society and the environment, and directs the process of speech;
   - YI 意 contains the library of intent, images, traces, ideas and words accumulated since birth.[362]

Water-ZHI 志 nourishes and strengthens Wood-HUN 魂 - the urge to speak in order to meet and communicate with the environment. ZHI 志 connects us to the desires, intent, experiences and discoveries of our ancestors. The ability to speak comes from the personal and

---

359 See page 43
360 Wieger, Lesson 59
361 See page 116 Chapter 4
362 See page 115 Chapter 4

social experiences of our ancestors and links the generations. ZHI 志 continuously prompts Liver and Gallbladder in deciding to use verbal ability, to move the vocal cords and diaphragm.

Anger injures ZHI 志 and impairs the ability of Gallbladder to organize and regulate experiences and thus YI 意 loses memories.³⁶³ In anger, speech becomes confused - words are spoken without decision and intent, automatically, devoid of context. In anger, speech may be loud or whispered, and this is a sign of suffering from an inability to communicate. According to ZHUANG ZI, Chapter 2:

> *Words are not just wind* (breath).... FU YAN FEI CHUI YE 夫言非吹也
> *People suppose that words are different from the peeps of baby birds, but is there any difference, or isn't there?*³⁶⁴ QI YI WEI YI YU KOU YIN YI YOU BIAN HU 其以為異於鷇音亦有辯乎

In anger, following injury to ZHI 志, there is damage to SHEN 神, described as *'a person forgets the words spoken before'*. Words are said like *peeps of baby birds* without purpose, involuntarily, just like secretion of sweat, tears or saliva. *'A person forgets the words spoken before'* may be called damage to working memory, which causes difficulty in using language and injures extended consciousness (SHEN 神). According to Damasio:

> *Working memory is the system responsible for the transient holding and processing of new and already-stored information, and is an important process for reasoning, comprehension, learning and memory updating.*³⁶⁵
> Working memory is *the ability to hold information in mind over a period of many seconds and to operate on it mentally.*³⁶⁶
> Extended consciousness... *depends on conventional memory and working memory. When it attains its human peak, it is also enhanced by language.*³⁶⁷

---

363 See page 115
364 Translation by B. Watson
365 Wikipedia. *Working memory*
366 Damasio, A. R. Descartes' Error: Emotion, Reason, and the Human Brain, p.62
367 Damasio, A. R., *The Feeling of What Happens*, p.14

❖ LING SHU, Chapter 8-4, anger: *Lower back and spine (back) are not able to bend, straighten, curl up or stretch.*

In overflowing anger, speech problems are associated with difficulties in body movement: painful muscles and contractions along the spine prevent bending down and straightening up.

Overflowing anger injures bones (ZHI 志 and Kidney YIN) and muscles (Liver YIN). SU WEN, Chapter 62, associates ZHI 志 and bones:
ZHI 志 and YI 意 communicate with each other inside the body and connect with bone marrow. ZHI YI TONG NEI LIAN GU SUI 志意通內連骨髓
LING SHU, Chapter 46, associates stiffness of muscles with anger:
When muscles are stiff and tight there is a lot of anger, GANG JIANG DUO NU 剛則多怒

Muscle cramps and difficulty in movement are signs of loss of body liquids. Stiffness is the opposite of flexibility and adaptability, which symbolize Water Modality, essential for life. The 'irrigation' of bones and joints by internal body liquids (YE 液) is described in LING SHU, Chapter 30:

> *When the grains enter* (stomach) *and QI is abundant, when substantial moisture penetrates the bones, when joints and bones allow to bend and straighten, when moisture is distributed, and is abundant in the brain and bone marrow, when the skin* (epidermis and dermis) *is irrigated, this is called* YE 液.
> 穀入氣滿, 淖澤注于骨, 骨屬屈伸, 泄澤補益腦髓, 皮膚潤澤, 是謂液

Muscle stiffness in overflowing anger is caused by:
- *Excess Liver fire* which dries body liquids and Blood
- *Kidney deficiency* and injury to ZHI 志, which prevent circulation of body liquids

❖ LING SHU, Chapter 8-4, anger: *Body hair breaks off; the complexion shows signs of premature death. Death will come in the last month of summer* (end of July and beginning of August)

Injury to Kidney is reflected in Lung - breaking of body hair (reversed generation), and in complexion (Water does not control Fire). The end of summer, the last month of summer (end of July and beginning of

August), is ruled by Soil Modality. At the end of summer, Soil over-controls Water, and then Kidney, weakened by overflowing anger, stops functioning and the patient dies.

Syndromes in Chinese medicine which describe the damage to Kidney and ZHI 志 caused by overflowing anger, LING SHU, Chapter 8-4

1. Confused Speech	
1a. YIN *Deficiency and Blood Dryness*, YIN XU XUE ZAO 陰虛血燥	Ki3-Ki7-H7, BL15-BL17, **H5-CV23**
1b. *Liver QI Congested and Knotted*, GAN QI YU JIE, 肝氣鬱結368	LIV3-LIV14, Ki7/Ki8-Ki5, **H5-CV23**
1c. *Phlegm-fire*, TAN HUO 痰火369	LIV2-CV12-ST40-ST41-GB8-BL8, **H5-CV23**
1d. *Blood flow Congested and Obstructed*, XUE XING YU ZHI 血行鬱滯370	SP10-SP6-BL17-LI4-ST36, **H5-CV23**
1f. *Heart and Spleen Dual Deficiency*, XIN PI LIANG XU 心脾兩虛371	BL15-BL20-SP6-ST36, GV22, **H5-CV23**
2. 'Overflowing anger in Kidney' and modern psychiatry	
2a. Invasion of personal space	BL18-**LIV5-GB40**-GB36,GB20-GB1, Ki5/**Ki7/Ki9**, BL52
2b. Adolescent identity crisis	GV26-CV6-Ki16, GB8, **LIV5-GB40**-LIV6-GV19, SP4, GV12, GB29-BL61-BL62, **Ki7-Ki9**
2c. Schizophrenia	
• Schizophrenia - YIN outbursts	GV16-GV14-GV26,CV15-CV12,PC7-PC8-SP1-LU11
• Schizophrenia - YANG outbursts	H7-SP6-BL18-BL20-BL15-GB30, ST40-CV12
2d. Uncontrollable overflowing anger in epilepsy, XIAN 癇	
• *Liver Fire and Phlegm-heat*, GAN HUO TAN RE 肝火痰熱	LIV2-H7-ST40-CV15-PC6-GV24
• YIN *Deficiency and* YANG *Excess*, YIN XU YANG SHENG 陰虛陽盛	SP6-Ki6-H7-BL18-BL23-CV15-GV24
• *Blood Flow Congested and Obstructed*, XUE XING YU ZHI 血行鬱滯372	SP6-SP10-BL20-ST40-LI4-CV15-GV14

---

368 See footnote 341, page 303
369 See footnote 331, page 290
370 See pages 295, 309, 332, 343
371 See pages 282. 296, 313, 334 sadness, in sorrow and grief, LING SHU, 8-4
372 See footnote 370, above

1. Confused Speech - damage to Kidney and ZHI 志 caused by overflowing anger

Acupuncture points to release speech are: **CV23-H5**

name	function	action
CV23 LIAN QUAN 廉泉 Ridge Spring	meeting of SHAO YIN, meeting of REN MAI with YIN WEI MAI	release ascent of body liquids, release tongue muscles
H5 TONG LI 通里 Penetrating the Interior	LUO of Heart	purify Heart, calm SHEN, release QI congestion in throat, tongue and speech

Figure 56. Uncontrollable overflowing anger causes confused speech. YIN *Deficiency and Blood Dryness*

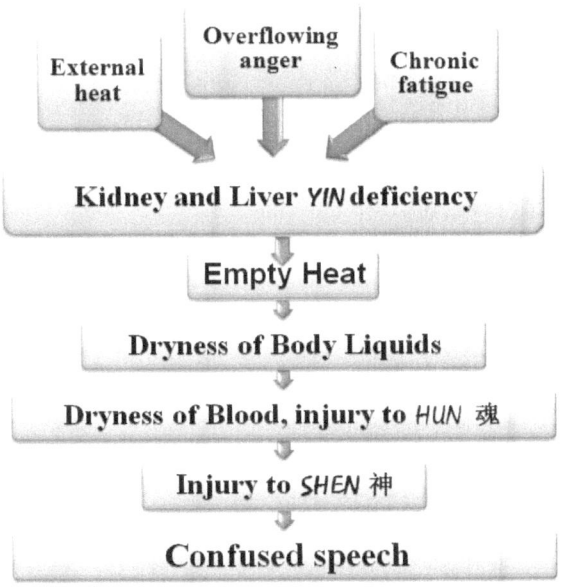

1a. Confused Speech, YIN *Deficiency and Blood Dryness,*
YIN XU XUE ZAO 陰虛血燥 - anger (Figure 56)

Etiology	Anger combined with external heat and/or chronic fatigue causes *Liver and Kidney* YIN *deficiency*. *Empty heat* dries body liquids and blood, thereby injuring SHEN and causing confused speech
Signs	confused speech, mental instability, anger, permanent conflict, alternating laughter and tears, exhaustion, palpitation, insomnia, fever in 'five palms', dry throat and night sweats
Tongue	red with dry coating
Pulse	thin (XI 細), wiry (XUAN 弦), fast (SHU 數)
Strategy	tonify YIN by SHAO YIN regulation, tonify Heart and Blood, release speech
Points	Ki3-Ki7-H7, BL15-BL17, **CV23-H5**

Acupuncture points to treat confused speech in *Kidney* YIN *Deficiency and Blood Dryness* - anger

name	function	action
Ki3-Ki7-H7 tonify YIN by regulation of SHAO YIN		
Ki3 TAI XI 太谿 Great Ravine	SHU-YUAN-Soil of Kidney	tonify Kidney YIN, release ascent of CHONG MAI and REN MAI, treat degenerative diseases, **tonify**
Ki7 FU LIU 復溜 Returning Current	JING-River-Metal of Kidney, tonify Water, enhance QI flow in Meridians from Ki. towards M.H. (PC)	tonify Kidney YIN, tonify Heart, reduce fire, tonify brain and bone marrow, improve coherence and decisiveness, calm anger
H7 SHEN MEN 神門 SHEN Gate	SHU-YUAN-Soil of Heart	calm SHEN, cool Heart, open Heart orifices

1b. Confused Speech, *Liver QI Congested and Knotted*,

GAN QI YU JIE, 肝氣鬱結 - anger

Compare overflowing anger (LING SHU, 8-3), melancholy and sadness, YU ZHENG (LING SHU, 8-4), ZANG ZAO and *Plum pit QI* in sorrow and grief (LING SHU, 8-4).

Confused speech and inability to communicate are characteristic of anger in Kidney.

Acupuncture points are: LIV3-LIV14, Ki7/Ki8-Ki5, **CV23-H5**

Acupuncture points to treat confused speech in *Liver QI Congested and Knotted* - anger

name	function	action
LIV3-LIV14 release congested Liver QI		
LIV3 TAI CHONG 太沖 Great Rush	SHU-YUAN-Soil of Liver	release and harmonize Liver
LIV14 QI MEN 期門 Cycle Gate	MU of Liver, regulate Liver YIN, meeting of Liv., Sp. Meridians and YIN WEI MAI	raise QI from abdomen to chest and release obstructions, benefit Gallbladder, circulate blood
Ki7/Ki8-Ki5 release and calm anger		
Ki7 FU LIU 復溜 Returning current	JING-River-Metal of Kidney, tonify Water, enhance QI flow in Meridians from Ki. towards M.H. (PC)	tonify Kidney YIN, brain and bone marrow, tonify Heart, reduce fire, improve coherence and decisiveness, calm anger
Ki8 JIAO XIN 交信 Intersecting Sincerity	XI of YIN QIAO MAI	clear heat, stimulate ZHI, improve coherence, decision ability, calm anger, drain damp from Lower JIAO
Ki5 SHUI QUAN 水泉 Water Spring	XI of Kidney	open Kidney obstruction, regulate CHONG MAI and REN MAI, treat menopause and andropause
BL15-BL17 tonify Heart and Blood		
BL15 XIN SHU 心俞 Heart SHU	SHU of Heart, regulate Heart YANG, release LUO of Heart	calm SHEN, move congestion of Heart blood, clear heat from Heart, tonify Heart YIN, **tonify**
BL17 GE SHU 膈俞 Diaphragm SHU	HUI-meeting of Blood, influence diaphragm	open chest, tonify and move blood, **tonify**

1c. Confused Speech, *Phlegm-fire*, TAN HUO 痰火 - anger

Compare Lily Bulb Disease, melancholy and sadness (LING SHU, 8-3), sorrow and grief, sorrow and grief causing ZANG ZAO (LING SHU, 8-4). Acupuncture points to disperse and purify *Liver fire*, dissolve *phlegm-fire* and release speech are: LIV2-CV12-ST40-ST41-GB8-BL8, **H5-CV23**

Acupuncture points to treat confused speech in *Phlegm-fire* - anger

name	function	action
LIV2-CV12-ST40-ST41-GB8-BL8 dissolve *phlegm-fire*, disperse and purify *Liver fire*		
ST40 FENG LONG 豐隆 Bountiful Bulge	LUO of Stomach	dissolve *phlegm-fire*, calm SHEN
ST41 JIE XI 解谿 Ravine Divide	JING-River-Fire of Stomach, tonify Soil	move fire congested in Stomach
CV12 ZHONG WAN 中脘 Central Venter	MU of Stomach, HUI-meeting of FU, 'knot' of TAI YIN, start of Lu. Meridian	move stagnations, regulate Stomach
LIV2 XING JIAN 行間 Moving Between	RONG-Fire of Liver	move YANG down, benefit G.B., stop wind, calm anger
GB8 SHUAI GU 率谷 Valley Lead	meeting of G.B. and Bl. Meridians	dissolve congested phlegm from brain
BL8 LUO QUE 絡卻 Declining Connection		clear sense organs, calm SHEN, transform phlegm, collect memory, disperse YANG from head

1d. Confused Speech, *Blood Flow Congested and Obstructed*, XUE XING YU ZHI 血行鬱滯 - anger

Compare melancholy and sadness - YU 鬱 of Blood (LING SHU, 8-4), KUANG in sorrow and grief, and joy and pleasure (LING SHU, 8-4).

Suppressed anger causes *Liver QI congestion* which obstructs the blood flow.

Confused speech appears after delivery or before menstruation in a woman physically and emotionally exhausted with a history of disease caused by 'heat' or menstrual disorders (Figure 57).

Acupuncture points to tonify Blood and QI and to release speech are: SP10-SP6-BL17-LI4-ST36, **H5-CV23**

Figure 57. Uncontrollable overflowing anger causes confused speech. *Blood Flow Congested and Obstructed*

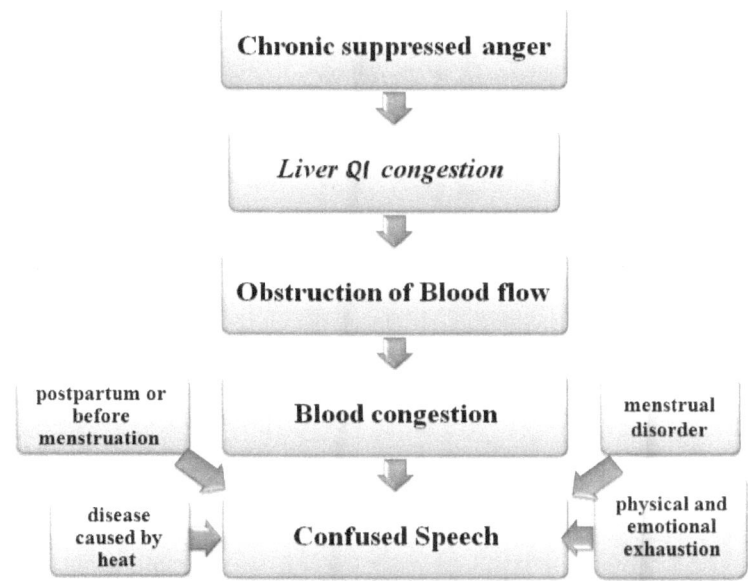

Acupuncture points to treat *Blood Flow Congested and Obstructed* -anger

name	function	action
SP10-SP6-BL17-LI4-ST36 tonify Blood and QI flow		
SP6 SAN YIN JIAO 三陰交 Meeting of Three YIN	meeting of Sp., Liv. and Ki. Meridians	tonify and nourish Blood, QI and YIN, move YIN up, nourish Spleen
SP10 XUE HAI 血海 Sea of Blood		invigorate and cool blood
BL17 GE SHU 膈俞 Diaphragm SHU	HUI-meeting of Blood, influence diaphragm	open chest, tonify and move blood
LI4 HE GU 合谷 Union Valley	YUAN of Large Intestine, entry point, command point of face and mouth	regulate QI, release excess YANG from head
ST36 ZU SAN LI 足三里 Leg Three Miles	HE-Soil of Stomach, tonify QI, Sea of Food point	regulate YANG deficiency above and YIN excess below: treat mental fatigue

1f. Confused Speech, *Heart and Spleen Dual Deficiency*,
XIN PI LIANG XU 心脾兩虛 - anger

Figure 58. Uncontrollable overflowing anger causes confused speech. *Heart and Spleen Dual Deficiency*

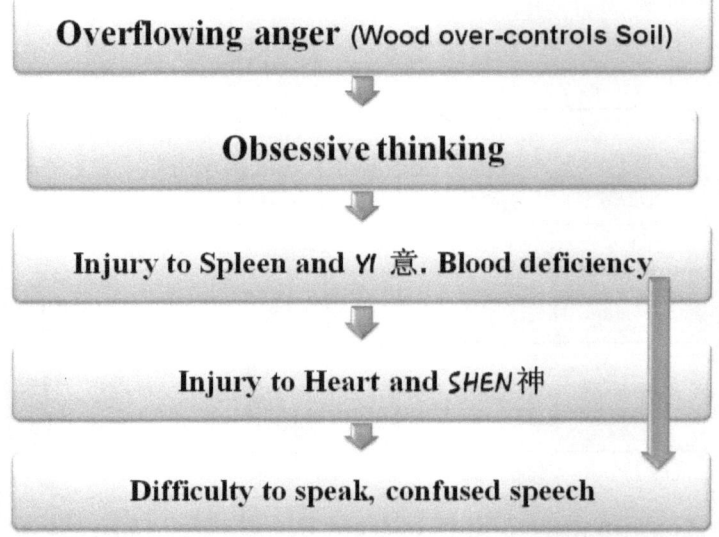

Compare melancholy and sadness (LING SHU, 8-3), apprehension, distress, obsessive thinking and worry (LING SHU, 8-4), YU ZHENG, melancholy and sadness (LING SHU, 8-), ZANG ZAO, sorrow and grief (LING SHU, 8-4).

In overflowing anger, Liver over-controls and depletes Spleen-YI 意. Spleen does not nourish Blood, resulting in *Blood deficiency* which injures Heart-SHEN, and this is expressed through difficulty in speaking, confused speech, a frightened, low voice (Figure 58). Acupuncture points for tonification of Spleen and Heart and to release speech are: BL15-BL20-SP6-ST36, GV22, **H5-CV23**.

Acupuncture points to treat *Heart and Spleen Dual Deficiency* - anger

name	function	action
BL15-BL20-SP6-ST36, GV22 tonify Spleen and Heart		
BL20 PI SHU 脾俞 Spleen SHU	SHU of Spleen, regulate Spleen YANG	tonify Spleen, **tonify**
BL15 XIN SHU 心俞 Heart SHU	SHU of Heart, regulate Heart YANG, release LUO of Heart	calm SHEN, tonify Heart YIN, **tonify**
SP6 SAN YIN JIAO 三陰交 Meeting of Three YIN	meeting of Sp., Liv. and Ki. Meridians	tonify and nourish Blood, QI and YIN, move YIN up, nourish Spleen, stop diarrhea, **tonify**
ST36 ZU SAN LI 足三里 Leg Three Miles	HE-Soil of Stomach, tonify QI, Sea of Food point, potentiate other points	regulate YANG deficiency above and YIN excess below, treat mental fatigue, **tonify**
GV22 XIN HUI 囟會 Fontanelle Meeting		strengthen JING, create new ideas

2. 'Overflowing anger in Kidney' and modern psychiatry
2a. 'Overflowing anger in Kidney' due to the invasion of personal space

Overflowing anger is an outburst of repressed anger emanating from cultural reasons or fear due to a continuous invasion of personal space with no possibility of escape.

Repressed anger is QI which is not a part of normal body QI, but obstructs ZHI 志-Kidney and HUN 魂-Liver-Gallbladder. This obstruction halts self-expression, and indirectly disturbs the relationship between YI 意 and ZHI 志. An outburst of violent anger disrupts contact with the environment and causes additional damage to the person. An outburst does not release anger, but continues to repress it, provoking degenerative diseases or cancer at menopause in women and in middle-aged men. Acupuncture points to release the congested QI of Liver, Kidney and Gallbladder obstructions are BL18-LIV5-GB40-GB36, GB20-GB1, Ki5/Ki7/Ki9-BL52

Acupuncture points to treat overflowing anger due to the invasion of personal space

name	function	action
BL18-LIV5-GB40-GB36 release congested Liver QI		
BL18 GAN SHU 肝俞 Liver SHU	SHU of Liver, regulate Liver YANG	move Liver QI and blood, **disperse**
LIV5 LI GOU 蠡溝 Woodworm Canal	LUO of Liver, start of LUO to genitals	calm and regulate Liver, benefit genitals, clear heat from Lower JIAO and Liver
GB40 QIU XU 丘墟 Hill Ruins	YUAN of Gallbladder, Group LUO of leg	disperse Gallbladder fire, regulate SHAO YANG
GB36 WAI QIU 外丘 Outer Hill	XI-Soil of Gallbladder	release anger, **needle in QI flow direction**
GB20-GB1 release Gallbladder		
GB20 FENG CHI 風池 Wind Pool	meeting of G.B., SAN JIAO meridian, YANG WEI MAI and YANG QIAO MAI	disperse heat and Liver wind, regulate QI and Blood, release YANG in back of neck and spine
GB1 TONG ZI LIAO 瞳子髎 Pupil Bone Hole	meeting of G.B., SAN JIAO and S.I. Meridians	clear excess heat
Ki5/Ki7/Ki9-BL52 release Kidney		
Ki5 SHUI QUAN 水泉 Water Spring	XI of Kidney	open Kidney obstruction, regulate CHONG MAI and REN MAI, treat menopause and andropause
Ki7 FU LIU 復溜 Returning current	JING-River-Metal of Kidney, tonify Water, enhance QI flow in Meridians from Ki. towards M.H. (PC)	tonify Kidney YIN, tonify Heart, reduce fire, move dampness, calm anger, improve coherence and decisiveness
Ki9 ZHU BIN 築賓 Guest House	XI and start of YIN WEI MAI, start of Ki.-Bl. JING BIE	cut harmful hereditary transfers (S. de Morand, page 519), purify Heart, calm SHEN, calm rage, insults, swearing, hate
BL52 ZHI SHI 志室 ZHI Chamber	influence ZHI, gather JING	warm QI, tonify Kidney, ZHI and JING

2b. 'Overflowing anger in Kidney' in adolescent identity crisis

Puberty is rapid and natural changes in Liver-HUN 魂 and Kidney-ZHI 志. When HUN 魂 and PO 魄, symbolizing father and mother, are not balanced, ZHI 志 is unstable. When YI 意 (ideas and images) is in disorder and is supported by unstable ZHI 志, disruptions occur in self-image and in the image of the environment, causing suffering.

Treatment of adolescent identity crisis is to release *Congested Liver QI* and HUN 魂, calm anger and treat addictions. Acupuncture points are: GV26-CV6-Ki16, GB8, LIV5-GB40-LIV6-GV19, SP4, GV12, GB29-BL61-BL62, Ki7-Ki9

Acupuncture points to treat adolescent identity crisis

name	function	action
LIV5-GB40-LIV6-GV19 release congested Liver QI and HUN 魂		
LIV5 LI GOU 蠡溝 Woodworm Canal	LUO of Liver, start of LUO to genitals	calm and regulate Liver, benefit genitals, clear heat from Lower JIAO and Liver
GB40 QIU XU 丘墟 Hill Ruins	YUAN of Gallbladder, Group LUO of leg	disperse *Gallbladder fire*, regulate SHAO YANG
LIV6 ZHONG DU 中都 Capital center	XI of Liver	sedate and regulate Liver, release Liver QI and blood
GV19 HOU DING 後頂 Behind the Vertex	influence HUN 魂	regulate YANG, calm *Liver fire rising* and HUN 魂
SP4 ,GV12, GB29-BL61-BL62, Ki7-Ki9 (see above) calm the anger		
SP4 GONG SUN 公孫 Grandfather-Grandson	opening of CHONG MAI, LUO of Spleen	raise Spleen QI through CHONG MAI, regulate neurohormonal system in adolescent [373]
GV12 SHEN ZHU 身柱 Body Pillar		calm uncontrollable hatred and desire to kill, purify Heart and Lung
GB29 JU LIAO 居髎 Squatting Bone Hole	meeting of G.B. Meridian, YANG WEI MAI and YANG QIAO MAI	strengthen lumbar region, clear heat
BL61 PU CAN 僕參 Subservient Visitor	meeting of YANG QIAO MAI and Bl. Meridian	calm brain, treat mental immaturity
BL62 SHEN MAI 申脈 SHEN Hour Vessel	open YANG QIAO MAI	purify head and eyes, restore presence and vigilance
GV26-CV6-Ki16 treat alcohol addiction, GB8 treat drug addiction		
GV26 SHUI GOU 水溝 Water Through	open LUO channels in face region	calm SHEN, open Heart orifices, purify head and brain
CV6 QI HAI 氣海 Sea of QI	MU of QI	tonify QI and especially Source QI, move congested QI, treat depression with desire to die (S. de Morand, page 615)
Ki16 HUANG SHU 肓俞 Membrane SHU	meeting of CHONG MAI and Ki. Meridian	treat feeling of emotional rejection
GB8 SHUAI GU 率谷 Valley Lead	meeting of G.B. and Bl. Meridians	dissolve congested phlegm from brain, treat drug addiction

---

[373] Influence the axis hypothalamus- pituitary-adrenal, according to Bossy

Frustrations, accumulated during the disordered construction of the personality, congest Liver QI. *Congested Liver QI*, together with unstable HUN 魂 and ZHI 志, cause *Liver fire rising*: an identity crisis, aggression, anger and violence. Alcohol and drug abuse complicate the situation and increase the instability of BEN SHEN 本神. The adolescent outburst of anger, coming from frustration and suffering, constitutes a powerful and uncontrollable hatred, with a tendency to curse and insult, to break, and a desire to kill.

2c. 'Overflowing anger in Kidney' - Schizophrenia

Schizophrenia is a mental disorder characterized by abnormal social behavior, failure to recognize what is real, disorganized thinking and speech. In Traditional Chinese medicine schizophrenia is part of DIAN KUANG 癲狂[374] In Modern China schizophrenia is called 'separation and rupture of JING and SHEN' (JING SHEN FEN LI 精神分裂). Between outbursts, schizophrenia may correspond to the following syndromes of Traditional Chinese Medicine:

- *Liver QI Congested and Knotted*, GAN QI YU JIE 肝氣鬱結[375]
- *Phlegm and QI Congested and Knotted*, TAN QI YU JIE 痰氣鬱結[376]
- *Phlegm-Dampness and QI Deficiency*, TAN SHI QI XU 痰濕氣虛[377]
- *Phlegm-Fire*, TAN HUO 痰火[378]
- *Heart and Spleen Dual Deficiency*, XIN PI LIANG XU 心脾兩虛[379]
- *YIN Deficiency and YANG Excess*, YIN XU YANG SHENG 陰虛陽盛[380]
- *Blood Flow Congested and Obstructed*, XUE XING YU ZHI 血行鬱滯[381]

Outbursts of schizophrenia alternate between the extremes of 'blazing fire' caused by HUN 魂 and 'freezing' caused by PO 魄, obstructing the Water-Fire axis and producing phlegm (TAN 痰).

---

374 See page 352
375 See footnote 341, page 303
376 See page 293, melancholy and sadness, LING SHU, 8-4
377 See page 283
378 See pages 307, 312, 317, 332 LING SHU, 8-3, LING SHU, 8-4
379 See footnote 342, page 303
380 See page 342
381 See pages 295, 332, 343

- YANG outburst of schizophrenia ('blazing fire' caused by HUN 魂, corresponding to 'overflowing anger in Kidney') is a serious obstruction of SHEN 神, expressed in restlessness and confusion of speech and thought (YI 意).
- YIN outburst of schizophrenia ('freezing' caused by PO 魄) imprisons SHEN 神, and is expressed in sadness, depression, withdrawal, lack of communication with the environment.

Overflowing anger in Kidney, YANG outbursts of schizophrenia

Signs	*QI excess*; agitation, rage, hallucinations; difficulty in thinking consistently; strange, extrovert and eccentric behavior with shouting; red complexion and eyes, dry stool
Tongue	red with yellow coating
Pulse	wiry (XUAN 弦), fast (SHU 數) with force (YOU LI 有力)
Strategy	calm excess YANG, dissolve *phlegm-fire*
Points	H7-SP6-BL18-BL20-BL15-GB30, ST40-CV12

Acupuncture points to treat YANG outbursts of schizophrenia, Overflowing anger in Kidney

name	function	action
H7-SP6-BL18-BL20-BL15-GB30 calm excess YANG		
H7 SHEN MEN 神門 SHEN Gate	SHU-YUAN-Soil of Heart	calm SHEN, cool Heart, open Heart orifices
SP6 SAN YIN JIAO 三陰交 Meeting of Three YIN	meeting of Sp., Liv. and Ki. Meridians	tonify and nourish Spleen, Blood, QI and YIN, move YIN up
BL18 GAN SHU 肝俞 Liver SHU	SHU of Liver, regulate Liver YANG	calm Liver
BL20 PI SHU 脾俞 Spleen SHU	SHU of Spleen, regulate Spleen YANG	tonify Spleen
BL15 XIN SHU 心俞 Heart SHU	SHU of Heart, regulate Heart YANG	calm SHEN, clear heat from Heart, tonify Heart YIN
GB30 HUAN TIAO 環跳 Jumping Round	meeting of G.B. and Bl. Meridians	calm and regulate YANG, **tonify**
ST40-CV12 dissolve *phlegm-fire*		
ST40 FENG LONG 豐隆 Bountiful Bulge	LUO of Stomach	dissolve *phlegm-fire*, calm SHEN, **disperse**
CV12 ZHONG WAN 中脘 Central Venter	MU of Stomach, HUI-meeting of FU, 'knot' of TAI YIN, start of Lu. Meridian	move stagnations, regulate Stomach, dissolve phlegm

Overflowing anger in Kidney - YIN outbursts of schizophrenia alternate with YANG outbursts

Signs	QI *deficiency*: exhaustion, no physical strength, mute; motionless in bizarre postures, slow reaction, difficulty in thinking, 'loose spirit', no will to live (ZHI 志), dark or pale complexion
Tongue	pale
Pulse	thin (XI 細), sinking (CHEN 沉)
Strategy	activate REN MAI and DU MAI, dissolve phlegm from Heart
Points	GV16-GV14-GV26, CV15-CV12, PC7-PC8-SP1-LU11

Acupuncture points to treat YIN outbursts of schizophrenia

name	function	action
GV16-GV14-GV26, CV15-CV12 activate REN MAI and DU MAI		
GV16 FENG FU 風府 Wind Mansion	meeting of DU MAI with YANG WEI MAI, point of bone marrow	move Source QI and JING up to brain, treat confusion, **gentle superficial tonification**
GV14 DA ZHUI 大椎 Big Mallet	meeting of DU MAI with six YANG Meridians	regulate QI and YANG flow to head and Heart, release excess heat and damp-heat from upper body
GV26 SHUI GOU Water Trough 水溝	open LUO channels in face region	calm SHEN, open Heart orifices, purify head and brain
CV15 JIU WEI 鳩尾 Turtledove Tail	LUO of REN MAI, YUAN of GAO - liquid fat	restore communication between inside and outside in divided consciousness, schizophrenia
CV12 ZHONG WAN 中脘 Central Venter	MU of Stomach, HUI-meeting of FU, 'knot' of TAI YIN, start of Lu. Meridian	move stagnations, regulate Stomach, dissolve phlegm
GB30 HUAN TIAO 環跳 Jumping Round	meeting of G.B. and Bl. Meridians	calm and regulate YANG
PC7-PC8-SP1-LU11 dissolve phlegm from Heart, assist other points		
PC7 DA LING 大陵 Big Mound	SHU-YUAN-Soil of Master of Heart	calm and purify SHEN
PC8 LAO GONG 勞宮 Labor Palace	RONG-Fire of Master of Heart	purify Heart, awaken SHEN
SP1 YIN BAI 隱白 Hidden White	JING-Well-Wood of Spleen	anchor a person to earth, give clarity of thought
LU11 SHAO SHANG 少商 Lesser Merchant	JING-Well-Wood of Lung	calm

2d. Overflowing anger in Kidney - epilepsy (XIAN 癇)

The character epilepsy-XIAN 癇 shows the radical 疒 'disease' and the phonetic 閒 'gap'. Epilepsy is a group of neurological diseases characterized by seizures.

Epileptic seizures are episodes that can vary from brief and nearly undetectable to prolonged, vigorous shaking, and are the result of excessive and abnormal nerve cell activity in the brain cortex.

The brain, Sea of Bone Marrow, is also one of the six Organs of Extraordinary Longevity (QI HENG ZHI FU 奇恒之腑) – storage of JING 精 governed by Kidney.

Epileptic seizures, which include loss of consciousness, convulsions, tongue biting and loss of bladder control, are signs of injury to Kidney. Some types of epilepsy include violent behavior, rage and aggression. In another type of epilepsy, there is a cessation of awareness: if the attack comes while the person is talking, he stops talking and afterwards does not remember the attack.

Overflowing anger in epilepsy - *Liver Fire and Phlegm-heat*, GAN HUO TAN RE 肝火痰熱

Signs	Rage in epilepsy with restlessness, frustration, insomnia, dry mouth, bitter taste in mouth, cough with yellow sputum, constipation
Tongue	red with yellow thin coating
Pulse	slippery (HUA 滑) or wiry (XUAN 弦), fast (SHU 數)
Strategy	dissolve *phlegm-heat* and calm *Liver Fire*
Points	LIV2-H7-ST40-CV15-PC6-GV24

Acupuncture points to treat overflowing anger in epilepsy
Liver Fire and Phlegm-heat

name	function	action
LIV2-H7-ST40-CV15-PC6-GV24 dissolve *phlegm-heat* and calm *Liver fire*		
H7 SHEN MEN 神門 SHEN Gate	SHU-YUAN-Soil of Heart	calm SHEN, cool Heart, open Heart orifices
LIV2 XING JIAN 行間 Moving Between	RONG-Fire of Liver	benefit Gallbladder, move YANG down, stop wind, calm anger
ST40 FENG LONG 豐隆 Bountiful Bulge	LUO of Stomach	dissolve *phlegm-fire* (heat), calm SHEN, **disperse**
CV15 JIU WEI 鳩尾 Turtledove Tail	LUO of REN MAI, YUAN of GAO - liquid fat	restoration of communication between inside and outside, in divided consciousness, epilepsy
PC6 NEI GUAN 內關 Inner Barrier	LUO of Master of Heart, open YIN WEI MAI	release three YIN, open chest, remove congestion between pelvis and chest, regulate QI, awaken SHEN
GV24 SHEN TING 神庭 SHEN Court	meeting of DU MAI with the Bl. and St. Meridians	communicate between orifices, calm SHEN, regulate mental restlessness

Overflowing anger in epilepsy - YIN *Deficiency and* YANG *Excess,* YIN XU YANG SHENG 陰虛陽盛

Signs	Rage during several days before an epileptic seizure, memory problems, low back pain, tinnitus, insomnia, heat in 'five palms', constipation
Tongue	red with peeled coating
Pulse	thin (XI 細), fast (SHU 數)
Strategy	nourish YIN, regulate YANG
Points	SP6-Ki6-H7-BL18-BL23-CV15-GV24

Acupuncture points to treat overflowing anger in epilepsy
YIN *Deficiency and* YANG *Excess*

name	function	action
SP6-Ki6-H7-BL18-BL23-CV15-GV24 nourish YIN, regulate YANG		
SP6 SAN YIN JIAO 三陰交 Meeting of Three YIN	meeting of Sp., Liv. and Ki. Meridians	tonify and nourish Blood, QI and YIN, move YIN up, nourish Spleen
Ki6 ZHAO HAI 照海 Shining Sea	open YIN QIAO MAI, ascent of YIN in SHAO YIN	calm SHEN, treat insomnia
H7 SHEN MEN 神門 SHEN Gate	SHU-YUAN-Soil of Heart	calm SHEN, cool Heart, open Heart orifices, treat insomnia
BL18 GAN SHU 肝俞 Liver SHU	SHU of Liver, regulate Liver YANG	tonify Liver YIN, move Liver QI and blood stagnation down from head, **disperse**
BL23 SHEN SHU 腎俞 Kidney SHU	SHU of Kidney, regulate Kidney YANG	tonify Kidney YIN
CV15 JIU WEI 鳩尾 Turtledove Tail	LUO of REN MAI, YUAN of GAO - liquid fat	restoration of communication between inside and outside, in divided consciousness, epilepsy
GV24 SHEN TING 神庭 SHEN Court	meeting of DU MAI with Bl. And St. Meridians	communicate between orifices, calm SHEN, regulate mental restlessness

Overflowing anger in epilepsy - *Blood Flow Congested and Obstructed*, XUE XING YU ZHI 血行鬱滯

Compare melancholy and sadness, sorrow and grief, joy and pleasure, and rage (LING SHU, 8-4).

Epilepsy in this case may originate from any kind of head injury, including injuries during childbirth. Its signs are: prolonged stabbing headache in a permanent location, aggravated at night, and rage before an epileptic seizure. Acupuncture points to circulate blood in head: SP6-SP10-BL20-ST40-LI4-CV15-GV14

Acupuncture points to treat overflowing anger in epilepsy - *Blood Flow Congested and Obstructed*

name	function	action
SP6-SP10-BL20-ST40-LI4-CV15-GV14 tonify blood flow in head		
SP10 XUE HAI 血海 Sea of Blood		invigorate and cool blood
SP6 SAN YIN JIAO 三陰交 Meeting of Three YIN	meeting of Sp., Liv. and Ki. Meridians	tonify and nourish Blood, QI and YIN, move YIN up, nourish Spleen
BL20 PI SHU 脾俞 Spleen SHU	SHU of Spleen, regulate Spleen YANG	tonify Spleen
ST40 FENG LONG 豐隆 Bountiful Bulge	LUO of Stomach	dissolve *phlegm-fire*/heat, calm SHEN
LI4 HE GU 合谷 Union Valley	YUAN of Large Intestine, entry point, command of face and mouth	regulate QI, release excess YANG from head
CV15 JIU WEI 鳩尾 Turtledove Tail	LUO of REN MAI, YUAN of GAO - liquid fat	restore communication between inside and outside in divided consciousness, epilepsy
GV14 DA ZHUI 大椎 Big Mallet	meeting of DU MAI with six YANG Meridians	regulate QI and YANG flow to head and heart, release excess heat and *damp-heat* from upper body

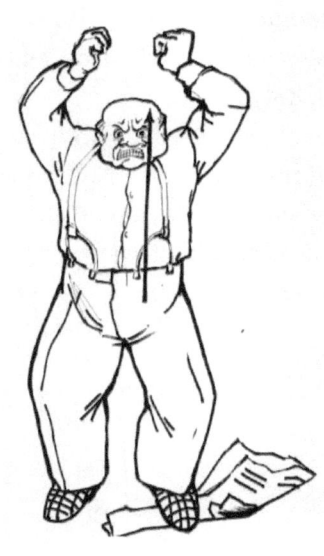

F. Damage to Kidney, JING 精 and bones caused by fear and dread (KONG JU 懼恐), LING SHU, Chapter 8-4

恐 KONG	fear	精 JING		是 SHI	be	而 ER	then
懼 JU	dread	傷 SHANG	injure	故 GU	thus	陰 YIN	
而 ER	then	則 ZE	this	五 WU	5	虛 XU	deficiency
不 BU	not	骨 GU	bone	藏 ZANG	organ	陰 YIN	
解 JIE	loose	痠 SUAN	pain	主 ZHU	direct	虛 XU	deficiency
則 ZE	this	痿 WEI	paralysis	藏 CANG	store	則 ZE	this
傷 SHANG	injure	厥 JUE	exhaust	精 JING		無 WU	no
精 JING		精 JING		者 ZHE	comma	氣 QI	
		時 SHI	occasion	也 YE	period	無 WU	no
		自 ZI	by itself	不 BU	not	氣 QI	
		下 XIA	descend	可 KE	able	則 ZE	then
				傷 SHANG	injure	死 SI	death
				傷 SHANG	injure	也 YE	period
				則 ZE	this		
				失 SHI	lose		
				守 SHOU	conserve		

Fear and dread (KONG JU 懼恐) *without release* (BU JIE 不解) *injure* JING 精.

Injury to JING 精 *causes pain in the bones, obstructions* (muscular flaccidity or atrophy of the limbs with motor impairment, WEI 痿), *and fatigue* (JUE 厥).

Sometimes JING 精 *flows down spontaneously.*

Indeed, the five ZANG *direct the* JING 精 *storage. They* (ZANG) *should not be harmed. If ZANG are harmed they lose their ability to conserve. Then* YIN *is deficient.* YIN *deficiency causes loss of* QI 氣. *Loss of* QI 氣 *is death.*

Five BEN SHEN 本神, the 'treasures' stored in the five ZANG, direct the JING 精 storage, and control Source and acquired JING, but it is Kidney-ZHI 志 that is directly responsible for JING storage. Kidney YIN accumulates JING through Source QI (YUAN QI 原氣/元氣). Kidney YANG (MING MEN 命門) controls the flow of vital QI (JING QI 精氣, QI carrying JING) to the other four ZANG. Kidney is the root of human existence and continuation of life. Source QI connects my Kidney with Kidney of my mother and Kidney of my father at conception.

All types of fear (apprehension, distress and dread) are emotions of Kidney. LING SHU, Chapter 8, gives a central place to fear in damage to JING 精. Chapters 8-3 and 8-4, begin and end with a description of damage caused by different types of fear.

> LING SHU, Chapter 8-3: *So apprehension, distress, obsessive thinking and worry (contemplation) injure SHEN. The injury to SHEN is expressed as fear and dread* (KONG JU 懼恐). *(JING 精) flows down, overflows and cannot stop.*[382]
>
> *In fear and dread* (KONG JU 懼恐) *SHEN is restless and scared away, and the person cannot be himself.*[383]
>
> LING SHU, Chapter 8-4: *When apprehension, distress, obsessive thinking and worry invade Heart, SHEN is injured. The injury to SHEN is expressed as fear and dread* (KONG JU 懼恐) *and loss of self.*[384]

Human life is accompanied throughout by a fear of death and a desire to live, which are the roots of motivation and actions. Kidney is the source of the paradox of human existence: fear of death related to a desire to live allows life, but fear accompanies a man throughout his life and shortens it.

❖ LING SHU, Chapter 8-4: *Fear and dread* (KONG JU 懼恐) *without release* (BU JIE 不解) *injure JING 精*

In LING SHU, Chapter 8-4, fear and dread are constantly present without the possibility of release (BU JIE 不解). The character JIE 解 is translated as 'release', 'loosen', 'untie', 'unfasten', and shows the

---

[382] See page 216
[383] See page 266
[384] See page 280

radicals 角 'horn', 牛 'ox' and 刀 'knife'. The character JIE 解 reminds us of the story of cutting an ox in ZHUANG ZI, Chapter 3. When the cook is cutting up an ox, his SHEN guides the knife through the intervals between tendons and joints without touching bones.

When fear and dread are constantly present without any possibility of release, Kidney is damaged and the JING reserves are deficient. SU WEN, Chapter 39, presents a connection between fear and JING:
> Fear (KONG 恐) makes JING 精 retreat. When JING retreats Upper JIAO closes. When (Upper JIAO) is closed, QI reverses its flow (descends toward the pelvis). (When QI) reverses its flow, the Lower JIAO inflates. So QI does not circulate.[385]

Fear and dread without release empty Kidney and Lower JIAO, causing obstruction of Upper JIAO. When Upper JIAO is obstructed, body liquids cannot rise, leading to swelling in hips, legs and abdomen.

In fear and dread, Water-Kidney does not control Fire-Heart, provoking conflict between Kidney YIN (Source QI and JING 精 storage) and Original/Source Fire-Kidney YANG (MING MEN 命門, the root of SAN JIAO).

❖ LING SHU, Chapter 8-4, fear and dread: *Injury to JING 精 causes pain in the bones, obstructions* (WEI 痿) *and fatigue* (JUE 厥).

Fear and dread deplete JING 精 in bone marrow and bones - Organs of Extraordinary Longevity (QI HENG ZHI FU 奇恒之腑). Kidney JING deficiency causes Kidney YIN deficiency, resulting in fatigue (JUE 厥), bone pain and QI flow obstruction (WEI 痿).

WEI 痿 is muscular flaccidity or atrophy of the limbs with motor impairment in the lower part of the body, expressed as dysfunction of muscle and tendons, weakness, atrophy or paralysis in the legs, and erectile dysfunction. Bone pain can also be an expression of WEI 痿.

---

385 See page 187

Body liquids (JIN YE 津液) and JING 精 participate in the production of the liquid fat (GAO 膏) that maintains bone marrow, bones, brain and the central nervous system (which store JING 精) and sperm (JING YE 精液, body liquids which transfer and emit JING 精). LING SHU, Chapter 36, relates the production of body liquids to liquid fat (GAO 膏) and to bones. JING 精 deficiency causes depletion of the liquid fat necessary for the maintenance of bones, and bones become painful:

> *The external and internal body liquids (JIN YE 津液) of five ZANG merge, gather and form liquid fat (GAO 膏). (Liquid fat) penetrates and strengthens bones and fills the brain and bone marrow, and flows down towards YIN (genitals) and legs.*
>
> *Imbalance of YIN and YANG increases the downward flow of YE 液 towards the genitals. The amount of YE 液 intended for bone marrow decreases and dries. Excessive descent of YE 液 leads to deficiencies which cause pain in hips, kidneys and the back of the neck.*

Muscular flaccidity or atrophy of the limbs with motor impairment (WEI 痿) results from the dysfunction of Muscle of Ancestors (ZONG JIN 宗筋). ZONG JIN is the center of the perineum, site of the attachment of the abdominal muscles, and allows the functioning of penis (erection) and clitoris.

> SU WEN, Chapter 44: *Muscle of Ancestors (ZONG JIN 宗筋) directs the gathering of bones and allows the function of joints. When Muscle of Ancestors is not irrigated, it dries and is obstructed.*

Further on, SU WEN Chapter 44 describes the deterioration of Muscle of Ancestors from weakness to paralysis:

> *Thoughts and reflections without limit, unsatisfied desires, intentions oriented towards the outside, exaggerated visits to the bedroom* (exaggeration in sex), (these) *relax Muscle of Ancestors (ZONG JIN 宗筋) which is expressed as WEI 痿* (muscular flaccidity or atrophy with motor impairment) *of tendons and vaginal secretions. The Classics said: the paralysis of tendons comes from Liver following an exaggeration in sex.*

When Water does not control Fire, the bones dry, bone marrow is depleted, legs do not carry the body, the condition shows WEI 痿 *of bones* (atrophy of limbs with motor impairment).

思想無窮所願不得意淫於外入房太甚宗筋弛縱發為筋痿及為白淫故《下經》曰：筋痿者生於肝使內也... 今水不勝火，則骨枯而髓虛，故足不任身，發為骨痿

Kidney YIN *deficiency causes empty heat.* SU WEN, Chapter 44, also describes WEI 痿 of bones caused by Kidney heat:

腎	SHEN	kidney	骨	GU	bones	發	FA	develop
氣	QI		枯	KU	dry	為	WEI	call
熱	RE	heat	髓	SUI	bone marrow	骨	GU	bone
則	ZE	this	減	JIAN	diminish	痿	WEI	atrophy
腰	YAO	hips						
脊	JI	back						
不	BU	not						
舉	JU	rise						

When heat QI *is in Kidney, hips and back cannot rise,*
Bones dry and bone marrow diminishes.
The situation develops into atrophy (WEI 痿) *of bones.*

LING SHU, Chapter 22, describes a relationship between chronic depression (DIAN 癲) and bones - a condition similar to JING 精 deficiency that causes pain in the bones:

> *When* DIAN 癲 *disease is in bones, points* (of acupuncture) *in the flesh in the interval between the upper jaw and teeth* (gums) *are swollen. Bones are prominent. There is sweating and apathy* (depression). *When there is a lot of vomiting and foamy saliva,* QI *spreads downward and there is no treatment for the disease.*[386]

---

386 See page 370

❖ LING SHU, Chapter 8-4, fear and dread: *Sometimes JING 精 flows down spontaneously.*

A medical text from the QING dynasty, *Encyclopedia of Ancient and Modern Medical Systems* (GE JIN YI TONG DA QUAN 古今醫統大全) describes a process of JING 精 loss resulting from loss of communication between Water and Fire:

Heart shapes Fire-governor, Kidney shapes Fire-minister. By order of destiny (MING 命) or Fire-governor, Fire-minister circulates JING 精. Indeed, when Kidney is sick, responsibility (for JING circulation) *is transmitted to Heart. Heart indeed rules SHEN 神. When SHEN suddenly becomes restless, JING 精 dissipates.*

Fear and dread injure communication between Water and Fire, causing an additional loss of JING 精 from the lower part of the body through spermatorrhea, vaginal discharge and constant liquid diarrhea.

❖ LING SHU, Chapter 8-4, fear and dread: *The five ZANG direct JING 精 storage. They (ZANG) should not be harmed. If ZANG are harmed, they lose their ability to conserve, and then YIN is deficient. YIN deficiency causes loss of QI. Loss of QI is death.*

According to SU WEN, Chapter 6:

Whatever does not emerge out of Earth is called 'based in YIN' and is called YIN in the center of YIN. Whatever emerges out of Earth is called YANG in the center of YIN. YANG gives the direction but YIN rules.

未出地者,命曰陰處,名曰陰中之陰;則出地者,命曰陰中之陽。陽予之正,陰為之主

Fear and dread cause JING 精 deficiency in Kidney and interfere with the distribution of JING 精 to ZANG. The resulting JING 精 deficiency in ZANG, which then cannot conserve YIN, provokes Kidney YIN deficiency, which causes YANG to lose root and direction. Therefore *empty fire* is released, harms the five ZANG and causes obstructions in the QI flow (WEI 痿):

- *Empty fire* in Heart dries blood,
- *Empty fire* in Liver causes contractions and muscular dystrophy,
- *Empty fire* in Spleen causes a feeling of numbness in flesh,
- *Empty fire* in Lung dries body fluids, and prevents the cooling and dissipation of QI and further dries Kidney (Lung does not nourish Kidney),
- *Empty fire* in Kidney 'burns' body liquids, bones, bone marrow, JING and causes death.

LING SHU, Chapter 8-4, in the last phrase, emphasizes the importance of BEN SHEN 本神 in acupuncture treatment:

是	SHI	be	以	SHI	in order	五	WU	5
故	GU	thus	知	ZHI	know	者	ZHE	comma
用	YONG	use	精	JING		以	YI	in order
鍼	ZHEN	needle	神	SHEN		傷	SHANG	damage
者	ZHE	comma	魂	HUN		鍼	ZHEN	needle
察	CHA	observe	魄	PO		不	BU	not
觀	GUAN	examine	之	ZHI	of	可	KE	able
病	BING	sick	存	CUN	presence	以	YI	in order
人	REN	man	亡	WANG	absence	治	ZHI	treat
之	ZHI	of	得	DE	obtain	之	ZHI	
態	TAI	state	失	SHI	lose	也	YE	period
			之	ZHI	of			
			意	YI				

Therefore, when using needles, observe and examine the condition of the patient in order to distinguish the presence or absence of JING, SHEN, HUN and PO 精神魂魄, *and the existence or loss of YI* 意 (intent).

If these five (JING, SHEN, HUN, PO, YI) are damaged, the person cannot be treated with needles.

9

LING SHU, Chapter 22, DIAN KUANG BING 癲狂病, madness and insanity

LING SHU, Chapter 22, presents treatments for severe mental disorders. This chapter is interesting and important, but also condensed and complicated to understand since definitions of diseases are vague and lack precision. However, it must be remembered that in ancient China definitions of diseases were not the same as those current today. When translating DIAN KUANG it should also be noted that definitions of mental diseases in ancient China were different from those used by modern psychiatry. Psychologists and psychiatrists are invited to compare the conditions described in LING SHU, Chapter 22, with modern definitions of mental diseases.

The title of LING SHU, Chapter 22, DIAN KUANG BING 癲狂病, may be interpreted in several ways: insanity and madness, depression and manic disease, quiet and agitated mental disorders, YIN madnesses and YANG madnesses. The character DIAN 癲 shows the radical 疒 'disease', and the phonetic 顛 'top of the head'.[387] DIAN 癲 means a disease that strikes the top of the head and is translated as 'madness', 'depression', 'mental (personality, mood swings) disorders', 'quiet, introverted YIN psychoses'. DIAN also includes a YIN type of restlessness which is not expressed outwardly.

The character KUANG 狂 shows the radical 犭[388] 'dog' and the phonetic 王 'king'. KUANG 狂 means 'a dog who thinks he is a king' and is translated as 'madness', 'insanity', 'mental or personality disorders' or 'agitated, extraverted and violent YANG type psychoses'.

Two of the classical commentaries on LING SHU, those of ZHANG JING YUE and ZHANG ZHI CANG, are used here for better understanding of

---

387 Wieger, Lesson 160
388 Radical 94 犬

LING SHU, Chapter 22. Methods of treatment are presented according to LEI JING and according to the clinical experience of Dr. J.M. Eyssalet.

LING SHU, Chapter 22, describes various, mostly severe, mental diseases accompanied by changes in body function (muscles, bones, nervous system, body liquids, Blood) and gives valuable instructions for treatment of:
1. DIAN 癲 – body-mind-spirit 'quiet' (YIN) disorders: mental (personality) disorders, psychoses (withdrawal, dysthymia, depression),
2. KUANG 狂 – body-mind-spirit 'agitated' (YANG) disorders: mental (personality) disorders, psychoses (mania, schizophrenia),
3. NI 逆 – rebel or counterflow QI, which flows either in a contrary direction or in an exaggerated fashion in the correct direction, causing congestion and obstruction.

LING SHU, Chapter 22, includes:
1. Eye examination (SHEN 神 is reflected in the eyes), (22-1)

2. Treatment of DIAN 癲 disease - quiet (YIN) body-mind-spirit disorders
   A. First signs of the onset of DIAN 癲 disease (22-2)
   B. Onset of DIAN 癲 disease together with restlessness and facial muscle contractions (22-3)
   C. Onset of DIAN 癲 disease together with muscle rigidity and backache (22-4)
   D. Observation of blood coagulation in crisis of DIAN 癲 disease with signs of excess (22-5)
   E. GU DIAN 骨癲, DIAN disease in bones together with depression and loss of body liquids (22-6)
   F. JIN DIAN 癲筋, DIAN disease in tendons and muscles together with loss of body liquids (22-7)
   G. MAI DIAN 癲脈, DIAN disease in MAI - blood vessels, channels and nervous system (22-8)
   H. DIAN 癲 disease develops into KUANG 狂 disease (22-9)

3. Treatments of KUANG 狂 disease, agitated (YANG) body-mind-spirit disorders
   I. Onset of KUANG 狂 disease - sorrow, stress and hunger causing memory loss, anger and fear (22-10)
   J. Onset of KUANG 狂 disease develops into a manic episode accompanied by insomnia, loss of appetite, excessive self-esteem, agitation and cursing (22-11)
   K. KUANG 狂 disease caused by fear, accompanied by agitation and euphoria, (22-12)
   L. KUANG 狂 disease, caused by QI deficiency, accompanied by screaming and visual and auditory hallucinations (22-13)
   M. KUANG 狂 disease caused by excessive joy, with bulimia and seeing ghosts (22-14)
   N. KUANG 狂 disease - acute psychotic episode (22-15)

4. Treatments of NI 逆, rebel or counterflow QI, which flows either in a contrary direction or in an exaggerated fashion in the correct direction, provoking congestion and obstruction.
   O. Congestion of cold and edema of limbs due to invasion of rebel wind FENG NI 風逆 (22-16)
   P. Sudden internal cold due to rebel QI (JUE NI 厥逆) in Kidney Meridian (22-17)
   Q. Internal cold in trunk due to rebel QI (JUE NI 厥逆) (22-18)
   R. Lower JIAO obstruction and urinary retention due to rebel afflux (22-19)
   S. Liver rebel QI 氣逆 invades Spleen (22-20)
   T. Obstructions of QI flow in SHAO YIN (Source QI) and YANG MING (acquired QI) in severe diseases (22-21)
   U. Two types of Kidney JING 精 deficiency (22-22)

1. Eye examination (SHEN 神 is reflected in the eyes),
LING SHU, Chapter 22-1

目	MU	eye	在	ZAI	located	上	SHANG	upper
眥	ZI	corner	內	NEI	interior	為	WEI	called
外	WAI	exterior	近	JIN	near	外	WAI	exterior
決	JUE	determine	鼻	BI	nose	眥	ZI	eye corner
於	YU	towards	者	ZHE	this	下	XIA	lower
面	MIAN	face	為	WEI	called	為	WEI	called
者	ZHE	this	內	NEI	interior	內	NEI	interior
為	WEI	called	眥	ZI	eye corner	眥	ZI	eye corner
銳	RU	exterior						
眥	ZI	eye corner						

The outer cantus (edge of the eye, MU ZI 目眥) *near the temple is called the external cantus.*

The inner cantus (edge of the eye, MU ZI 目眥) *near the nose is called the internal cantus.*

The upper part (of the eye) *belongs to the external cantus. The lower part* (of the eye) *belongs to the internal cantus.*

Surprisingly, LING SHU, Chapter 22, starts with the patient's eye examination, apparently to emphasize the connection between changes in the eye and changes of the patient's SHEN 神, since SHEN is reflected in the eyes. According to ZHANG JING YUE, the commentator on LING SHU, Chapter 22:[389]

> *The chapter's subject is mental diseases* DIAN KUANG BING 癲狂病. *If the eye cantus* (edge, MU ZI 目眥) *is mentioned here, it is because it is related to* (mental disease) ... *It should be noted that to treat the mental disease, one has to observe* SHEN QI 神氣, *and to start an examination from the eyes. The outer cantus, inner cantus and the upper and lower parts of the eye are associated with different* (meridians), *and* (help to) *diagnose which meridian is damaged. The chapter begins in this way to demonstrate what needs to be known, in order of priority.*

---

[389] ZHANG JING YUE (1563-1640), LEI JING

Eyes are the doors of SHEN, as expressed in LING SHU, Chapter 89:

五	WU	5	精	JING	
藏	ZANG	organs	之	ZHI	of
六	LIU	6	窠	CHAO	nest
府	FU	organs of transit	為	WEI	shape, form
之	ZHI	are	眼	YAN	eye
精	JING				
氣	QI				
皆	JIE	all			
上	SHANG	ascend			
注	ZHU	flow			
於	YU	towards			
目	MU	eye			
而	ER	so			
為	WEI	shape, form			
之	ZHI	of			
精	JING				

JING QI 精氣 *of all five ZANG and six FU ascend, flow to the eyes and form JING* 精.
Nesting of JING 精 *forms eyes.*

Eyes are the most important intersection of JING QI 精氣 flow in meridians towards the brain (one of the six Organs of Extraordinary Longevity which store JING). JING QI 精氣, QI which carries JING, necessary for brain functioning, flows to the eyes through many meridians:

A. Eight of the Twelve Meridians JING MAI 經脈,
B. Three divergent channels JING BIE 經別,
C. Five tendino-muscular channels (meridians) JING JIN 經筋,
D. Three longitudinal connecting channels (divergent LUO) LUO BIE 絡別,
E. Four of the Eight Extraordinary Meridians QI JING BA MAI 奇經八脈,
F. Extra-meridian point TAI YANG 太陽 (Great YANG), located in the center of each temple, is one of the important points associated with eye function.

A. JING MAI 經脈 (meridians) which flow around the eye:
   1. Gallbladder Meridian (DAN JING MAI) starts near the external cantus, GB1,
   2. Small Intestine Meridian (XIAO CHANG JING MAI) flows from ST12 through SI18 to the external cantus (GB1) and then to SI19; another branch of Small Intestine JING MAI flows from SI18 to the internal cantus - BL1.
   3. The branch of SAN JIAO Meridian (SAN JIAO JING MAI) flows to the external cantus, GB1, and another branch ends at the outer edge of the eyebrow, TW23.
   4. The internal section of Liver Meridian (GAN JING MAI) flows under the eye and ascends to GV20, located at the top of the head.
   5. The internal branch of Heart Meridian (XIN JING MAI) flows through the throat to the eyes.
   6. Stomach Meridian (WEI JING MAI) starts under the eye - ST1.
   7. The internal branches of Large Intestine Meridian (DA CHANG JING MAI) flow from LI20 to BL1 and to ST1.
   8. Bladder Meridian (PANG GUANG JING MAI) starts from internal cantus - BL1.

B. Divergent channels/meridians JING BIE 經別 which flow around the eye:
   1. Liver and Gallbladder JING BIE connects to GB1.
   2. Spleen and Stomach JING BIE bypasses the eye, flows through BL1 and connects to ST1.
   3. Heart and Small Intestine JING BIE connects to BL1.

C. Tendino-muscular channels/meridians JING JIN 經筋 which flow around the eye:
   1. Gallbladder JING JIN flows to the external cantus, following the flow of Gallbladder JING MAI.
   2. Small Intestine JING JIN flows to the external cantus following the flow of the internal branch of Small Intestine JING MAI from SI18 to GB1, and then ascends to the head.
   3. Large Intestine JING JIN passes the external cantus and continues to the head.

4. Stomach JING JIN ascends to the external cantus and a branch covers the entire lower eyelid.
5. The central branch of Bladder JING JIN ends in the forehead in BL1, and a branch covers the entire upper eyelid.

D. Longitudinal connecting channels/meridians (divergent LUO) LUO BIE 絡別 which flow around the eye:
   1. Heart LUO BIE flows from the tongue to the eye and forehead.
   2. Bladder LUO BIE flows towards the internal cantus.
   3. Stomach LUO BIE flows towards the head through the throat, and passes the external cantus

E. Extraordinary Meridians (QI JING BA MAI 奇經八脈) which flow around the eye:
   1. Two symmetrical branches of REN MAI 任脈 start from CV24 and flow to ST1 and eyes.
   2. One branch of DU MAI 督脈 passes through ST1 and ends in the center of the eye; another branch of DU MAI follows Bladder JING JIN to BL1.
   3. YIN QIAO MAI 陰蹻脈 ends at the internal cantus - BL1.
   4. YANG QIAO MAI 陽蹻脈 meets with YIN QIAO MAI at the internal cantus - BL1, and then flows to GB20.

2. Treatment of DIAN 癲 disease - quiet (YIN) body-mind-Spirit disorders, LING SHU, Chapter 22

DIAN 癲 is translated as 'madness', 'depression', 'mental (personality, mood swings) disorders', 'quiet, introverted YIN psychoses'. Epilepsy is called DIAN XIAN 癲癇. LING SHU, Chapter 22, describes one type of DIAN as cramps and seizures resembling epilepsy.

LING SHU, Chapter 22, describes seven clinical manifestations of DIAN 癲 disease and also gives a diagnostic method to identify the location of the QI obstruction by observing blood clotting.

DIAN 癲 is accompanied by changes in body functioning: facial muscle contractions, disorders of muscles, tendons, bones, respiratory system, heart rate, body liquids and blood, and may include a YIN type of restlessness which is not expressed outwardly.

Onset of DIAN 癲 disease is accompanied by:
- Loss of joy of life together with unfocused eyes (22-2)
- Muscle contractions around the mouth, crying and screaming respiratory distress and palpitation (22-3)
- Muscle stiffness and backache (22-4)

DIAN 癲 disease damages:
- Bones and body liquids (22-6)
- Tendons, muscles and body liquids (22-7)
- Channels, vascular and nervous systems (22-8)

LING SHU, Chapter 22, recommends observing the patient's complexion during the acupuncture treatment of DIAN 癲 disease: *when there is a change in complexion (XUE BIEN 血變) stop the treatment.*

The character XUE 血, usually translated as 'blood', is translated in this text as 'complexion'. Heart 'opens' in the face, and a change of complexion is the sign of the change of blood flow in the heart. The change of complexion (XUE BIEN 血變) in the patient should be observed, especially in the area between the eyebrows - the meeting place between YIN and YANG in the body, which corresponds to the extra-meridian point YIN TANG 印堂. Any change in complexion between the eyebrows can be a sign of a troubled mental state or personality disorder.

DIAN 癲, the body-mind-spirit imbalance of YIN type, may develop into
- Clinical depression, or
- YANG type agitated insanity - KUANG.

A. First signs of the onset of DIAN 癲 disease, LING SHU, Chapter 22-2

癲	DIAN		甚	SHEN	considerably	取	QU	puncture
疾	JI	disease	作	ZUO	make	手	SHOU	hand
始	SHI	begin	極	JI	extreme	太	TAI	great
生	SHENG	generate	已	YI	already	陽	YANG	
先	XIAN	first	而	ER	so	陽	YANG	
不	BU	no	煩	FAN	tormented	明	MING	bright
樂	LE	joy	心	XIN	heart	太	TAI	great
頭	TOU	head	候	HOU	observe	陰	YIN	
重	ZHONG	heavy	之	ZHI		血	XUE	complexion
痛	TONG	ache	於	YU	auxiliary words	變	BIAN	change
視	SHI	look	顏	YAN	complexion	為	WEI	has
舉	JU	upwards				止	ZHI	stop
目	MU	eye						
赤	CHI	red						

Onset of DIAN 癲 disease manifests as unhappiness (BU LE 不樂), 'heavy head', headache, gaze fixed upwards and redness of the eyes. When the situation becomes extreme, (the patient's) heart is troubled. Observe the complexion (of the patient).
Puncture (points on) Arm TAI YANG (Small Intestine), Arm YANG MING (Large Intestine) and Arm TAI YIN (Lung). When there is a change in complexion, stop the treatment.

The first signs of the onset of DIAN disease manifest as:
a. Unhappiness (loss of joy of life), which may be a sign of depression following a prolonged imbalance of the QI flow, or an expression of personality disorder. Unhappiness reflects the separation of man from his environment and presents damage to the Heart-Kidney (Fire-Water/SHEN 神 - ZHI 志) axis.

b. A feeling of heaviness in the head, headache, a fixed gaze upwards and redness of the eyes - signs of YANG/*fire rising*, following the separation between Fire and Water (Water does not control Fire). The location of the redness in the eyes shows which meridian is suffering from *excess fire*.

c. Trouble and suffering of Heart-Consciousness (FAN XIN 煩心) is reflected in changes of mood: sadness, disgust, apathy, irritability. Suffering of Heart-Consciousness is expressed as palpitation and arrhythmia (extra-systoles) which correspond to the signs of the syndrome *Heart Fire Rising*.

NAN JING, difficulty 59, describes a similar onset of DIAN disease:
At the onset of DIAN *disease, intent is joyless* (YI BU LE 意不樂); (the patient) *is lying on his back gazing straight* 癲疾始發, 意不樂, 直視僵仆.

Acupuncture points to treat DIAN disease at its onset, Chapter 22-2

Meridian	release excess YANG/*fire* from Heart and Lung
	Strategy of treatment and points
Arm TAI YANG, Small Intestine - FU (transit organ) YANG of Fire-Heart, '*turbid* of the *turbid*'[390]	Disperse *fire*: SI7-SI8, **disperse** Calm restlessness: SI7-PC6-GV26
Arm YANG MING, Large Intestine - FU (transit organ), YANG of Metal-Lung	Save Metal over-controlled by Fire: LI6-LI7
Arm TAI YIN, Lung	Disperse heat from chest by tonification of Metal YIN and moving Lung QI down: LU9-LU7 Dissolve mucus from Lung: LU9-ST40-CV22.

---

390 See page 43

Acupuncture points to treat DIAN disease at onset, LING SHU, Chapter 22-2

name	function	action
SI7 ZHI ZHENG 支正 Upright Branch	LUO of Small Intestine	clear heat, calm SHEN, disperse desires interrupting QI flow, treat feeling of emptiness, emotionality, mental pain, memory loss,[391] **disperse**
SI8 XIAO HAI 小海 Small Sea	HE-Soil of Small Intestine, sedation point	clear Heart heat, release phlegm-fire, regulate Blood and QI, treat melancholy, insomnia, restlessness, **disperse**
Calm restlessness: SI7-PC6-GV26		
PC6 NEI GUAN 內關 Inner Barrier	LUO of Master of Heart, open YIN WEI MAI	release three YIN, open chest, remove congestion between pelvis and chest, regulate QI, awaken SHEN
GV26 SHUI GOU Water Trough 水溝	open LUO channels in facial region	calm SHEN, open Heart orifices, purify head and brain
Save Metal over-controlled by Fire: LI6-LI7		
LI6 PIAN LI 偏歷 Veering Passageway	LUO of Large Intestine	open and regulate water passages, clear heat from YANG MING, move Lung QI down
LI7 WEN LIU 溫溜 Warm Flow	XI of Large Intestine	clear YANG MING fire, release Metal attacked by fire, calm SHEN: hypersensitivity, hallucinations, confused speech
Release Metal YIN: LU9-LU7; dissolve mucus from Lung: LU9-ST40-CV22		
LU9 TAI YUAN 太淵 Supreme abyss	SHU-YUAN-Soil of Lung, tonify Metal, HUI-meeting of vessels	purify heat, release and tonify Lung, resolve phlegm, treat insomnia with restlessness, treat confusion, release wind originating from internal fire
LU7 LIE QUE Broken Sequence	LUO of Lung, open REN MAI	treat rebel QI, move Lung QI and liquids down, release throat
ST40 FENG LONG 豐隆 Bountiful Bulge	LUO of Stomach	dissolve phlegm-fire, calm SHEN
CV22 TIAN TU 天突 Celestial Chimney	Minor Celestial Window, meeting of REN MAI with YIN WEI MAI	dissolve mucus from throat, benefit throat

---

391 S. de Morand, page 474

B. Onset of DIAN 癲 disease together with restlessness and facial muscle contortion, LING SHU, Chapter 22-3

癲 DIAN		候 HOU	control	左 ZUO	left	血 XUE	complexion
疾 JI	disease	之 ZHI	of	強 QIANG	rigid	變 BIAN	change
始 SHI	onset	手 SHOU	hand	者 ZHE	comma	為 WEI	is
作 ZUO	manifest	陽 YANG		攻 CONG	operate	止 ZHI	stop
而 ER	then	明 MING	bright	其 QI	its		
引 YIN	twitch	太 TAI	great	右 YOU	right		
口 KOU	mouth	陽 YANG		強 QIANG	rigid		
啼 TI	weep			者 ZHE	comma		
呼 HU	cry			攻 CONG	operate		
喘 CHUAN	gasp			左 ZUO	left		
悸 JI	palpitation						
者 ZHE	comma						

Onset of DIAN 癲 *disease manifests as contortions around the mouth, crying, shouting, shortness of breath and palpitation.*
Puncture (points on) *Arm* TAI YANG (Small Intestine) *and Arm* YANG MING (Large Intestine). *If the body is stiff on the left side, puncture the right. If the body is stiff on the right side, puncture the left. When there is a change in complexion, stop the treatment.*

LING SHU, Chapter 22-2, describes an unusual type of DIAN 癲 with extraverted behavior and shouting. The signs of the onset of DIAN disease here are:
- Contortions (tics) around the mouth
- Restlessness
- Crying and shouting - a sign of an imbalance between Liver and Lung
- Shortness of breath and palpitation - signs of anxiety

Contortions, convulsions and tics of muscles around the mouth are the signs of a disturbance of the tendino-muscular channels of Stomach, Large Intestine and Small Intestine, and correspond to *Startling (fright) Wind* or *Fright Seizures* (JING FENG 驚風) with three possible etiologies:

a. *Wind-Phlegm* obstructs Qi flow in the face
b. *Phlegm-Heat Obstructs Heart Orifices* (facial orifices)
c. *Liver Blood Deficiency Generates Wind.* GAN XUE XU SHENG FENG 肝血虛生風

a. Onset of DIAN 癲 together with restlessness and facial muscle contortion - *wind-phlegm* obstructs Qi flow in the face

Congested Liver Qi and Spleen Qi deficiency cause *wind-phlegm* and internal wind (release of congested Liver Qi). Spleen deficiency causes a disruption of the flow of body liquids, which stagnate and form phlegm. Wind moves phlegm up to the facial region where it obstructs Qi flow, provoking seizures around the mouth (Figure 59).

Figure 59. Onset of DIAN 癲 **disease.** *Wind-phlegm* **obstructs** Qi **flow in face**

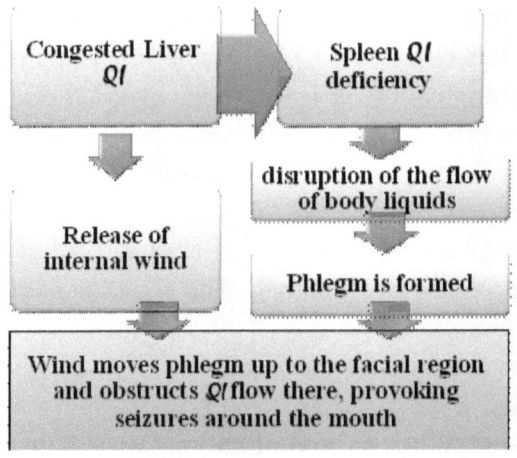

b. Onset of DIAN 癲 together with restlessness and facial muscle contortion - *Phlegm-Heat Obstructs Heart Orifices* (facial orifices)

Overeating of hot and spicy food causes the formation of phlegm-heat. Extreme anger causes the rise of *Liver fire* which moves phlegm up to the face and obstructs orifices, causing seizures around the mouth. All facial orifices are ruled by their respective ZANG but supervised by Heart, and are therefore called Heart orifices.

c. Onset of DIAN 癲 together with restlessness and facial muscle contortion - *Liver Blood Deficiency Generates Wind*, GAN XUE XU SHENG FENG 肝血虛生風

Chronic bleeding associated with chronic Kidney weakness depletes Blood reserves and causes *Liver Blood Deficiency*, which causes a release of internal wind ('empty' Liver QI) upwards, provoking seizures around the mouth.

According to LING SHU, Chapter 22-3, the treatment of DIAN with seizures around the mouth resulting from *Startling (fright) Wind* (JING FENG 驚風) is to disperse wind by puncturing points on Small Intestine (Arm TAI YANG) and Large Intestine Meridians (Arm YANG MING), combined with points on Stomach Meridian (Leg YANG MING): SI3-GV26-GV14, LI4-ST4-ST6. The treatment of distortions on the left side is to puncture points on the right side and vice versa.

Acupuncture points to treat DIAN together with seizures around the mouth caused by *Startling Wind* (JING FENG 驚風), LING SHU, Chapter 22-3

name	function	action
SI3-GV26-GV14, LI4-ST4-ST6 puncture meridians of non-affected side		
HOU XI SI3 後谿 Back Ravine	SHU -Wood of Small Intestine, open DU MAI	calm SHEN, expel wind-fire, treat epilepsy and muscle contractions, regulate orifices
GV26 SHUI GOU Water Trough 水溝	open LUO channels in facial region	calm SHEN, open Heart orifices, purify head and brain, treat muscle spasms, *lips moving like a worm crawling* (according to ZHEN JIU DA CHANG)
GV14 DA ZHUI 大椎 Big Mallet	meeting of DU MAI with six YANG Meridians	regulate QI and YANG flow to head and heart, release wind-fatigue, release excess heat and damp-heat from upper body, treat spasms in DIAN
LI4 HE GU 合谷 Union Valley	YUAN of Large Intestine, entry point, command point of face and mouth	regulate QI, release excess YANG from head
ST4 DI CANG 地倉 Earth Granary	meeting ST., L.I. Meridians, YANG QIAO MAI and REN MAI	expel wind from face, treat muscle spasms around mouth and eye
ST6 JIA CHE 頰車 Jaw Bone		expel wind

C. Onset of DIAN 癲 disease together with muscle rigidity and backache, LING SHU, Chapter 22-4

癲 DIAN	disease	候 HOU	control	血 XUE	complexion
疾 JI	disease	之 ZHI	of	變 BIAN	change
始 SHI	begin	足 ZU	leg	為 WEI	has
作 ZUO	generate	太 TAI	great	止 ZHI	stop
先 XIAN	first	陽 YANG			
反 FAN	turn	陽 YANG			
僵 JIANG	contract	明 MING	bright		
因 YIN	so	太 TAI	great		
而 ER	then	陰 YIN			
脊 JI	back	手 SHOU	hand		
痛 TONG	ache	太 TAI	great		
		陽 YANG			

Onset of DIAN 癲 *disease manifests as body stiffness; turning causes back pain.*
Treat Leg TAI YANG *(Bladder), Leg* YANG MING *(Stomach), Leg* TAI YIN *(Spleen), and Arm* TAI YANG *(Small Intestine).*
When there is a change in complexion, stop the treatment.

According to LING SHU, Chapter 22-4, back muscle stiffness and back pain are signs of the onset of DIAN disease. Back muscle stiffness may develop into opisthotonos, a state of severe hyperextension and spasticity in which an individual's head, neck and spinal column enter into a complete 'bridging' or 'arching' position. Etiology of muscle stiffness may be:
- *Liver Wind* (internal excess)
- *Empty Heat* caused by *Liver and Kidney* YIN *Deficiency*
- *Phlegm-Heat Obstructing Heart Orifices* - seizures and epilepsy

Treatment of DIAN together with muscle stiffness and backache is by puncturing points on TAI YANG (Bladder and Small Intestine) and YANG MING (Stomach) Meridians:
- Treat back stiffness and pain, opisthotonos: BL58-BL62
- Treat seizures: BL62-GV20-GB20-SI3-BL15, or BL63-BL61-BL60-H7-ST41, (according to SHEN JIU JING LUN)

- Treat TAI YANG excess in head and back: BL5, stiffness of spine: BL2, BL47
- Nourish body liquids in muscles and tendons: GV8-ST28 (according to BAI ZHENG FU)

Acupuncture points to treat DIAN together with muscle stiffness and backache, LING SHU, Chapter 22-4

name	function	action
DIAN with back stiffness, pain, opisthotonos: BL58-BL62		
BL62 SHEN MAI 申脈 SHEN Hour Vessel	open YANG QIAO MAI	purify head and eyes, treat inability to bend or straighten up and redness of internal eye cantus [392]
BL58 FEI YANG 飛陽 Taking Flight	LUO of Bladder	treat protruding tongue, back muscle contractions (opisthotonos) in DIAN, treat muscle pain and leg weakness [393]
DIAN with seizures - treat muscle contractions: BL62-GV20-GB20-SI3-BL15		
GV20 BAI HUI 百會 Hundred Meetings	meeting of DU MAI with six YANG Meridians	move YANG down through QI flow of DU MAI, purify head and brain, calm Liver wind, treat restlessness and heavy head
GB20 FENG CHI 風池 Wind Pool	meeting of G.B., SAN JIAO Meridians, YANG WEI MAI and YANG QIAO MAI	disperse heat and Liver wind, regulate QI and Blood, release YANG in back of neck and spine
HOU XI SI3 後谿 Back Ravine	SHU-Wood of Small Intestine, open DU MAI	calm SHEN, expel wind-fire, treat epilepsy and muscle contractions
BL15 XIN SHU 心俞 Heart SHU	SHU of Heart, regulate Heart YANG	calm SHEN, release LUO of Heart, treat back stiffness and pain in DIAN [394]
DIAN with seizures, treat muscle contractions: BL63-BL61-BL60-H7-ST41		
BL63 JIN MEN 金門 Golden Gate	XI of Bladder, start with YANG WEI MAI	relax tendons, calm brain, treat seizures in DIAN, **moxa**
BL61 PU CAN 僕參 Honored Servant	meeting with YANG QIAO MAI	calm brain, treat seizures and shouts that sound horse-like
BL60 KUN LUN 昆侖 Mountain	JING-River-Fire of Bladder	relax tendons
H7 SHEN MEN 神門 SHEN Gate	SHU-YUAN-Soil of Heart	calm SHEN, cool Heart (insomnia, stress), open Heart orifices
ST41 JIE XI 解谿 Ravine Divide	JING-River-Fire of Stomach, tonify Soil	move fire congested in Stomach, treat released or trembling SHEN

---

392 according to YI XUE RU MEN
393 according to JIA JI JING YI and XUE RU MEN
394 according to ZHEN JIU XUE JIAN BIAN

Acupuncture points to treat muscle stiffness and backache in DIAN, LING SHU, Chapter 22-4 continued

Treat contractions of muscles and tendons BL5, BL2-BL47, GV8-ST28		
BL47 HUN MEN 魂門 HUN Gate	regulate HUN 魂, gather Liver JING	spread Liver QI, treat muscle contractions of spine
BL2 ZAN ZHU 攢竹 Bamboo Gathering		treat muscle contractions of spine in DIAN
BL5 WU CHU 五處 Fifth Place		treat TAI YANG excess in head, back of neck and back
ST28 SHUI DAO 水道 Waterway		clear and regulate pathways of liquids in muscles and tendons
GV8 JIN SUO 筋縮 Sinew Contraction		calm SHEN, treat spasms of tendons and muscles (especially in back)

D. Observation of blood coagulation in DIAN 癲 disease crises with signs of excess, LING SHU, Chapter 22-5

治 ZHI	treat	病 BING	disease	至 ZHI	reach	不 BU	not
癲 DIAN		至 ZHI	reach	其 QI	his	動 DONG	move
疾 JI	disease	視 SHI	observe	發 FA	issue	灸 JIU	moxa
者 ZHE	comma	之 ZHI	it	時 SHI	time	窮 QIONG	bone border
常 CHANG	constant	有 YOU	has	血 XUE	blood	骨 GU	GV1
與 YU	with	過 GUO	excess	獨 DU	alone	二 ER	20
之 ZHI	its	者 ZHE	comma	動 DONG	move	十 SHI	
居 JU	stay	寫 XIE	disperse	矣 YI	period	壯 ZHUANG	cones
察 CHA	observe	之 ZHI	it			窮 QIONG	bone border
其 QI	his	置 ZHI	take			骨 GU	GV1
所 SUO	where	其 QI	its			者 ZHE	is
當 DANG	have to	血 XUE	blood			骶 DI	coccyx
取 QU	puncture	於 YU	into			骨 GU	bone
之 ZHI	of	瓠 HU	gourd				
處 CHU	place	壺 HU					
		之 ZHI	of				
		中 ZHONG	center				

In order to treat DIAN 癲 *disease (the practitioner) should always be with the patient and observe him to determine which points to puncture.*

If in a crisis of (DIAN) *disease, there are signs of excess,* (the practitioner) *should disperse the meridians by draining blood into a container. In the crisis blood moves. If blood does not move, burn 20 moxas on Bone Border* (CHANG QIANG ,GV1). *Bone Border is located on the coccyx.*

LING SHU, Chapter 22-5, describes a diagnostic method for DIAN disease with signs of excess by observing blood coagulation, in order to determine the location of the disorder in QI flow.

According to ZHANG SHI's commentary on LING SHU:
Conserve the blood (of a patient) in a container made of the skin of gourd. If blood is agitated it is due to QI (present inside blood) call and answer. If the pernicious QI influences the Arm TAI YIN Meridian (Lung) and Arm TAI YANG Meridian (Small Intestine), then blood is agitated. It acts according to the cyclic movement of the Heaven and TAI YANG 太陽. If blood is not agitated, it is because that the disease entered the Water of the Earth. This is why one must apply 20 moxas on the coccyx.

The diagnosis and therapy of DIAN is according to the principle of distinction of the QI of 'Water'-YIN-Earth and QI of 'Fire'-YANG- Heaven:
- **Absence of blood coagulation** is a sign of fire/YANG excess in the upper body, due to the obstruction of YIN QI flow in Arm TAI YIN Meridian and Arm TAI YANG Meridian (Small Intestine and Lung Meridians), which (like all arm meridians) are connected to Heaven. Blood flow is associated with Heaven and the sun (Great YANG, TAI YANG 太陽). Fire/YANG excess in the upper body causes the blood in the container to move (agitate), preventing blood coagulation.

- **Blood coagulation** is a sign of fire trapped in the lower body and the penetration of pernicious QI into Leg TAI YIN and Leg TAI YANG (Bladder and Spleen Meridians) obstructing the blood flow. The treatment is to move YANG towards the upper body by strengthening the root of YANG: burning 20 moxa cones on the acupuncture point GV1 (CHANG QIANG 長強, *Always Strong*, the first point on Governing Vessel - DU MAI, the father of YANG). GV1 is the beginning of the longitudinal LUO of DU MAI, which helps to expel pernicious QI, and also the meeting point with Conception Vessel (REN MAI 任脈). This method of YANG release by burning moxa cones is also effective in different types of schizophrenia.

E. GU DIAN 骨癲, DIAN disease in bones together with depression and loss of body liquids, LING SHU, Chapter 22-6

骨	GU	bone	而	ER	then	嘔	OU	vomit
癲	DIAN		骨	GU	bone	多	DOU	much
疾	JI	disease	居	JU	protruding	沃	WO	saliva
者	ZHE	comma	汗	HAN	sweat	沫	MO	foam
顑	KAN	protruding	出	CHU	exit	氣	QI	
齒	CHI	teeth	煩	FAN	torment	下	XIA	descend
諸	ZHU	all	悗	MIAN	apathy	泄	XIE	disperse
腧	SHU	point				不	BU	not
分	FEN	interval				治	ZHI	cure
肉	ROU	flesh						
皆	JIE	all						
滿	MAN	swollen						

When DIAN disease is in bones (GU DIAN 骨癲), all the acupuncture points (SHU 腧) in the interval below the upper jaw and teeth (gums) are swollen,
Bones are protruding; there is sweating, suffering and apathy (depression).
When there is a lot of vomiting and foamy saliva, QI disperses downward and there is no cure for the disease.

Signs of DIAN disease in bones (GU DIAN 骨癲) are:
- Insufficiency of body liquids and injury to their circulation (Kidney, Spleen and Lung function is damaged):
  - Swelling of face, swelling below the upper jaw, swelling of gums - a sign of the stagnation of body liquids,
  - Sweat - loss of body liquids (dehydration),
  - Prominent bones - a sign of loss of flesh and body liquids,
- Suffering and apathy - signs of depression.

DIAN disease in bones, caused by poor irrigation by the body liquids, damages Kidney-ZHI 志 and Lung-Large-Intestine-PO 魄 (related to body formation and bones).[395]

---

395 See page 29

There is no cure for DIAN disease in bones in cases where there is additional loss of body liquids and QI resulting in further injury to Kidney and Lung function, through:
- Vomiting – a sign of YANG weakness in Middle JIAO. Stomach does not retain liquids therefore Spleen does not absorb liquids and cannot provide nourishing moisture for the body.
- Excretion of foamy saliva - a sign of damage to Kidney liquids.

However, the situation may be improved by puncture of points which:
- Tonify bones and body liquids: BL28, BL42, BL43-GV14, BL22/BL23, BL20
- Treat facial swelling: CV24-GV26, LI9, ST37-BL11-GB39-Ki3,

Acupuncture points to treat DIAN disease in bones, LING SHU, Chapter 22-6

name	function	action
Tonify bones and body liquids in DIAN: BL28, BL42, BL43-GV14, BL22 or BL23, BL20		
BL20 PI SHU 脾俞 Spleen SHU	SHU of Spleen, regulate Spleen YANG	improve absorption and circulation of body liquids, stop vomiting, tonify **with hot needle**
BL22 SAN JIAO SHU 三焦俞	SHU of SAN JIAO	open and regulate water passages, **tonify with hot needle**
BL23 SHEN SHU 肾俞 Kidney SHU	SHU of Kidney, regulate Ki. YANG	open and regulate water passages
BL28 PANG GUANG SHU 膀胱俞 Bladder SHU	SHU of Bladder, regulate Bl. YANG	open and regulate water passages, calm bone pain
BL42 PO HU 魄戶 PO Door	regulate PO 魄	treat suffering, restlessness, depression, loss of reality, bone and vertebrae pain, vomiting, **tonify**
BL43 GAO HUANG SHU 膏肓俞 SHU of Liquid Fat	gather JING in Upper JIAO	calm SHEN, strengthen Source QI, Ki., Sp., brain and bone marrow, **moxa**
GV14 DA ZHUI 大椎 Big Mallet	meeting of DU MAI with 6 YANG Meridians	treat chronic bone and bone marrow diseases accompanied by spine pain and vomiting

Acupuncture points to treat DIAN disease in bones, LING SHU, Chapter 22-6, continued

Treat facial swelling in DIAN: CV24-GV26, LI9, ST37-BL11-GB39-Ki3, GB13		
CV24 CHENG JIANG 承漿 Sauce Receptacle	meeting REN MAI, DU MAI, L.I. and St. Meridians	treat facial edema and excessive salivation in DIAN
GV26 SHUI GOU 水溝 Water Trough	open LUO channels in facial region	calm SHEN, open Heart orifices, purify head and brain, treat facial swelling and excessive salivation in DIAN
LI9 SHOU SHANG LIAN 手上廉 Hand Upper Ridge		treat bones and bone marrow with difficulty in limb movement
ST37 SHANG JU XU 上巨虛 Great Deficiency Above	Lower HE of Large Intestine, Lower Body Sea of Blood (with ST39, BL11)	treat pain in bone marrow caused by cold, diarrhea with loss of appetite and sweat, limb weakness
BL11 DA ZHU 大杼 Great Shuttle	HUI-meeting of Bones, Sea of Blood, Spine Rectitude SHU (LING SHU, Chapter 15), meeting of Bl., S.I, S.J., G.B., Sp. and Lu. Meridians	benefit bones, irrigate Wood (muscles and tendons)
GB39 XUAN ZHONG 懸鍾 Suspended Bell	HUI-meeting of bone marrow, meeting of Leg 3 YANG	move YANG QI from the upper body down, tonify bones and bone marrow, nourish JING, **tonify**
Ki3 TAI XI 太谿 Great Ravine	SHU-YUAN-Soil of Kidney	tonify Kidney YIN, release ascent of CHONG MAI and REN MAI, treat degenerative diseases, nourish bones, **tonify**
GB13 BEN SHEN 本神 Root of SHEN	meeting of G.B. Meridian with YANG WEI MAI	treat vomiting, phlegm in brain and excessive salivation in DIAN

F. JIN DIAN 筋癫, DIAN **disease in tendons and muscles together with loss of body liquids,** LING SHU, Chapter 22-7

筋	JIN	tendons	刺	CI	needle	嘔	OU	vomit
癫	DIAN		項	XIANG	neck	多	DUO	much
疾	JI	disease	大	DA	big	沃	WO	saliva
者	ZHE	comma	經	JING	meridian	沫	MO	foam
身	SHEN	body	之	ZHI	of	氣	QI	
倦	JUAN	curled up	大	DA	Big Shuttle BL11	下	XIA	descend
攣	LUAN	cramp	杼	ZHU		泄	XIE	disperse
急	JI	spasm	脈	MAI	vessel	不	BU	not
大	DA	big				治	ZHI	cure

When DIAN disease is in tendons/muscles (JIN DIAN 筋癫), the patient is curled up and suffers greatly from cramps and spasms (of muscles), Puncture DA ZHU 大杼 (Great Shuttle, BL11) on the great meridian which flows on the neck (TAI YANG, Bladder Meridian)
When there is much vomiting and foamy saliva, QI disperses downward and there is no cure for the disease.

JIN DIAN 筋癫 in tendons/muscles is expressed as spasms, cramps and convulsions of muscles and tendons, and inability to move.

Both JIN DIAN 筋癫 and GU DIAN 骨癫 (disease in bones) result from 'poor irrigation' by body liquids.

There is no cure for DIAN disease in tendons/muscles when there is additional loss of body liquids and QI through vomiting and excretion of foamy saliva, bringing further damage to Kidney and Lung function.

However the situation may be improved through puncture of points on Bladder Meridian: BL11-BL39-BL47-BL46.

Acupuncture points to treat DIAN disease in tendons and muscles together with loss of body liquids, LING SHU, Chapter 22-7

name	function	action
Tonify tendons (muscles) in DIAN: BL11-BL39-BL47-BL46		
BL11 DA ZHU 大杼 Great Shuttle	HUI-meeting of Bones, Sea of Blood, Spine Rectitude SHU (LING SHU, Chapter 15), meeting of Bl., S.I, S.J., G.B., Sp. and Lu. Meridians	benefit bones, irrigation of Wood (muscles and tendons)
BL39 WEI YANG 委陽 Bent YANG	Lower HE of SAN JIAO	improve irrigation of spine and tendons /muscles in DIAN
BL47 HUN MEN 魂門 HUN Gate	regulate HUN 魂, gather Liver JING	spread Liver QI, treat muscle contractions along spine
BL46 GE GUAN 膈關 Diaphragm Pass		treat muscle contractions, pain in bones and excessive salivation

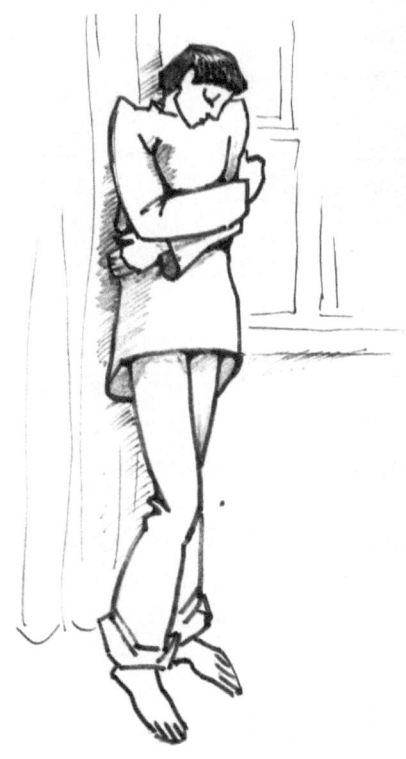

G. MAI DIAN 脈癲, DIAN disease in blood vessels, channels (meridians) and nervous system, LING SHU, Chapter 22-8

脈	MAI	vessels	脈	MAI	vessels	不	BU	not	嘔	OU	vomit
癲	DIAN		滿	MAN	full	滿	MAN	full	吐	TU	spit
疾	JI	disease	盡	JIN	all	灸	JIU	moxa	沃	WO	saliva
者	ZHE	comma	刺	CI	needle	之	ZHI	on	沫	MO	foam
暴	BAO	sudden	之	ZHI	of	挾	XIE	under	氣	QI	
仆	PU	fall	出	CHU	exit	項	XIANG	neck	下	XIA	descend
四	SI	4	血	XUE	blood	太	TAI	great	泄	XIE	disperse
肢	ZHI	limbs				陽	YANG		不	BU	not
之	ZHI	of				灸	JIU	moxa	治	ZHI	cure
脈	MAI	vessels				帶	DAI	Belt			
皆	JIE	all				脈	MAI	Vessel, GB26			
脹	ZHANG	swollen				於	YU	on			
而	ER	and				腰	YAO	waist			
縱	ZONG	lax				相	XIANG	mutual			
						去	QU	distance			
						三	SAN	3			
						寸	CUN	distance measure			
						諸	ZHU	all			
						分	FEN	division			
						肉	ROU	flesh			
						本	BEN	base			
						腧	SHU	point			

When DIAN disease is in vessels (MAI DIAN 癲脈), the patient suddenly falls and faints, the blood vessels in all four limbs are swollen and limp. If the vessels are swollen, puncture to bleed all of them,

If the vessels are not swollen, burn moxa under the neck on TAI YANG (Bladder Meridian), burn moxa on DAI MAI 帶脈 (GB26), located on each side of the body on the waist three CUN (distance measures) (below the tip of the 11th rib), and on all divisions of flesh (points on the joints and between tendons).

When there is vomiting, coughing with sputum and foamy saliva, QI disperses downward, and there is no cure for the disease.

MAI DIAN 脈癲 describes damage to blood vessels, channels, meridians and the nervous system:
- Sudden fainting and falling corresponding to epilepsy, brain damage.
- Blood vessel/meridian trajectories on limbs are swollen (edema) and limp.

As with DIAN in bones and DIAN in tendons/muscles, there is no cure for MAI DIAN 脈癲 when there is a loss of body liquids and QI through vomiting, coughing with sputum and excretion of foamy saliva.

MAI DIAN 脈癲 corresponds to the following syndromes of Chinese Medicine:

1. *Wind in the Center* (ZHONG FENG 中風)	PC9, H9, LU11, LI1, TW1, SI1
2. *Wind Epilepsy* (FENG XIAN 風癇)	BL10 **moxa**
3. *'Tightening' (obstruction) of Belt Meridian* (DAI MAI 帶脈)	GB27, GB26: Ki3-BL62-BL11-LI13

1. *Wind in the Center* (wind penetrating straight to its aim) (ZHONG FENG 中風) characterized by sudden fainting, phlegm, locked jaws and inability to drink, may correspond to MAI DIAN 脈癲 **characterized by swelling** of blood vessels or meridian pathways. The treatment of this condition is by bleeding JING-Well[396] points on meridians the pathways of which are in the swollen area: PC9, H9, LU11, LI1 ,TW1,SI1.

Acupuncture points to treat MAI DIAN 脈癲 (swelling of blood vessels or meridian pathways), LING SHU, Chapter 22-8

name	function
Treat MAI DIAN with swelling of blood vessels: PC9, H9, LU11 ,LI1 ,TW1,SI1	
H9 SHAO CHONG 少衝 *Lesser Surge*	JING-Well-Wood of Heart
PC9 ZHONG CHONG 中衝 Central *Surge*	JING-Well-Wood of Master of Heart
LU11 SHAO SHANG 少商 *Lesser Merchant*	JING-Well-Wood of Lung
LI1 SHANG YANG 商陽 YANG *Merchant*	JING-Well-Metal of Large Intestine
TW1 GUAN CHONG 關衝 *Surge Pass*	JING-Well-Metal of SAN JIAO
SI1 SHAO ZI 少澤 *Lesser* Marsh	JING-Well-Metal of Small Intestine

396 According to QIAN KUN SHENG YI

2. *Wind Epilepsy* (FENG XIAN 風癇) characterized by a sudden fall and seizures, pain at the back of the neck, the rolling of eyes and confused speech, may correspond to MAI DIAN 脈癲 **without prominent swelling** in blood vessels or on the meridian pathways. The recommended treatment is to burn seven moxa cones on the acupuncture point located on the back of the neck, on Bladder Meridian (BL10, TIAN ZHU 天柱, *Celestial Pillar*, Major Celestial Window Point).

3. *'Tightening'* (obstruction) *of* DAI MAI 帶脈 (*Belt Meridian* - one of Eight Extraordinary Meridians) inhibiting QI flow in those meridians whose trajectories pass through the waist. The recommended treatment is the burning of moxa cones on the acupuncture point GB26 (DAI MAI 帶脈). Belt Meridian (DAI MAI 帶脈) may also be treated by puncturing GB27 and GB26 and points on joints and tendons: Ki3-BL62-BL11-LI13

name	function	action
Treat DAI MAI obstruction in DIAN: GB26, GB27-GB28		
GB26 DAI MAI 帶脈	meeting with DAI MAI	drain damp, regulate DAI MAI, moxa
GB27 WU SHU 五樞 Fifth Pivot	meeting with DAI MAI	transform stagnation, regulate DAI MAI
GB28 WEI DAO 維道 Linking Path	meeting with DAI MAI	transform stagnation, regulate DAI MAI
Treat points on joints and tendons in DAI MAI obstruction in DIAN: Ki3-BL62-BL11-LI13		
Ki3 TAI XI 太谿 Great Ravine	SHU-YUAN-Soil of Kidney	tonify Kidney YIN, release ascent of CHONG MAI and REN MAI, treat degenerative diseases
BL62 SHEN MAI 申脈 SHEN Hour Vessel	open YANG QIAO MAI	purify head and eyes, restore presence and vigilance, **tonify**
BL11 DA ZHU 大杼 Great Shuttle	HUI- meeting of Bones, Sea of Blood, Spine Rectitude SHU (LING SHU, Chapter 15), meeting of Bl., S.I, S.J., G.B., Sp. and Lu. Meridians	benefit bones, irrigation of Wood (muscles and tendons), **tonify**
LI13 SHOU WU LI 手五里 Arm Five LI		treat articular rheumatism of limbs or joint pains, lack of force in limbs, **tonify**

H. DIAN 癲 disease develops into KUANG 狂 disease, LING SHU, Chapter 22-9

癲	DIAN	
疾	JI	disease
者	ZHE	comma
疾	JI	disease
發	FA	develop
如	RU	like
狂	KUANG	
者	ZHE	comma
死	SI	death
不	BU	no
治	ZHI	cure, treatment

When DIAN 癲 disease develops into KUANG 狂 disease, it causes death and is incurable.

DIAN 癲 disease, quiet introverted YIN body-mind-spirit disorders, may develop into KUANG 狂 disease - agitated, extraverted and violent YANG body-mind-spirit disorders (psychoses, madness, insanity, mental or personality disorders).[397]

2. Treatments of KUANG 狂 disease, agitated (YANG) body-mind-spirit disorders, LING SHU, Chapter 22

LING SHU, Chapter 22, after presenting DIAN 癲 disease, continues by presenting KUANG 狂 disease - agitated, extraverted and violent YANG psychoses, madness, insanity, mental or personality disorders, manic or schizophrenic attacks. KUANG 狂 disease may occur due to the development of DIAN 癲 disease or as a result of a deep injury to YIN and YANG.

According to NAN JING, Difficulty 59:

> *In onset of KUANG 狂 a person does not sleep or eat, glorifies himself, his abilities and his height, laughs and sings inappropriately, is happy without reason, restless without order and without end.*[398]

---

397 See page 352, for the character KUANG 狂
398 See Chapter 8, page 289

LING SHU, Chapter 22, describes onset of KUANG 狂 disease as:
- Memory loss, anger and fear caused by sorrow, stress and hunger (22-10),
- A manic episode together with insomnia, loss of appetite, excessive self-esteem, agitation, swearing (22-11).

LING SHU, Chapter 22, then presents several expressions of KUANG 狂 disease similar to psychotic episodes and characterized by:
- Agitation and euphoria caused by fear (22-12)
- Screaming with visual and auditory hallucinations caused by QI deficiency (22-13)
- Bulimia and seeing ghosts, caused by excessive joy (22-14)
- Acute psychotic episode (22-15)

I. Onset of KUANG 狂 disease: sorrow, stress, hunger, memory loss, anger and fear, LING SHU, Chapter 22-10

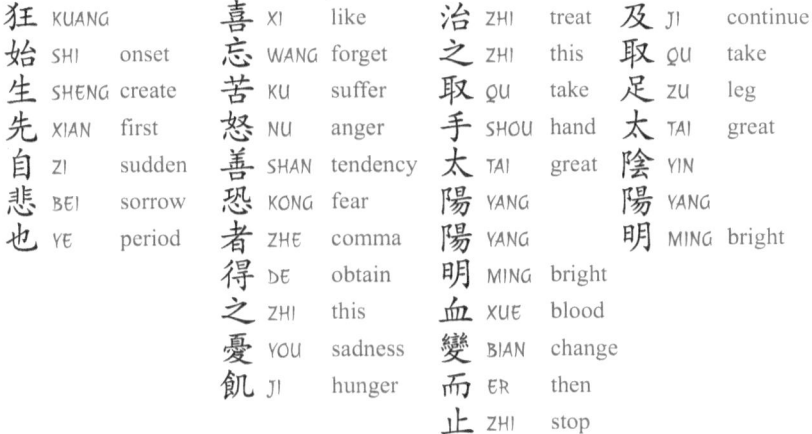

狂	KUANG		喜	XI	like	治	ZHI	treat	及	JI	continue
始	SHI	onset	忘	WANG	forget	之	ZHI	this	取	QU	take
生	SHENG	create	苦	KU	suffer	取	QU	take	足	ZU	leg
先	XIAN	first	怒	NU	anger	手	SHOU	hand	太	TAI	great
自	ZI	sudden	善	SHAN	tendency	太	TAI	great	陰	YIN	
悲	BEI	sorrow	恐	KONG	fear	陽	YANG		陽	YANG	
也	YE	period	者	ZHE	comma	陽	YANG		明	MING	bright
			得	DE	obtain	明	MING	bright			
			之	ZHI	this	血	XUE	blood			
			憂	YOU	sadness	變	BIAN	change			
			飢	JI	hunger	而	ER	then			
						止	ZHI	stop			

KUANG 狂 manifests at the beginning as sudden sorrow (ZI BEI 自悲). There is memory loss, suffering (KU 苦), anger (NU 怒) and a tendency to fear (KONG 恐), all of which come from sadness together with worry (YOU 憂) and hunger.

The treatment is to puncture (the points) on Arm TAI YANG (Small Intestine) and YANG MING (Large Intestine). When there is a change in complexion, stop the treatment.

Continue (the treatment) by puncturing (the points) on Leg TAI YIN (Spleen) and YANG MING (Stomach).

KUANG 狂 starts with sudden sorrow (ZI BEI 自悲). Sorrow (BEI 悲) compresses the chest (Upper JIAO), causing heat which interferes with the function of Heart, Master-of-Heart and Lung. Damage caused by sorrow (BEI 悲) is described in:

> SU WEN, Chapter 39: *Sorrow (BEI 悲) compresses the communication system of Heart... Nourishing QI and Defensive QI are not distributed, and QI of heat settles in the center.*[399]

> LING SHU, Chapter 8-3: *So sorrow and grief* (BEI AI 悲哀) *agitate the center* (of man). *There are fatigue and interruptions, and life is lost.*[400]

> LING SHU, Chapter 8-4: *When sorrow and grief* (BEI AI 悲哀) *invade Liver, there is restlessness in the centre and this injures* HUN 魂. *Injury to* HUN 魂 *results in* KUANG, *memory loss and lack of* JING 精. *Lack of* JING 精 *is the loss of rectitude.*[401]

Heat in the chest in the onset of KUANG disease is expressed as:
- Sorrow (BEI 悲) develops into sadness together with worry, stress, oppression, suffering, and preoccupation (YOU 憂)[402] and heat in the chest.
- A feeling of hunger - a sign of Stomach heat, caused by heat spreading from Upper JIAO to Middle JIAO.

A feeling of hunger and sadness (YOU 憂) are both cause and effect of heat in the chest, provoking:
- Memory loss and suffering (KU 苦) caused by heat injuring Heart and Master of Heart (the communication system of Heart with the environment).
- Anger (NU 怒), caused by *Liver heat* which spreads from Master-of-Heart. Both Liver and Master of Heart Meridians belong to the JUE YIN 厥陰 layer of QI flow (one of Six Layers, LIU JING 六經).

---

399 See page 181
400 See page 223
401 See page 298
402 See page 52, for the character YOU 憂

- Fear (KONG 恐), caused by deficiency of Kidney JING 精 and body liquids as a result of heat injuring Lung function: JING 精 is not absorbed from the air and body liquids do not descend.

Treatment of the onset of KUANG disease is similar to the treatment of the onset of DIAN 癲 disease (LING SHU, 22-2).[403] When there is a change in complexion, stop the treatment.

- Release *Heart fire* by dispersing its YANG, Small Intestine Meridian, Arm TAI YANG: SI7-SI8
- Release *Lung fire* by dispersing its YANG, Large Intestine Meridian, Arm YANG MING: LI6-LI7
- Disperse heat obstructing chest by tonification of Lung YIN, and improve Lung function of lowering by puncturing points on Lung Meridian, Arm TAI YIN: LU9-LU7
- Since Fire generates Soil, it is possible to pull fire from Heart Meridian down to the legs by puncturing points on Spleen-Soil Meridian, Leg TAI YIN: SP1-SP4

name	function	action
SP1 YIN BAI 隱白 Hidden White	JING-Well-Wood of Spleen	anchor a person into soil, give clarity of thought, return sleep, treat dissatisfaction, nightmares, 'does not know people', shyness, fear [404]
SP4 GONG SUN 公孫 Grandfather-Grandson	opening of CHONG MAI, LUO of Spleen	move Spleen QI up through CHONG MAI, calm restlessness with abdominal swelling, treat hallucinations, insomnia and fear

- When QI of Leg YANG MING (Stomach) descends, QI of Leg SHAO YIN (Kidney) ascends: tonify Kidney indirectly by puncturing points on Stomach Meridian. ST36-ST41.

---

403 See page 365
404 S. de Morand, page 497

name	function	action
ST36 ZU SAN LI 足三里 Leg Three Miles	HE-Soil of Stomach, tonify QI, Sea of Blood point, potentiate other points	regulate YANG deficiency above and YIN excess below, regulate WEI QI, strengthen SHEN, treat prolonged melancholy, mental fatigue, lack of vitality or body disorders caused by emotions (S. de Morand, page 438)
ST41 JIE XI 解谿 Ravine Divide	JING-River-Fire of Stomach, tonify Soil, potentiate ST36	move fire congested in Stomach, treat released or trembling SHEN

J. KUANG 狂 disease onset develops into a manic episode accompanied by insomnia, loss of appetite, excessive self-esteem, agitation and cursing, LING SHU, Chapter 22-11

狂 KUANG		自 ZI	self	治 ZHI	treat	視 SHI	observe
始 SHI	onset	辯 BIAN	clever	之 ZHI	this	之 ZHI	this
發 FA	develop	智 ZHI	wisdom	取 QU	take	盛 SHENG	full
少 XIAO	little	自 ZI	self	手 SHOU	hand	者 ZHE	is
臥 JI	sleep	尊 ZUN	honor	陽 YANG		皆 JIE	all
不 BU	not	貴 GUI	value	明 MING	bright	取 QU	take
飢 JI	hunger	也 YE	period	太 TAI	great	之 ZHI	this
自 ZI	self	善 SHAN	tendency	陽 YANG		不 BU	not
高 GAO	high	罵 MA	curse	太 TAI	great	盛 SHENG	full
賢 XIAN	ability	詈 LI	curse	陰 YIN		釋 SHI	select
也 YE	period	日 RI	day	舌 SHE	tongue	之 ZHI	this
		夜 YE	night	下 XIA	below	也 YE	period
		不 BU	not	少 XIAO	small		
		休 XIU	rest	陰 YIN			

When KUANG 狂 onset develops into insomnia, anorexia and excessive self-esteem, the patient praises his cleverness, his wisdom, his skills and his nobility, cursing all the time, and does not rest during day or night.

The treatment is to puncture (points on) Arm YANG MING (Large Intestine), TAI YANG (Small Intestine), TAI YIN (Lung) and SHAO YIN (Heart) under the tongue.

If excess is observed, puncture (points) on all (these meridians). If there is no excess, then choose (which meridian to treat).

LING SHU, Chapter 22-11, describes the development of KUANG disease as a manic episode: insomnia, anorexia, excessive self-esteem, cursing and restlessness, corresponding to YANG/fire excess syndromes:
- Insomnia is caused by fire excess preventing the entering of Defensive QI into the body to allow sleep.
- Anorexia is caused by Spleen deficiency since overactive Fire-*Heart YANG* does not nourish Soil-Spleen.
- *Excessive self-esteem* expressed by overestimation of one's *cleverness, wisdom, skills and nobility* is a sign of damage to self-identity, social values and communication with the environment caused by heat injuring Heart and SHEN.
- Restlessness, agitation, curses are caused by YANG /fire rising to the head.

Treatment of KUANG disease development is the same as treatment of the onset of KUANG disease and of DIAN 癲 disease (LING SHU, 22-2):[405]
- Release *Heart fire* by dispersing its YANG, Small Intestine Meridian, Arm TAI YANG: SI7-SI8
- Release *Lung fire* by dispersing its YANG, Large Intestine Meridian, Arm YANG MING: LI6-LI7
- Disperse heat obstructing chest by tonification of Lung YIN, and improve Lung function of lowering by puncturing points on Lung Meridian, Arm TAI YIN: LU9-LU7
- H5 TONG LI 通里, *Penetrating the Interior*, LUO point on Heart Meridian, which purifies Heart, calms SHEN, treats schizophrenia and agoraphobia

Chinese medicine syndromes describing the development of KUANG disease (manic episode) of LING SHU, Chapter 22-11, are: [406]

1. *Phlegm-fire Harasses Upper Body*, TAN HUO SHANG RAO 痰火上擾	GV14-GV26-LI8-PC9, ST40-TW2-TW10-GV19
2. *Excess Fire in YANG MING*, YANG MING HUO SHENG 陽明火盛	LI11-ST42-ST40-GV14-TW6-PC8

---

405 See page 365
406 See pages 307, 308, KUANG caused by sorrow and grief, LING SHU, 8-4

1. KUANG 狂 disease - *Phlegm-fire Harasses the Upper Body*, TAN HUO SHANG RAO 痰火上擾, LING SHU, Chapter 22-11

Compare KUANG following sorrow and grief (LING SHU, Chapter 8-4).
Treatment points are: GV14-GV26-LI8-PC9, ST40-TW2-TW10-GV19

name	function	action
GV14-GV26-LI8-PC9 open Heart orifices, dissipate *fire*/YANG from head, calm SHEN		
GV26 SHUI GOU Water Trough 水溝	open LUO channels in facial region	calm SHEN, open Heart orifices, purify head and brain
GV14 DA ZHUI 大椎 Big Mallet	meeting of DU MAI with six YANG Meridians	regulate QI and YANG flow to head and heart, release excess heat and damp-heat from upper body
LI8 XIA LUAN 下廉 Lower Ridge		calm SHEN, clear heat, open Heart orifices, disperse
PC9 ZHONG CHONG 中衝 Central Surge	JING-Well-Wood of Master of Heart, tonify Fire	cool heat, open Heart orifices
ST40-TW2-TW10-GV19 purify phlegm		
ST40 FENG LONG 豐隆 Bountiful Bulge	LUO of Stomach	dissolve *phlegm-fire*, calm SHEN
TW2 YE MEN 液門 Body Fluids Gate	RONG-Water of SAN JIAO	enhance flow of body liquids, treat fear and anxiety
TW10 TIAN JING 天井 Celestial Well	HE-Soil of SAN JIAO, communicate between LUO	calm SHEN, cool blood, purify heat, dissolve phlegm, treat *affliction, sadness and insomnia* (S. de Morand. p. 539)
GV19 HOU DING 後頂 Behind Vertex	influence HUN 魂	regulate YANG, calm *Liver fire rising* and HUN 魂

2. KUANG 狂 disease - *Excess Fire in* YANG MING, YANG MING HUO SHENG 陽明火盛, LING SHU, Chapter 22-11

Compare KUANG following sorrow and grief or excessive joy (LING SHU, Chapter 8-4).

Acupuncture points to release heat from YANG MING, treat constipation, calm SHEN are: LI11-ST42-ST40-GV14-TW6-PC8

name	function	action
LI11-ST42-ST40-GV14-TW6-PC8		
LI11 QU CHI 曲池 Pool at the Bend	HE-Soil of Large Intestine	balance QI and Blood, dissipate heat from upper body
ST40 FENG LONG 豐隆 Bountiful Bulge	LUO of Stomach	dissolve *phlegm-fire*, calm SHEN
ST42 CHONG YANG 衝陽 Surging YANG	YUAN of Stomach	calm SHEN, dissipate heat from St. Meridian, treat constant elation, treat walking and climbing up to high places
GV14 DA ZHUI 大椎 Big Mallet	meeting of DU MAI with 6 YANG Meridians	regulate QI and YANG flow to head and heart, release excess heat and damp-heat from upper body
TW6 ZHI GOU 支溝 Branch Ditch	JING-River-Fire of SAN JIAO	regulate QI of SAN JIAO, treat constipation and clear heat from skin
PC8 LAO GONG 勞宮 Labor Palace	RONG-Fire of Master of Heart	clear heat from JUE YIN, purify Heart, awaken SHEN, cool blood

K. KUANG 狂 disease caused by fear, accompanied by agitation and euphoria, LING SHU, Chapter 22-12

狂	KUANG		妄	WANG	absurd	治	ZHI	treat
言	YAN	words	行	XING	walk	之	ZHI	this
驚	JING	startle	不	BU	not	取	QU	take
善	SHAN	tendency	休	XIU	rest	手	SHOU	hand
笑	XIAO	laugh	者	ZHE	this	陽	YANG	
好	HAO	love	得	DE	obtain	明	MING	bright
歌	GE	sing	之	ZHI	of	太	TAI	great
樂	LE	elation	大	DA	big	陽	YANG	
			恐	KONG	fear	太	TAI	great
						陰	YIN	

In KUANG 狂 *disease the patient's speech is delirious; he likes to laugh, loves to sing and is elated, walks around aimlessly and without rest. The condition comes from great fear* (DA KONG 大恐).

The treatment is to puncture (points on) *Arm* YANG MING (Large Intestine), TAI YANG (Small Intestine) *and* TAI YIN (Lung).

LING SHU, Chapter 22-12, presents KUANG as a psychotic episode provoked by great fear (DA KONG 大恐). Fear is a sign of *Kidney YIN and Kidney JING* 精 *deficiency* impairing the control of Fire-Heart by Water-Kidney. According to LING SHU, Chapter 8-3: *In fear and dread* (KONG JU 恐懼) SHEN *is restless and scared away, and the person cannot be himself*.[407] In KUANG 狂 *Heart fire/YANG* rises and SHEN is restless causing:

- Laughter, elation and joy without reason, incoherent speech, strange behavior - an expression of *Heart fire/YANG*
- A desire to sing and walk around aimlessly - a sign of Spleen injury by *Heart fire/YANG* (Fire does not generate Soil)

Treatment of KUANG, a psychotic episode caused by fear, is similar to that described previously for KUANG (22-11, 22-10) and for DIAN 癲 disease onset (LING SHU, 22-2):[408]

- Release *Heart fire* by dispersing its YANG, Small Intestine Meridian, Arm TAI YANG: SI7-SI8, SI5
  SI5 YANG GU 陽谷 YANG *Valley*, JING-River-Fire of Small Intestine; puncture (using dispersion technique) to disperse *Heart fire* and treat incoherent speech and laughter
- Release *Lung fire* by dispersing its YANG, Large Intestine Meridian, Arm YANG MING: LI6-LI7
- Disperse heat obstructing chest by tonification of Lung YIN, and improve Lung function of lowering by puncturing points on Lung Meridian, Arm TAI YIN: LU9-LU7

KUANG described in LING SHU, Chapter 22-12, may correspond also to *No Interaction between Heart and Kidney* (XIN SHEN BU JIAO 心腎不交).[409] In KUANG due to fear, the characteristic signs are agitation, overreaction, hyperactivity, elation with fear, horror and inconsistency. The treatment points are: BL23-Ki7, Ki5-ST27 (tonify), BL44-PC7-H7.

---

407 See page 266
408 See page 365
409 See pages 236, 251, 285, LING SHU, 8-3; LING SHU, 8-4

Acupuncture points to treat KUANG 狂 disease, *No Interaction between Heart and Kidney*,
XIN SHEN BU JIAO 心腎不交, LING SHU, Chapter 22-12

name	function	action
BL23-Ki7 tonify Kidney		
BL23 SHEN SHU 腎俞 Kidney SHU	SHU of Kidney, Kidney YANG regulation	tonify Kidney YIN, **tonify**
Ki7 FU LIU 復溜 Returning Current	JING-River-Metal of Kidney, tonify Water, enhance QI flow in meridians from Ki. towards M. H. (PC)	tonify Kidney YIN, tonify Heart, reduce fire, tonify brain and bone marrow, improve coherence and decisiveness, calm anger
Ki5-ST27 regulate SHAO YIN – YANG MING. When QI in YANG MING descends, QI in SHAO YIN ascends[410]		
Ki5 SHUI QUAN 水泉 Water Spring	XI of Kidney	open Kidney obstructions, **tonify**
ST27 DA JU 大巨 Great Gigantic	passage of YANG from chest to abdomen	tonify Kidney and JING, calm SHEN, disperse QI in Middle JIAO, treat fear with insomnia, **tonify**
BL44-PC7-H7 tonify Heart		
PC7 DA LING 大陵 Big Mound	SHU-YUAN-Soil of Master of Heart	calm and purify SHEN, cool Heart palpitation, cool blood, purify RONG QI
H7 SHEN MEN 神門 SHEN Gate	SHU-YUAN-Soil of Heart	calm SHEN, cool Heart (insomnia, stress), open Heart orifices
BL44 SHEN TANG 神堂 Spirit Hall	stabilize SHEN	stabilize SHEN, calm Heart, regulate QI, treat excess in chest, move down QI rising in panic (S. de Morand, page 593)

---

410 See page 411

L. KUANG 狂 disease caused by QI deficiency, accompanied by screaming and visual and auditory hallucinations,
LING SHU, Chapter 22-13

狂	KUANG	少	XIAO	little	治	ZHI	treat	陽	YANG
目	MU	eye	氣	QI	之	ZHI	this	明	MING	bright
妄	WANG	false	之	ZHI	of	取	QU	take	足	ZU	leg
見	JIAN	visions	所	SUO	in	手	SHOU	hand	太	TAI	great
耳	ER	ear	生	SHENG	origin	太	TAI	great	陰	YIN	hand
妄	WANG	false	也	YE	period	陽	YANG		頭	TOU	head
聞	TING	hear				太	TAI	great	兩	LIANG	2
善	SHAN	tendency				陰	YIN		顑	KAN	cheek
呼	HU	scream								
者	ZHE	comma								

In KUANG 狂 a patient has visual and auditory hallucinations and tends to scream; the condition comes from QI deficiency.
The treatment is to puncture (points on) *Arm YANG MING* (Large Intestine), (Arm) *TAI YIN* (Lung) *and* (Arm) *TAI YANG* (Small Intestine), *Leg TAI YIN* (Spleen) *and head on both cheeks.*

LING SHU, Chapter 22-13, describes KUANG 狂 as a psychotic episode or schizophrenic attack provoked by QI deficiency. QI deficiency causes *Kidney QI deficiency* which develops into *Liver and Heart fire/YANG rising* (Kidney does not control Heart and does not nourish Liver), expressed as:
- Auditory hallucinations and visual hallucinations, caused by JING deficiency in eyes (Liver) and ears (Heart, Kidney), resulting from uncontrolled YANG ascent to the head.
- Release of *Liver fire* provoking restlessness of HUN 魂 expressed outwardly as screaming.

The treatment for KUANG caused by QI deficiency (accompanied by screaming, visual and auditory hallucinations) is similar to the treatment described previously for KUANG (22-10, 22-11, 22-12) and for DIAN 癲 disease onset (22-2):[411]

---

411 See page 365

- Release *Heart fire* by dispersing its YANG, Small Intestine Meridian, Arm TAI YANG: SI7-SI8.
- Disperse heat from the chest by tonification of Lung YIN and improve the Lung function of lowering by puncturing points on Lung Meridian, Arm TAI YIN: LU9-LU7.
- Release *Lung fire* by dispersing its YANG, Large Intestine Meridian, Arm YANG MING: LI6-LI5.
  LI5 YANG XI 陽谿, *Small YANG Valley*, JING-River-Fire point of Large Intestine Meridian, which purifies fire from Metal.
- Since Fire generates Soil, it is possible to pull fire from Heart Meridian down to the legs by puncturing points on Spleen-Soil Meridian, Leg TAI YIN: SP1-SP4.[412]
- Treat visual and auditory hallucinations: SI19-BL8-BL61-ST5 (ST5 is located on the cheek, on the jaw joint).

name	function	action
SI19 TING GONG 聽宮 Auditory Palace	exit point, meeting of SAN JIAO, S.I. and G.B. Meridians	treat auditory hallucinations
BL8 LUO QUE 絡卻 Declining Connection.		clear sense organs, calm SHEN, collect memory, disperse YANG from head, treat visual and auditory hallucinations in KUANG (JIA JI JING)
BL61 PU CAN 僕参 Honored Servant	meeting of Bl. Meridian with YANG QIAO MAI	calm brain, treat hallucinations in KUANG
ST5 DA YING 大迎 Great Reception		regulate contractions of eyes, ears and vocal cords

---

412 See page 381

M. KUANG 狂 disease, caused by excessive joy, accompanied by bulimia and seeing ghosts, LING SHU, Chapter 22-14

狂	KUANG	得	DE	obtain	治	ZHI	treat	後 HOU then
者	ZHE comma	之	ZHI	this	之	ZHI	this	取 QU take
多	DUO much	有	YOU	has	取	QU	take	手 SHOU hand
食	SHI eat	所	SOU	from	足	ZU	leg	太 TAI great
善	SHAN tendency	大	DA	big	太	TAI	great	陰 YIN
見	JIAN see	喜	XI	joy	陰	YIN		太 TAI great
鬼	GUI ghost				太	TAI	great	陽 YANG
神	SHEN spirit				陽	YANG		陽 YANG
喜	XI joy				陽	YANG		明 MING bright
笑	XIAO laugh				明	MING	bright	
而	ER and							
不	BU not							
發	FA issue							
於	YU of							
外	WAI exterior							
者	ZHE comma							

In KUANG 狂 *the patient is bulimic; he sees ghosts and spirits, is joyful and laughs without external reason.* (The condition) *comes from great joy* (DA XI 大喜).

The treatment is to puncture (points on) *Leg* TAI YIN (Spleen), *Leg* TAI YANG (Bladder) *and Leg* YANG MING (Stomach).

Then puncture (points on) *Arm* TAI YIN (Lung), *Arm* TAI YANG (Small Intestine) *and Arm* YANG MING (Large Intestine).

LING SHU, Chapter 22-14, presents KUANG, a psychotic episode caused by great joy (DA XI 大喜) with the following symptoms:
- Laughter for no reason due to *Blazing Heart-fire.*
- Bulimia resulting from damage to Metal-PO 魄 by Heart fire (Fire over-controls Metal). Injured PO 魄 attempts to strengthen and build the body and cool Lung and Heart fire through eating.
- Seeing celestial spirits (SHEN 神), and earth spirits (demons, ghosts) (GUI 鬼) occurs when Fire-Heart does not nourish Soil-Spleen-YI 意. Intent and ideas lose contact with reality.

- Over-control of Metal-skin by Fire-Heart may manifest as 'burning of the skin': eczema or psoriasis.[413]

According to LING SHU, Chapter 8-4, joy and pleasure cause KUANG:
When joy and pleasure (XI LE 喜樂) without limit invade Lung, this injures PO 魄. Injury to PO 魄 results in KUANG 狂. In KUANG, YI 意 loses its ability to acknowledge the existence of others.[414]

The treatment of KUANG, a psychotic episode caused by excessive joy according to LING SHU, Chapter 22-14:
- Since Fire generates Soil, it is possible to pull fire from Heart Meridian down to the legs by puncturing points on Spleen-Soil Meridian, Leg TAI YIN: SP1-SP4. [415]
- Release *Heart fire* by puncturing points on Leg TAI YANG (Bladder): BL63-BL61.

name	function	action
BL63 JIN MEN 金門 Golden Gate	XI of Bladder, meeting of Bladder Meridian with YANG WEI MAI	calm brain
BL61 PU CAN 僕參 Honored Servant	meeting of Bladder Meridian with YANG QIAO MAI	calm brain, treat hallucinations in KUANG

KUANG 狂 treatment according to LING SHU, Chapter 22-14, is similar to the treatment described previously for KUANG and DIAN 癲 disease onset:[416]
- Release Heart fire by dispersing its YANG, Small Intestine Meridian, Arm TAI YANG: SI7-SI8
- Disperse heat from the chest by tonification of Lung YIN and improve the Lung function of lowering by puncturing points on Lung Meridian, Arm TAI YIN: LU9-LU7
- Release *Lung fire* by dispersing its YANG, Large Intestine Meridian, Arm YANG MING: LI6-LI5.[417]

---

413 See page 321, and pleasure in LING SHU, Chapter 8-4
414 See page 318
415 See page 381
416 See page 365
417 See page 389, for LI5

Chinese Medicine syndromes that describe KUANG 狂 disease, caused by excessive joy, with bulimia and seeing ghosts are:

1. *Liver and Gallbladder Fire Flaring Upwards,* GAN DAN HUO SHANG YAN 肝膽火上炎[418] following *Liver QI Congestion* — PC7-PC8-LIV2-GB43, GV14-GV24
2. *Blood Flow Congested and Obstructed,* XUE XING YU ZHI 血行鬱滯[419] — SP10-SP6-BL14, LI11-ST25-GV14
3. *Confusion of Heart and SHEN,* XIN SHEN HUO LUAN 心神惑亂[420] — BL15-SP6-LIV3-PC5-GV22-LIV14-CV14

1. KUANG 狂 caused by excessive joy - *Liver and Gallbladder Fire Flaring Upwards,* GAN DAN HUO SHANG YAN 肝膽火上炎 following *Liver QI Congestion*

Compare overflowing anger (LING SHU, 8-3). 420 KUANG following excessive joy causes an 'explosion' of Congested *Liver QI*, expressed as *Liver and Gallbladder Fire Flaring Upwards* with bulimia, irritability with laughter for no reason and hallucinations. The treatment is to calm *Liver and Gallbladder fire*, and disperse heat from the head: PC7-PC8-LIV2-GB43, GV14-GV24.

name	function	action
PC7-PC8-LIV2-GB43 disperse and purify *Liver and Gallbladder fire*		
LIV2 XING JIAN 行間 Moving Between	RONG-Fire of Liver	move YANG down, benefit G.B., calm anger
GB43 XIA XI 俠谿 Pinched Ravine	RONG-Water of Gall-bladder, tonify Wood	purify head, ears and eyes, return order and mental uprightness, cool *Gallbladder fire*
PC7 DA LING 大陵 Big Mound	SHU-YUAN-Soil of Master of Heart	calm and purify SHEN, cool Heart palpitation, cool blood
PC8 LAO GONG 勞宮 Labor Palace	RONG-Fire of Master of Heart	disperse heat from JUE YIN, purify Heart, awaken SHEN, cool blood, treat anger, **disperse**
GV14-GV24 disperse heat from head		
GV14 DA ZHUI 大椎 Big Mallet	meeting of DU MAI with six YANG Meridians	regulate QI and YANG flow to head and heart, release excess heat from upper body
GV24 SHEN TING 神庭 SHEN Court	meeting of DU MAI with Bl. and St. Meridians	communicate between orifices, calm SHEN, regulate restlessness

---

418 See page 262, LING SHU, 8-3
419 See footnote 370
420 See pages 265, 297

2. KUANG 狂 caused by excessive joy - *Blood Flow Congested and Obstructed*, XUE XING YU ZHI 血行鬱滯

Compare melancholy and sadness (depression), in sorrow and grief, and in overflowing anger (LING SHU, 8-4).

KUANG caused by excessive joy obstructs the blood flow and damages the nervous system and sense organs (eyes and ears), which results in hallucinations, erratic behavior and emotional instability: hyperexcitability with laughter and curses, memory loss.

The treatment is to tonify the Blood flow and release excess YANG: SP10-SP6-BL14, LI11-ST25-GV14.

name	function	action
SP10-SP6-BL14 tonify blood flow		
SP6 SAN YIN JIAO 三陰交 Meeting of 3 YIN	meeting of Sp., Liv., and Ki. Meridians	tonify and nourish Blood, QI and YIN, move YIN up, nourish Spleen
SP10 XUE HAI 血海 Sea of Blood.		invigorate and cool Blood
BL14 JUE YIN SHU 厥陰俞	SHU of Master of Heart	clear heat
release excess YANG: LI11-ST25-GV14		
LI11 QU CHI 曲池 Pool at the Bend	HE-Soil of Large Intestine	balance QI and Blood, cool Blood, dissipate heat from upper body
ST25 TIAN SHU 天樞 Celestial Axis	MU of Large Intestine	dissolve phlegm, calm SHEN, regulate HUN 魂 and PO 魄
GV14 DA ZHUI 大椎 Big Mallet	meeting of DU MAI with six YANG Meridians	regulate QI and YANG flow to head and heart, release excess heat from upper body

3. KUANG 狂 caused by excessive joy - *Confusion of Heart and SHEN*, XIN SHEN HUO LUAN 心神惑亂

Compare overflowing anger (LING SHU, 8-3) and melancholy and sadness (LING SHU, 8-4).

KUANG caused by excessive joy is due to prolonged injury to YIN by *Liver QI congestion* which results in *Heart Blood and YIN Deficiency* and *Liver Fire*. The characteristic signs in this manifestation of *Confusion of Heart and* SHEN are rage alternating with joy, restlessness, detachment from reality, curses, lack of contact with reality, hallucinations and bulimia. The treatment is to nourish Heart YIN: BL15-SP6-LIV3-PC5-GV22-LIV14-CV14.

name	function	action
LIV3 TAI CHONG 太沖 Great Rush	SHU-YUAN-Soil of Liver	release and harmonize Liver
SP6 SAN YIN JIAO 三陰交 Meeting of 3 YIN	meeting of Sp., Liv. and Ki. Meridians	tonify and nourish Blood, QI and YIN, move YIN up, nourish Spleen
BL15 XIN SHU 心俞 Heart SHU	SHU of Heart, Heart YANG regulation	calm SHEN, clear heat from Heart, release LUO of Heart
PC5 JIAN SHI 間使 Interval Envoy	JING-River-Metal of Master of Heart - JUE YIN, Group LUO of 3 arm YIN	regulate YIN deficiency above and YIN stagnation below, open chest, calm SHEN, calm SHAO YANG, calm suffering and stop the crying
LIV14 QI MEN 期門 Cycle Gate	MU of Liver, regulate Liver YIN, meeting of Liv., Sp. Meridians and YIN WEI MAI	move QI up from abdomen to chest, spread Liver QI, invigorate Blood, harmonize Liver and Stomach
GV22 XIN HUI 囟會 Fontanelle Meeting		strengthen JING, create new ideas
CV14 JU QUE 巨闕 Great Tower Gate	MU of Heart, regulate Heart YIN	calm SHEN and Heart, dissolve phlegm, open chest, move *turbid* QI down

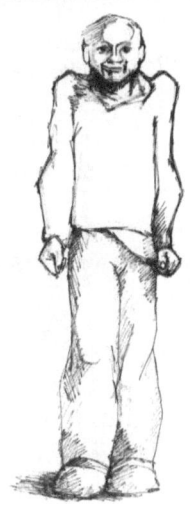

N. KUANG 狂 disease - acute psychotic episode, LING SHU, 22-15

狂 KUANG		先 XIAN	first	動 DONG	move	不 BU	not
而 ER	then	取 QU	take	脈 MAI	vessel	已 YI	recover
新 XIN	recent	曲 QU	bent	及 JI	if	以 YI	then
發 FA	issue	泉 QUAN	spring	盛 SHENG	full	法 FA	system
未 WEI	not	右 YOU	right	者 ZHE	comma	取 QU	take
應 YING	respond	左 ZUO	left	見 JIAN	look	而 ER	then
如 RU	like	者 ZHE	comma	血 XUE	blood	灸 JIU	moxa
此 CI	these above			有 YOU	has	骨 GU	bone
者 ZHE	comma			頃 QING	easy	骶 DI	coccyx
				已 YI	recover	二 ER	20
						十 SHI	
						壯 ZHUANG	cone

When KUANG is acute and does not match signs described before, first puncture QU QUAN 曲泉 (Spring at the Bend, LIV8), on the left and the right sides. If there is an excess in blood vessels then bleed. Relief occurs immediately.

If there is no immediate relief after this method, burn 20 moxa cones on the coccyx (GV1).

LING SHU, Chapter 22-15, describes treatment for KUANG with sudden onset. Acute episodes of KUANG are caused by *Empty Liver YANG rising* due to *Kidney and Liver YIN deficiency*.

The treatment is to puncture LIV8 (QU QUAN 曲泉, *Spring at the Bend*): LIV8 is HE-Water point, which strengthens and cools Liver without exhausting it.

Liver YANG/fire causes the swelling of blood vessels in the area of LIV8, at the medial end of the transverse popliteal crease. It is recommended to bleed these swollen blood vessels, using a lance needle, to release the communication between Liver Meridian and its inner pathway, and to expel *empty Liver YANG* outward to prevent Liver YANG invading Heart.

When puncturing and bleeding of LIV8 does not help, it is recommended to burn 20 moxa cones on the tailbone, GV1, CHANG QIANG 長強,[421] which is the meeting point between Governing Vessel (DU MAI) and Conception Vessel (REN MAI), and the beginning of the longitudinal LUO of DU MAI; this point helps to expel pernicious QI. Heating GV1 strengthens the root of YANG, allowing ascent of YIN - JING QI 精氣 to cool blood and pacify Liver YANG/fire.

4. Treatment of rebel QI (NI 逆) which provokes QI congestion and obstruction, LING SHU, Chapter 22

LING SHU, Chapter 22, continues with a description of damage caused by rebel QI (NI 逆) which flows either in a contrary direction or in an exaggerated fashion in the correct direction, and thereby prevents the balanced (natural or right) QI flow, provoking congestion, obstruction and disturbance of body functions. Balanced QI flow is an expression of the proper functioning of ZANG:

- Liver and Gallbladder direct the 'smooth' QI flow upwards and outwards
- Heart governs QI flow in all directions, and also communication within the body and between man and the environment
- Spleen moves QI upwards to the chest; Stomach and Intestines move QI downwards
- Lung moves QI downwards and gathers QI from the skin inwards, helping Kidney to store QI
- Kidney stores Source QI: with the help of Liver, Kidney moves JING QI 精氣 upwards to the head, and together with Bladder moves QI downwards

LING SHU, Chapter 22, describes seven obstructions caused by NI 逆, rebel QI:

- Congestion of cold and edema of limbs due to rebel wind (FENG NI 風逆)
- Sudden internal cold due to rebel QI (JUE NI 厥逆) in Kidney Meridian

---

[421] See page 269

- Internal cold in trunk due to rebel QI (JUE NI 厥逆)
- Lower JIAO obstruction and urinary retention due to rebel afflux
- Liver rebel QI (QI NI 氣逆) invades Spleen
- Obstruction of QI flow in SHAO YIN (Source QI) and YANG MING (acquired QI) in severe diseases
- Two cases of Kidney JING 精 deficiency

O. Congestion of cold and edema of limbs caused by invasion of rebel wind (FENG NI 風逆), LING SHU, 22-16

風 FENG	wind	唏 XI	moan	取 QU	take	肉 ROU	flesh
逆 NI	rebel	然 RAN	such	手 SHOU	arm	清 QING	cold
暴 BAO	sudden	時 SHI	moment	太 TAI	great	取 QU	take
四 SI	4	寒 HAN	cold	陰 YIN		滎 RONG	point
肢 ZHI	limbs	飢 JI	hunger	表 BIAO	exterior	骨 GU	bone
腫 ZHONG	swell	則 ZE	then	裏 LI	interior	清 QING	cold
身 SHEN	body	煩 FAN	depress	足 ZU	leg	取 QU	take
漯 LUO	chills	飽 BAO	full	少 SHAO	small	井 JING	point
漯 LUO	shivers	則 ZE	then	陰 YIN		經 JING	point
		善 SHAN	tend	陽 YANG		也 YE	period
		變 BIAN	change	明 MING	bright		
				之 ZHI	of		
				經 JING	meridian		

Rebel wind (FENG NI 風逆) causes sudden swelling of the four limbs, chills and shivers, the patient moans from cold, when hungry he is depressed, when satiated he is restless.

The treatment is to puncture (points on) Arm TAI YIN (Lung) according to the exterior-interior method (BIAO LI 表裏), then Leg SHAO YIN (Kidney) and Leg YANG MING (Stomach).

When cold is in flesh puncture RONG 滎 points. When cold is in bones, puncture JING-Well 井 and JING-River 經 points.

LING SHU, Chapter 22-16, describes an acute condition caused by external and harmful rebel wind (FENG NI 風逆) causing a sudden congestion of QI and disruption of the flow of body liquids and QI:

- Disruption in the flow of body liquids occurs due to impaired Kidney, Spleen and Lung function. When the external rebel wind invades Lung, it obstructs the descent of body liquids, causing edema (swelling) of hands. When the external rebel wind invades Kidney and Spleen, it obstructs the rise of body liquids, causing edema in the legs.
- QI flow is slow and deficient causing a feeling of cold with chills and shivers resulting from:
  - injury to Stomach and Spleen, caused by excessive control of Soil by Wood-wind, leading to Nourishing QI deficiency
  - injury to Lung, which regulates QI flow in meridians
  - deficiency of Nourishing QI, which causes depression when the patient is hungry; deficiency of Spleen QI, which leads to QI congestion in Middle JIAO after eating, causing restlessness

Treatment of rebel wind is by:
- Regulation between exterior-interior (BIAO LI 表裏), using LUO-YUAN points of Arm TAI YIN (Lung) and YANG MING (Large Intestine): LU7-LI4
- Moving body liquids down by tonifying Lung: BL13-LU5-LI7
- Tonification of Leg SHAO YIN (Kidney Meridian): Ki7-Ki3
- Regulation of flow of body liquids: ST28-SP9, SP7-BL22-BL27
- Dispersion of cold from muscles (flesh) by RONG 榮 points on Spleen Meridian (YIN) SP2 and SAN JIAO Meridian (YANG) - TW2
- Dispersion of cold from bones by JING-Well 井 and JING-River 經 points on Leg YIN Meridians: SP1-SP5, Ki1-Ki7, LIV1-LIV4 and Leg YANG Meridians: ST41-ST45, BL60-BL67, GB38-GB44

Acupuncture points to treat congestion of cold and edema of limbs, caused by invasion of rebel wind, LING SHU, 22-16

name	function	action
Regulate exterior-interior using LUO-YUAN points of Metal		
LU7 LIE QUE 列缺 Broken Sequence	LUO of Lung, open REN MAI	treat rebel QI, move Lung QI and liquids down
LI4 HE GU 合谷 Union Valley	YUAN of Large Intestine, entry point, command point of face and mouth	regulate QI, release excess YANG from head
move body liquids down by tonification of Lung: BL13-LU5-LI7		
BL13 FEI SHU 肺俞 Lung SHU	SHU of Lung, regulate Lung YANG	release Lung
LU5 CHI ZE 尺澤 Cubit Marsh	HE-Water of Lung, disperse Metal	release Lung QI and TAI YIN, treat depression
LI7 WEN LIU 溫溜 Warm Flow	XI of Large Intestine	release Metal
Tonification of Leg SHAO YIN (Kidney): Ki7-Ki3		
Ki3 TAI XI 太谿 Great Ravine	SHU-YUAN-Soil of Kidney	tonify Kidney YIN, release ascent of CHONG MAI and REN MAI, treat degenerative diseases, tonify
Ki7 FU LIU 復溜 Returning Current	JING-River-Metal of Kidney, tonify Water, enhance QI flow in meridians from Ki. towards M.H. (PC)	tonify Kidney YIN
Regulation of body liquids flow: ST28-SP9, SP7-BL22-BL27		
ST28 SHUI DAO 水道 Water Way		clear and regulate flow of body liquids
SP9 YIN LING QUAN 陰陵泉 YIN Mound Spring	HE-Water of Spleen	tonify Spleen YANG, regulate flow of body liquids
SP7 LOU GU 漏谷 Leaking Valley		strengthen Spleen, invigorate QI and blood flow, reduce swelling, purify RONG QI
BL22 SAN JIAO SHU 三焦俞	SHU of SAN JIAO	open and regulate water passages
BL27 XIAO CHANG SHU 小腸俞 Small Intestine SHU	SHU of Small Intestine, regulate YANG of S.I.	regulate Bladder, tonify Lower JIAO
Disperse cold from muscle by RONG 榮 points on Spleen Meriidian - SP2 and SAN JIAO Meridian - TW2		
SP2 DA DU 大都 Great Metropolis	RONG-Fire of Spleen, tonify Soil	regulate Spleen and Middle JIAO, drain damp, regulate body liquids, **tonify**
TW2 YE MEN 液門 Body Liquids Gate	RONG-Water of SAN JIAO	enhance flow of body liquids, disperse cold from limbs, **disperse**

Acupuncture points to treat congestion of cold and edema of limbs caused by invasion of rebel wind, LING SHU, 22-16, continued

Disperse cold from bones by JING-Well 井 and JING-River 經 points of Leg YIN and YANG Meridians: SP1-SP5, Ki1-Ki7, LIV1-LIV4, ST41-ST45, BL60-BL67, GB38-GB44	
SP1 YIN BAI 隱白 Hidden White	JING-Well-Wood of Spleen
SP5 SHANG QIU 商丘 Merchant Hill	JING-River-Metal of Spleen
Ki1 YONG QUAN 湧泉 Gushing Spring	JING-Well-Wood of Kidney
Ki7 FU LIU 復溜 Returning Current	JING-River-Metal of Kidney
LIV1 DÀ DUN 大敦 Large Pile	JING-Well-Wood of Liver
LIV4 ZHONG FENG 中封 Mound Center	JING-River-Metal of Liver
ST45 LI DUI 厲兌 Severe Mouth	JING-Well-Metal of Stomach
ST41 JIE XI 解谿 Ravine Divide	JING-River-Fire of Stomach
BL67 ZHI YIN 至陰 Reaching YIN	JING-Well-Metal of Bladder
BL60 KUN LUN 昆侖 Mountain KUN LUN	JING-River-Fire of Bladder
GB44 ZU QIAO YIN 足竅陰 Foot Orifice YIN	JING-Well-Metal of Gallbladder
GB38 YANG FU 陽輔 YANG Assistance	JING-River-Fire of Gallbladder

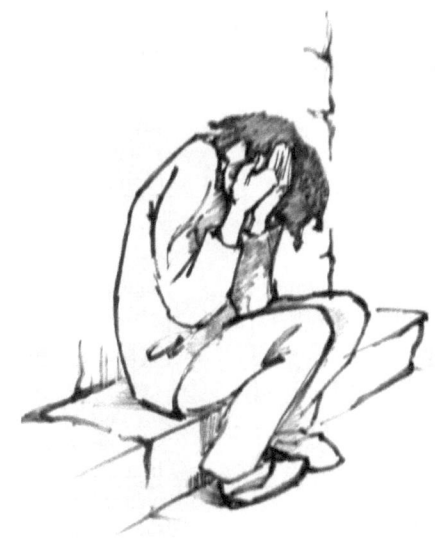

P. Sudden internal cold caused by rebel QI (JUE NI 厥逆) in Kidney Meridian, LING SHU, 22-17

厥	JUE	tired	煩	FAN	oppress	暖	NUAN	warm
逆	NI	rebel	而	ER	and	取	QU	take
為	WEI	recent	不	BU	not	足	ZU	leg
病	BING	disease	得	DE	obtain	少	SHAO	small
也	YE	period	食	SHI	eat	陰	YIN	
足	ZU	leg	脈	MAI	pulse	清	QING	cold
暴	BAO	sudden	大	DA	big	取	QU	take
清	QING	cold	少	SHAO	small	足	ZU	leg
胸	XIONG	thorax	皆	JIE	all	陽	YANG	
若	RUO	like	澀	SE	choppy	明	MING	bright
將	JIANG	almost						
裂	LIE	explode						
腸	CHANG	intestine						
若	RUO	like						
將	JIANG	almost						
以	YI	by						
刀	DAO	knife						
切	QIE	cut						
之	ZHI	this						

清 QING	cold	
則 ZE	then	
補 BU	tonify	
之 ZHI	them	
溫 WEN	warm	
則 ZE	then	
寫 XIE	disperse	
之 ZHI	them	

When the disease is caused by rebel (QI) (JUE NI 厥逆), there is sudden cold in legs, a sensation of bursting of the thorax and intestinal pain as if stabbed by a knife.

The patient is anxious and cannot eat; his pulse is alternately large or small and choppy,

Puncture (points on) *Leg SHAO YIN* (Kidney) *if the patient's body is warm; puncture* (points on) *Leg YANG MING* (Stomach) *if the patient's body is cold.*

When the patient's body is cold, tonify the points. When the patient's body is warm, disperse the points.

Rebel QI (JUE NI 厥逆) in Kidney Meridian (Leg SHAO YIN) may be caused by injury to Kidney from:
- Repetitive fear
- Continuous accumulation of emotional and sexual frustrations
- Source QI (YUAN QI 原氣/元氣) deficiency due to age or a weak constitution

LING SHU, Chapter 22-17, describes JUE NI 厥逆 as a congestion of internal cold which starts in the legs and spreads to the abdomen and chest following the pathways of Kidney Meridian and Extraordinary Meridian CHONG MAI 衝脈. Cold disrupts the function of CHONG MAI: ascent and distribution of YUAN QI, JING QI 精氣 (QI carrying JING), Blood and Defensive QI (WEI QI 衛氣).

Signs of rebel QI (JUE NI 厥逆) in Kidney Meridian (Leg SHAO YIN) are:
- Sudden cold in legs (a sign of congested cold disturbing Kidney Meridian)
- Sensation of the thorax bursting (a sign of congested cold in Kidney Meridian and in CHONG MAI)
- Intestinal pain as if stabbed by a knife (sign of cold congestion in Kidney Meridian and in CHONG MAI)
- Restlessness with an inability to eat (a sign of congested cold in Leg SHAO YIN, Kidney Meridian, which prevents descent of Leg YANG MING, Stomach Meridian) [422]
- Choppy, alternating large and small pulse (sign of cold and obstruction of the flow of Blood and QI)

LING SHU, in Chapters 38 and 62, describes the pathway of the descending branch of CHONG MAI, which follows Kidney Meridian to the leg and is responsible for heating the feet:

> ...then from there (QI JI, QI CHONG, ST30) *it runs alongside SHAO YIN meridian on the inner thigh to permeate the 3 YIN channels, and its anterior branch runs inwards and exits at the hill and*

---

[422] Ascent of SHAO YIN regulates descent of YANG MING, see page 411

unites with it, descends following the top of the foot and penetrates into the space of the great toe, where it permeates and heats up the muscles and tendons. In the event of congestion of these little vessels, the artery (pedal) stops beating and the absence of pulse at the level of the top of the foot is the indicator of JUE NI 厥逆 (afflux), *origin of cold* (of the feet).

NAN JING, Difficulty 29, connects the internal cold with rebel QI in CHONG MAI:

If CHONG is diseased, the QI will counterflow (rebel) *and in the interior* (of the body) *there will be tension* (cramps)[423]

衝之為病逆氣而裏急

Treatment of JUE NI 厥逆 in Kidney Meridian is:
- Treatment of cold in legs by points on Leg SHAO YIN, Kidney Meridian: Ki3-Ki7 [424]
- Treatment of abdominal contraction when a body is warm by points on Leg SHAO YIN, Kidney Meridian: Ki16-Ki14
- Treatment of rebel afflux (JUE NI 厥逆) when a body is warm by points on Leg SHAO YIN, Kidney Meridian and CHONG MAI: Ki22-Ki24-SP4
- Treatment of rebel afflux (JUE NI 厥逆) when the body is cold by points on Leg YANG MING, Stomach Meridian: ST25-ST27-ST37-ST41. Tonify points on Stomach Meridian if the whole body is cold. Disperse points on Stomach Meridian if there is a sensation of cold with hot flashes (empty heat) in the thorax, for example in menopause.

---

423 *The Classic of Difficulties:* A Translation of the Nan Jing by Bianque, Bob Flaws
424 See page 399

Acupuncture points to treat sudden internal cold caused by rebel QI (JUE NI 厥逆) in Kidney Meridian, LING SHU, 22-17

name	function	action
Treat abdominal contraction when a body is warm: Ki16-Ki14		
Ki16 HUANG SHU 肓俞 Membrane SHU	meeting of Ki. Meridian with CHONG MAI	treat abdominal pain caused by cold (According to ISHIMPO and JIA JI JING), **puncture perpendicularly**
Ki14 XI MAN 四滿 Fourfold Fullness	meeting of Ki. Meridian with CHONG MAI	treat cold and Kidney stones BEN TUN (with spastic pain), **puncture perpendicularly**
Treat cold in chest when a body is warm: Ki22-Ki24-SP4		
Ki22 BU LANG 步廊 Corridor Walk	meeting with CHONG MAI	move rebel Lung and Stomach QI down, release rebel QI from chest, **puncture perpendicularly**
Ki24 LING XU 靈墟 Large Hill of LING (Spirit)	meeting with CHONG MAI	move rebel Lung and Stomach QI down, release congestion and pain in chest by moving rebel QI down through CHONG MAI, **puncture perpendicularly**
SP4 GONG SUN 公孫 Grandfather-Grandson	opening of CHONG MAI, LUO of Spleen	treat pain and contractions of abdomen
Dispersion of rebel JUE NI when body is cold: ST25-ST27-ST37-ST41		
ST25 TIAN SHU 天樞 Celestial Axis	MU of Large Intestine, meeting with CHONG MAI	move YANG towards YIN from middle of body, dissolve phlegm and obstructions, calm SHEN, treat cold in center of body, **moxa**
ST27 DA JU 大巨 Great Gigantic	passage of YANG from chest to abdomen	tonify Kidney and JING, calm SHEN, disperse QI in Middle JIAO, separate *clear* and *turbid* of Small Intestine, **tonify**
ST37 SHANG JU XU 上巨虛 Great Deficiency Above	Lower HE of Large Intestine, Lower Body Sea of Blood (with ST39, BL11)	treat diarrhea with loss of appetite and sweat, weakness in limbs, **tonify**
ST41 JIE XI 解谿 Ravine Divide	JING-River-Fire of Stomach, tonify Soil	move fire congested in Stomach, treat depression accompanied by anorexia, **tonify**

Q. Congestion in trunk caused by rebel QI (JUE NI 厥逆), LING SHU, Chapter 22-18

厥	JUE	tired	取	QU	take	與	YU	on
逆	NI	rebel	之	ZHI	of	背	BEI	back
腹	FU	abdomen	下	XIA	below	輸	SHU	points
脹	ZHANG	swollen	胸	XIONG	thorax	以	YI	use
滿	MAN	full	二	ER	2	手	SHOU	hand
腸	CHANG	intestines	脅	XIE	ribs	按	AN	press
鳴	MING	make sound	咳	KE	cough	之	ZHI	of
胸	XIONG	thorax	而	ER	and	立	LI	establish
滿	MAN	full	動	DONG	move	快	KUAI	fast
不	BU	not	手	SHOU	hand	者	ZHE	comma
得	DE	obtain	者	ZHE	comma	是	SHI	this
息	XI	breath				也	YE	period

When the disease is caused by rebel QI (JUE NI 厥逆), and there is fullness and swelling of abdomen, borborygmi in intestines, thoracic fullness with respiratory difficulties,
Puncture sub-thoracic points under the ribs on both sides (two hypochondria), *where movement while coughing can be felt with the hands.*
Treat back SHU 輸 points where the patient experiences quick relief with the pressure of the hand.

LING SHU, Chapter 22-18, describes damage caused by rebel QI (JUE NI 厥逆) obstructing regular QI flow in the trunk. QI loses its ability to descend, provoking congestion in the chest with respiratory distress, and congestion and swelling of the abdomen with borborygmi.

According to LING SHU, Chapter 59, congestion and swelling of the abdomen with borborygmi and respiratory distress are signs of the obstruction of Defensive QI (WEI QI 衛氣) flow:

When WEI QI 衛氣 detained in the middle of the abdomen, drags along, accumulates, and does not move. There it luxuriates and collects and is not fixed in a proper place. This causes congestion in man ribs and the middle of the stomach. There is panting and an unruliness in breathing 喘呼逆息.[425]

LING SHU, Chapter 59, also proposes a treatment for the condition: *When both upper (thorax) and lower (abdomen) are congested, treat both upper and lower and the point one CUN below the lowest rib* (eleventh rib, LIV13). *If the disease is severe, treat using the chicken foot* (three point star) *method of insertion* (puncture diagonally).[426]

Treatment of WEI QI 衛氣 obstruction described in LING SHU, Chapter 22-18:
- Release WEI QI flow: LIV13, LIV14
- Treat back SHU 輸 points to tonify Lung, Heart and Liver: BL13-BL15-BL18, and points on the back sensitive to touch.

name	function	action
Release WEI QI flow: LIV13, LIV14		
LIV13 ZHANG MEN 章門 Chapter Gate	MU of Spleen, HUI-meeting of five ZANG, meeting of Liv., Ki., H., Sp., Lu., G.B. Meridians	treat Upper JIAO obstruction and rebel QI obstructing WEI QI, *If the disease is severe, treat using the chicken foot* (three point star) *method of insertion* (puncture diagonally)
LIV14 QI MEN 期門 Cycle Gate	MU of Liver, regulate Liver YIN, meeting of Liv., Sp. Meridians and YIN WEI MAI	move QI from abdomen to chest, benefit Gallbladder, treat abdominal swelling
Treat back SHU 輸 points, tonify Lung, Heart and Liver: BL13-BL15-BL18		
BL13 FEI SHU 肺俞 Lung SHU	SHU of Lung, regulate Lung YANG	tonify Lung
BL15 XIN SHU 心俞 Heart SHU	SHU of Heart, regulate Heart YANG	calm SHEN, move congestion of Heart Blood, tonify Heart YIN, release LUO of Heart
BL18 GAN SHU 肝俞 Liver SHU	SHU of Liver, regulate Liver YANG	move Liver QI and Blood

---

425 Translated by WU JING-NUAN
426 Translated by WU JING-NUAN

R. Lower JIAO obstruction and urinary retention caused by rebel afflux, LING SHU, Chapter 22-19

內	NEI	interior	刺	CI	needle
閉	BI	close	足	ZU	leg
不	BU	not	少	SHAO	small
得	DE	obtain	陰	YIN	
溲	SOU	urinate	太	TAI	great
			陽	YANG	
			與	YU	on
			抵	DI	coccyx, sacrum
			上	SHANG	above
			以	YI	with
			長	CHANG	long
			鍼	ZHEN	needle

When the interior (obstruction) *prevents urination, puncture* (points on) *Leg* SHAO YIN (Kidney), *Leg* TAI YANG (Bladder) *and* (the point) *on the coccyx with a long needle.*

LING SHU, Chapter 22-19, describes Lower JIAO obstruction by rebel QI (JUE NI 厥逆) probably caused by fear. JUE NI 厥逆 obstructs Kidney QI causing urinary dysfunction (dysuria or anuria) and edema in the lower body. SU WEN, Chapter 39, explains how fear causes Lower JIAO swelling:

> *Fear makes* JING 精 *retreat. When* JING 精 *retreats Upper* JIAO *closes. When* (Upper JIAO) *is closed, QI reverses its flow* (descends toward the pelvis). (*When QI*) *reverses its flow, Lower JIAO inflates. So QI does not circulate.*[427]

LING SHU, Chapter 22-19, proposes a treatment for Lower JIAO obstruction and urinary retention due to rebel afflux:
- Treatment of urinary dysfunction and edema by puncturing points on Kidney (Leg SHAO YIN) and Bladder (Leg TAI YANG) Meridians: Ki7-Ki5, BL63, BL23; Ki4-BL64 (LUO-YUAN)

---

[427] See page 187

- Puncture (with a long needle) the point located on the coccyx (tailbone): GV1
- Treatment of urinary dysfunction according to LEI JING, the commentary on LING SHU: GV1, BL63, BL61, BL58, BL39, Ki9, Ki1

name	function	action
Treatment of urinary dysfunction and edema: Ki7-Ki5, BL63, BL23; Regulation of Kidney and Bladder Meridians (LUO-YUAN) Ki4-BL64,		
Ki5 SHUI QUAN 水泉 Water Spring	XI of Kidney	release Kidney obstruction, treat urinary dysfunction and edema
Ki7 FU LIU 復溜 Returning Current	JING-River-Metal of Kidney, Water tonification, enhance QI flow in meridians from Ki. towards M.H. (PC)	tonify Kidney YIN, tonify Heart, reduce fire, treat urinary dysfunction and edema, tonify
BL63 JIN MEN 金門 Golden Gate	XI of Bladder, meeting with YANG WEI MAI	treat urinary dysfunction and edema
BL23 SHEN SHU 腎俞 Kidney SHU	SHU of Kidney, regulate Kidney YANG	tonify Kidney YIN, treat urinary dysfunction and edema
Ki4 DA ZHONG 大鍾 Big Bell	LUO of Kidney, enhance QI flow in meridians from Ki. towards M.H.(PC)	open Upper JIAO, regulate inferior orifices, treat urinary dysfunction and edema
BL64 JING GU 京骨 Capital Bone	YUAN of Bladder	calm SHEN, treat urinary dysfunction and edema
Treatment of disuria according to LEI JING: GV1, BL61, BL58, BL39, Ki9, Ki1		
GV1 CHANG QIANG 長強, Always Strong	LUO of DU MAI, connecting to CV1, meeting of DU MAI, REN MAI, Ki. and G.B. Meridians	treat five types of painful urinary dysfunction[428]
BL61 PU CAN 僕參 Honored Servant	meeting of Bl. Meridian and YANG QIAO MAI	treat urinary dysfunction and edema
BL58 FEI YANG 飛陽 Taking Flight	LUO of Bladder	treat urinary dysfunction and edema
BL39 WEI YANG 委陽 Bent YANG	Lower HE of SAN JIAO	regulate urination
Ki9 ZHU BIN 築賓 Guest House	XI and beginning of YIN WEI MAI, beginning of Ki.-Bl. JING BIE	treat urinary dysfunction and edema
Ki1 YONG QUAN 湧泉 Gushing Spring	JING-Well-Wood of Kidney, root of SHAO YIN	move rebel QI and YANG down, open Heart orifices

---

428 Deadman (difficult urination, retention of urine, dark urine, seminal emission due to fear or fright)

S. Liver Rebel QI (QI NI 氣逆) invades Spleen, LING SHU, Chapter 22-20

氣	QI	
逆	NI	rebel
則	ZE	then
取	QU	take, puncture
其	QI	his
太	TAI	great
陰	YIN	
陽	YANG	
明	MING	bright
厥	JUE	exhausted
陰	YIN	

When disease is caused by rebel QI (QI NI 氣逆) puncture (points on) *TAI YIN* (Spleen), *YANG MING* (Stomach) *and JUE YIN* (Liver).

LING SHU, Chapter 22-20, presents, without clinical signs, a treatment for rebel Liver QI (QI NI 氣逆) invading Spleen (Wood over-controls Soil) by puncturing points on Stomach, Spleen and Liver Meridians.
- TAI YIN (Spleen Meridian): LIV13-SP1-SP4
- YANG MING (Stomach Meridian): ST36-ST41, ST40-ST44
- JUE YIN (Liver Meridian): LIV8-PC3-LIV14

Acupuncture points to treat Liver rebel QI (QI NI 氣逆) which invades Spleen, LING SHU, Chapter 22-20

name	function	action
treatment of rebel Liver QI invading Spleen by TAI YIN: LIV13-SP1-SP4		
LIV13 ZHANG MEN 章門 Chapter Gate	MU of Spleen, HUI- meeting of five ZANG, meeting of Liv., Ki., H., Sp., Lu., G.B. Meridians	treat Upper JIAO obstruction and rebel QI which obstructs WEI QI (LING SHU, 59)
SP1 YIN BAI 隱白 Hidden White	JING-Well-Wood of Spleen	move rebel QI in TAI YIN down
SP4 GONG SUN 公孫 Grandfather-Grandson	opening of CHONG MAI, LUO of Spleen	

Acupuncture points to treat Liver rebel QI (QI NI 氣逆) which invades Spleen, LING SHU, Chapter 22-20, continued

treatment of rebel Liver QI invading Spleen through YANG MING: ST36-ST41, if there is phlegm-heat: ST40-ST44		
ST36 ZU SAN LI 足三里 Leg Three Miles	HE-Soil of Stomach, Sea of Blood point, tonify QI, potentiate other points	regulate YANG deficiency above and YIN excess below, regulate WEI QI, move rebel QI down
ST41 JIE XI 解谿 Ravine Divide	JING-River-Fire of Stomach, tonify Soil	move fire congested in Stomach with ST36
ST40 FENG LONG 豐隆 Bountiful Bulge	LUO of Stomach	dissolve phlegm-fire, calm SHEN
ST44 NEI TING 內庭 Inner Courtyard	RONG-Water of Stomach	cool and move QI of YANG MING down, dissolve phlegm, move fire down from head
treatment of rebel Liver QI invading Spleen by JUE YIN: LIV8-PC3-LIV14		
LIV14 QI MEN 期門 Cycle Gate	MU of Liver, regulate Liver YIN, meeting of Liv., Sp. Meridians and YIN WEI MAI	treat abdominal swelling, move downwards rebel QI which causes painful cramps in abdomen (like a piglet running in abdomen) with fear
LIV8 QU QUAN 曲泉 Spring at the bend	HE-Water of Liver, tonify Wood	tonify Liver YIN (especially in *Kidney YIN deficiency*), move rebel Liver QI down, clear excess heat, move dampness, regulate Lower JIAO
PC3 QU ZE 曲澤 Marsh at the Crook	HE-Water of Master of Heart	dissipate heat from Upper JIAO, cool Blood and Heart, disperse stagnant blood, disperse toxins caused by stagnation

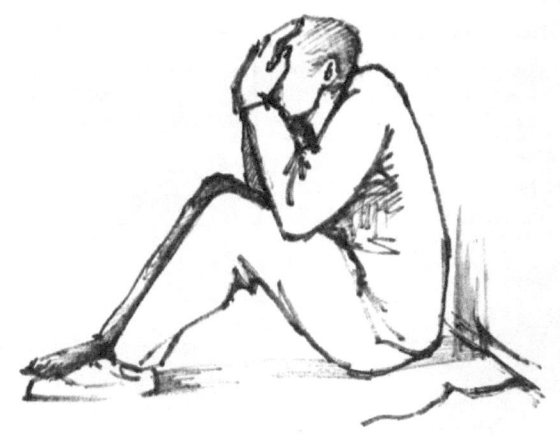

T. Obstructions of QI **flow in** SHAO YIN 少陰 (Source QI) **and** YANG MING 陽明 (acquired QI) **in severe diseases,** LING SHU, Chapter 22-21

甚	SHEN	extreme
取	QU	take
少	SHAO	small
陰	YIN	
陽	YANG	
明	MING	bright
動	DONG	move
者	ZHE	these
經	JING	meridians
也	YE	period

In severe diseases puncture (points on) SHAO YIN 少陰 (Kidney) *and* YANG MING 陽明 (Stomach) *to mobilize these meridians.*

Figure 60. **The flow in Six Layers** (LIU JING 六經)**: When** QI **descends in the** YANG MING 陽明 **layer, it helps the ascent of** QI **in the** SHAO YIN 少陰 **layer**

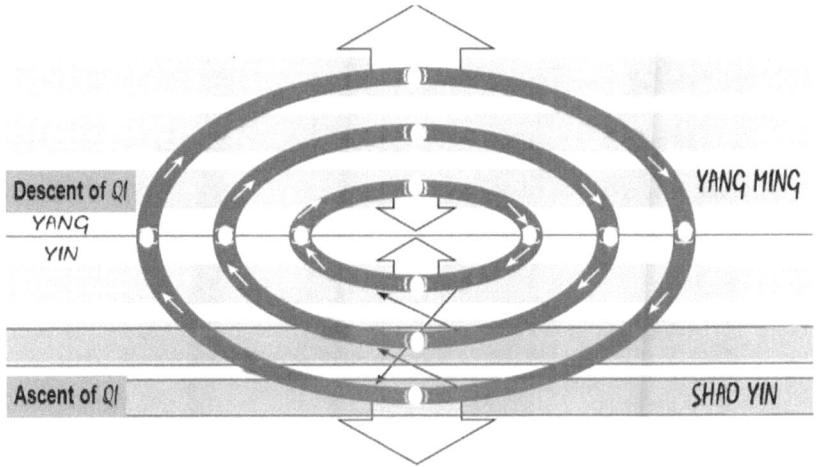

Chronic diseases deplete both inborn (Source, YUAN QI 原氣/元氣) and acquired QI, and then QI (NI 逆) rebels causing obstructions. LING SHU, Chapter 22-21, proposes (without presenting clinical signs) treating serious diseases by balancing acquired and Source QI (YUAN QI 原氣/元氣). The treatment is carried out by combining points on SHAO YIN (which includes Heart Meridian and Kidney Meridian) and YANG MING (which includes Large Intestine Meridian and Stomach Meridian). Kidney stores inborn Source QI (YUAN QI 原氣/元氣). Stomach contains food – a provider of acquired QI.

Of the Six Layers (LIU JING 六經), YANG MING is the lowest YANG layer and it communicates with the three YIN layers. SHAO YIN is the innermost layer of Six Layers and communicates with the interior of the body. QI in the YANG MING layer moves to the lower body. This descent of QI in the YANG MING layer is the indirect cause of the ascent of QI in the meridians of the SHAO YIN layer (Figure 60). The QI flow in Six Layers depends also on the balance between the descent of QI in the meridians of the YANG MING layer and the ascent of QI in the meridians of the SHAO YIN layer.

The treatment for regulating Source QI (SHAO YIN) and acquired QI (YANG MING) in severe disease is to mobilize:
- Descent of QI in YANG MING: ST36-ST4; when there is agitation: ST42-ST40 [429]
- Ascent of QI in SHAO YIN: Ki3-Ki7;[430] when there is *Kidney YIN deficiency*: Ki5-Ki10.

name	function	action
Ki10 YIN GU 陰谷 YIN Valley	HE-Water of Kidney	tonify Kidney YIN
Ki5 SHUI QUAN 水泉 Water Spring	XI of Kidney	open Kidney obstruction, regulate CHONG MAI and REN MAI, treat menopause and andropause

---

429 See page 285
430 See page 399

U. Two types of Kidney JING 精 deficiency, LING SHU, Chapter 22-22

少	SHAO	small	骨	GU	bone	短	DUAN	short	補	BU	tonify
氣	QI		痠	SUAN	pain	氣	QI		足	ZU	leg
身	SHEN	body	體	TI	body	息	XI	breath	少	SHAO	small
漯	LUO	shivers	重	ZHONG	heavy	短	DUAN	short	陰	YIN	
漯	LUO		懈	XIE	ankylosis	不	BU	not	去	QU	discard
也	YE	period	惰	DUO	inert	屬	ZHU	link	血	XUE	blood
言	YAN	speech	不	BU	not	動	DONG	move	絡	LUO	vessels
吸	XI	broken	能	NENG	able	作	ZUO	act	也	YE	period
吸	XI		動	DONG	move	氣	QI				
也	YE	period	補	BU	tonify	索	SUO	exhaust			
			足	ZU	leg						
			少	SHAO	small						
			陰	YIN							

When there is QI deficiency (SHAO QI 少氣), the body is very cold, speech is disrupted, bones ache and there is a sensation of heaviness and rigidity of the body and difficulty moving, tonify Leg SHAO YIN (Kidney).

When there is shortness of breath (QI DUAN 氣短) and dyspnea (XI DUAN 息短), (breath) without connection, agitation and exhaustion of QI, tonify Leg SHAO YIN (Kidney) and bleed congested connecting channels (LUO 絡) (obstructed capillaries).

LING SHU, Chapter 8-4, describes Kidney JING 精 deficiency caused by fear and dread (KONG JU 慄恐):
Injury to JING causes pain in the bones, obstructions (muscular flaccidity or atrophy of the limbs with motor impairment, WEI 痿) and exhaustion (JUE 厥). Sometimes JING 精 flows down spontaneously. [431]

LING SHU, Chapter 22-22, presents two cases of *Kidney JING 精 deficiency* causing rebel QI (QI NI 氣逆).

---

431 See page 345

In LING SHU, Chapter 22-22, the **first case** of *Kidney JING* 精 *deficiency* includes the following signs:

- *QI* deficiency (small *QI*) or small breath (SHAO QI 少氣)
- Extreme cold caused by inability of deficient Kidney YANG (MING MEN 命門) to heat the body [432]
- Disrupted speech caused by shortness of breath - a sign of Lung deficiency as a result of Kidney JING 精 deficiency
- Damage to bones expressed as pain in bones and difficulty in moving the joints (stiffness and heaviness of body) due to *Kidney JING* 精 *deficiency*. Bones are one of the six Organs of Extraordinary Longevity which store JING 精. *Kidney JING* 精 *deficiency* causes osteoporosis – *bones ache*.

Tonification of Leg SHAO YIN (Kidney Meridian) is the treatment for the first type of *Kidney JING* 精 *deficiency*:

- Strengthen JING and bones: **Ki3**-Ki4-BL40, BL52-BL43
- Treat severe pain in bones: **Ki3**-GB39-BL11
- Treat cold in bones: **Ki3**-Ki7-LI9/ST37

In LING SHU, Chapter 22-22, the **second case** of *Kidney JING* 精 *deficiency* includes the following signs:
- Shortness of breath (QI DUAN 氣短), with dyspnea (the feeling that one cannot breathe well enough) and temporary cessation of breath (XI DUAN 息短), indicates disruption of Kidney's function of grasping QI (inhale). Breath also *loses its connection* with SAN JIAO. Respiration occurs as a result of communication between Upper and Lower JIAO.
- Agitation is due to the progression of *Kidney JING* 精 *deficiency* to *Kidney YIN deficiency*.
- Exhaustion or extreme tiredness (SUO 索) is a consequence of the dysfunction of SAN JIAO and agitation.

---

432 See page 44

Treatment for the second type of *Kidney JING 精 deficiency* is tonification of Leg SHAO YIN (Kidney Meridian):
- Tonify the lower leg branch of CHONG MAI and improve the flow in the small connecting channels (LUO 絡): **Ki3**
- Treat the respiratory disorders (reestablish communication between Upper and Lower JIAO): Ki4-Ki7-Ki22-Ki27-BL22-TW8.
- Bleed small congested blood vessels in the region of the connecting channels (LUO 絡). Congested LUO 絡 cause obstruction of blood flow in capillaries. In long term blood and QI stagnation, small blood vessels may be observed under the skin on the pathway of Kidney Meridian as a consequence of hypoxia (lack of oxygen supply to the tissues).

LING SHU, Chapter 10, prescribes treatment for the invasion of pernicious external QI in the connecting channels (LUO 絡):

> LUO 絡 (*connecting/linking channels*) *are unable to flow through the great joints. They must move by alternate routes* (JUE DAO 絕 道) *to exit and to enter* (the joints); *then they come together again at the center of the skin. Their assemblage can be seen from the outside. Consequently, for puncturing* LUO 絡 *channels, one must needle their connections above* (on the surface) *where there may be an extreme amount* (knots, JIE 結) *of blood. If* (knots, JIE 結) *are allowed to remain,* BI 痺 (rheumatism, painful obstruction) *will ensue.*

LING SHU, Chapter 22-22, describes internal rebel QI (QI NI 氣逆) resulting from lack of communication between Lung and deficient Kidney, and causing overheating of Lung and disturbances in the descent of body liquids to bones and joints.

The situation may develop into weakness of the limbs, muscular flaccidity or atrophy of the limbs with motor impairment (WEI 痿), and then into WEI BI 痿痺 - severe motor impairment of joints, paralysis.

Acupuncture points to treat *Kidney* JING 精 *deficiency* accompanied by speech disorders, shortness of breath and pain in the bones, LING SHU, Chapter 22-22

name	function	action
strengthen JING and bones: **Ki3**-Ki4-BL40, BL52-BL43		
Ki3 TAI XI 太谿 Great Ravine	SHU-YUAN-Soil of Kidney	tonify Kidney YIN, release ascent of CHONG MAI and REN MAI, nourish bones, treat four limbs, cold dampness of bones, **tonify**
Ki4 DA ZHONG 大鍾 Big Bell	LUO of Kidney, enhance QI flow in meridians from Ki. towards M.H. (PC)	open Upper JIAO, treat spine rigidity
BL40 WEI ZHONG 委中 Bend Middle	HE-Soil of Bladder, Command Point for back	strengthen body and muscles and tendons through supply of body liquids and JING
BL52 ZHI SHI 志室 ZHI Chamber	influence ZHI, gather JING	warm QI, tonify Kidney, ZHI and JING, **tonify**
BL43 GAO HUANG SHU 膏肓俞 SHU of Liquid Fat	gather JING in Upper JIAO	strengthen Source QI, Kidney, Spleen, brain, bone marrow and Blood, **moxa**
treat severe pain in bones: **Ki3**-GB39-BL11, treat cold in bones: **Ki3**-Ki7-LI9/ST37		
BL11 DA ZHU 大杼 Great Shuttle	HUI-meeting of Bones, Sea of Blood, Spine Rectitude SHU,[433] meeting of Bl., S.I, S.J., G.B., Sp. and Lu. Meridians	benefit bones, irrigation of Wood (muscles and tendons)
GB39 XUAN ZHONG 懸鍾 Suspended Bell	HUI-meeting of bone marrow, meeting of Leg 3 YANG	move YANG QI down from the upper body, tonify bones and bone marrow, nourish JING, **tonify**
LI9 SHOU SHANG LIAN 手上廉 Hand Upper Ridge		treat bones and bone marrow in case of difficulty in limb movement
ST37 SHANG JU XU 上巨虛 Great Deficiency Above	Lower HE of Large Intestine, Lower Body Sea of Blood point	treat pain in bone marrow caused by cold, limb weakness, impotence
Ki7 FU LIU 復溜 Returning Current	JING-River-Metal of Kidney, tonify Water, enhance QI flow in meridians from Ki. towards M.H. (PC)	tonify Kidney YIN, tonify Heart, reduce fire, tonify brain and bone marrow

[433] LING SHU, Chapter 15

Acupuncture points to treat Kidney JING 精 deficiency accompanied by speech disorders, shortness of breath and pain in the bones, LING SHU, Chapter 22-22, continued

Treat respiratory disorders: Ki4-Ki7-Ki22-Ki27-BL22-TW8		
Ki22 BU LANG 步廊 Corridor Walk	meeting of Ki. Meridian with CHONG MAI	treat chest pain together with increased rate of breathing, release Lung QI through CHONG MAI and Ki. Meridian
Ki27 SHU FU 俞府 Transport Mansion	meeting point of all SHU	unbind chest
TW8 SAN YANG LUO 三陽絡 3 YANG Connection	intersection for three Arm YANG meridians	treat respiratory problems and speech difficulties
BL22 SAN JIAO SHU 三焦俞	SHU of SAN JIAO	open and regulate water passages, **tonify with hot needle**

Conclusion

The Ancient Chinese philosophical and medical texts do not separate body and mind, and they offer different pathways for the influence of emotional imbalance on the body.

Ancient Chinese thought and medicine identify the five *Roots of* SHEN (BEN SHEN 本神). BEN SHEN 本神 organize the specific life stages of each human being (integrating the physical body, emotions, thoughts) and the ability to realize inborn potential, starting from the moment of conception. Each BEN SHEN 本神 is related to one of the five ZANG 臟 (organ-functions).

This book has proposed regarding the emotions as the middle level of the Three Levels of Man organized according to the Trinity of Powers[434] (SAN CAI 三才) - Heaven, Man and Earth.
- Man is expressed on the subtle level of Heaven (Upper Level) as Five *Roots of* SHEN (BEN SHEN 本神): SHEN 神, HUN 魂, YI 意, PO 魄, ZHI 志. Five *Roots of* SHEN are responsible throughout man's existence for organizing, through the functioning of body and mind, the possibilities presented at the origin of life (heredity).
- Man at the level of Man (Middle Level) links subtle universal influences (Heaven) with 'substantial forms' (Earth) by means of expression of the five emotions, which express and regulate the individual.
- Man at the level of Earth (Lower Level) is expressed in 'substantial forms' by means of the five ZANG 臟: Heart, Liver, Spleen, Lung and Kidney, which build body tissues and the five emotions with the help of QI 氣, Blood, the five flavors and body liquids.

Emotions and passions occur during the interaction between the five ZANG containing the five BEN SHEN 本神, and the environment - the influence of the climate, nutrition, air, and especially of culture (moral or spiritual values).

---

434 Legge J.

The imbalance of BEN SHEN 本神 is one of the first influences at the root of generalized imbalance, generating long-lasting harmful emotions, especially when it occurs in the early stages of human life during the fetal development and birth.

Harmful emotions and passions may emerge:
• as an incident, due to an intense external event;
• as a continuum, often due to the effects of known or unknown problems in the patient's life, family and environment.

Harmful emotions and passions express the general imbalance of QI flow in man, leading to disease. It is therefore especially recommended to start with questions related to all periods of the patient's life when questioning him. The imprints of the initial stages of life are the most important to orientate the investigation. The patient does not always know the course of his mother's pregnancy, the circumstances of his birth and the early stages of his life. However, after asking parents and other family members, the patient sometimes obtains surprising results.

The patient should be asked about:
1. Fetal development, pregnancy. All problems in this stage of development injure PO 魄;
    • The patient's position in the family (eldest child, second, third, ..., youngest) influences SHEN 神, HUN 魂, PO 魄;
    • A small gap in age between the siblings may influence Kidney;
    • Whether a patient has a twin influences PO 魄, SHEN 神 and YI 意;
    • Any miscarriages of the patient's mother prior to his birth influence Kidney and ZHI 志;
    • His mother's body-mind-spirit state during pregnancy provides information about the mother's Kidney JING 精 and Master of Heart:
        • Fertility treatments influence YI 意 and ZHI 志
        • Complications of pregnancy injure PO 魄
        • Occupation/work at time of pregnancy (stressful, exhausting, physically tiring, frustrating) influence SHEN 神, YI 意 and ZHI 志

- Diseases the mother had before and during the pregnancy influence Kidney, PO 魄 and YI 意
- Stability and quality of life (change of residence, diseases and deaths in the family and other traumatic events) influence Master of Heart, SHEN 神 and ZHI 志
- Nutrition
- The attitude of the mother and those around her to the pregnancy (desirable or not)

2. Birth. All problems at this stage injure HUN 魂:
    - Whether premature, at term, or after term
    - Prolonged labor, labor induction, cesarean birth, vacuum or forceps delivery, anesthesia
    - Birth complications: fetal distress, breech birth, nuchal cord

3. Names form self-identity and are influenced by HUN 魂. What does the patient's name mean to him?
    - Whether the patient was named in memory of a sibling or relative who had died, which also influences SHEN 神 and Master of Heart
    - Whether the patient uses a nickname
    - Whether the patient changed his name (at what age and for what reason?), which also influences SHEN 神

4. Stages of childhood development:
    - The relationship with parents (too close, strained or lack of contact)
    - The father as a symbol of authority and communication with the environment influences HUN 魂 of his children
    - The mother as a symbol of body nourishment and ingathering influences PO 魄 of her children
    - Influence of the grandfathers, uncles, brothers (HUN 魂) and grandmothers, aunts, sisters (PO 魄)
    - Education: study in school, achievements and failures, learning disabilities, interests influence YI 意 - ZHI 志
    - Delayed speech or stuttering influence SHEN 神 and HUN 魂
    - Serious childhood diseases or recurring diseases

- Ear infections are usually a sign of Kidney and JING 精 deficiency
- Recurrent throat infections are usually a sign of Liver and Kidney dysfunction
- Recurrent cough or pneumonia is usually a sign of Lung and Kidney dysfunction
- Asthma and skin diseases are usually a sign of Lung, Liver, Heart or Kidney dysfunction
- Chronic diarrhea is usually a sign of Liver and Spleen dysfunction

5. Changes in the patient's life (physical and emotional):
   - Transition into adolescence or menopause influence HUN 魂 and ZHI 志
   - Grief, separations, abortion, influence Master of Heart, YI 意, HUN 魂 and PO 魄
   - Change of apartments, cities, states, influence YI 意 and PO 魄
   - Accidents and surgeries influence YI 意, PO 魄, ZHI 志, HUN 魂

We conclude with the recommendation from LING SHU, Chapter 8, BEN SHEN 本神, which we saw in the introduction: *The first law in the art of acupuncture is the necessity of rooting in SHEN (BEN YU SHEN 本于神)* - the therapist must develop above all the ability to listen to and communicate with the patient. The therapist questions. The patient replies. The **right question** emerges from this back and forth listening and communication.

This book invites Chinese medicine therapists to explore the ancient texts. The therapist is invited to regard the patient as a unity to be approached via the three levels Spirit - mind (emotions) – body and to explore the function of the acupuncture points, according to his clinical experience. The therapist is invited to listen to the patient, and in this listening may find his own personal approach to treatment for the specific and unique person before him.

List of Figures

Figure 1. On the TAI JI 太極 symbol space and time are described by YIN-YANG 陰陽 11

Figure 2. The character SHEN 神 'Individual Spirit' in ancient seal and classical script 13

Figure 3. SHEN 神 is a meeting between heredity (individual genes) and environment (air and food) 14

Figure 4. The vertical plane: SHEN 神 through Heart (XIN 心) links Heaven and Earth providing an awareness of the moment 15

Figure 5. The horizontal plane: time and space represented on the TAI JI symbol by four seasons and four regions 16

Figure 6. Five Modalities represented on the TAI JI symbol. In the figure to the left, Soil is located on the periphery between Fire and Metal, in the figure to the right Soil at the center of the circle 16

Figure 7. Law of Generation (SHENG 生) of Five Modalities 23

Figure 8. Law of Control (KE 尅) of Five Modalities 24

Figure 9. Relationship between Wood Modality and other Modalities 24

Figure 10. Abusive Relationship (Reversed Generation) (CHENG 乘) of Five Modalities 25

Figure 11. Insult Relationship (Reversed Control) (WU 侮) of Five Modalities 26

Figure 12. Man on Three Levels (Heaven-Man-Earth) expressed by Five Modalities. Emotions communicate between BEN SHEN 本神 and ZANG 臟 27

Figure 13. BEN SHEN 本神 - five aspects of SHEN 神, represented on the TAI JI symbol 28

Figure 14. The character PO 魄 - Metal Modality aspect of BEN SHEN 本神, purified terrestrial influences in ancient seal and classical script 29

Figure 15. The character HUN 魂 - Wood Modality aspect of BEN SHEN 本神, 'talking' terrestrial influence in ancient seal and classical script 32

Figure 16. The character ZHI 志 - Water Modality aspect of
BEN SHEN 本神 in ancient seal and classical script..................33
Figure 17. The character YI 意 - Soil Modality aspect of BEN SHEN 本神
in ancient seal and classical script..................................34
Figure 18. Interaction between BEN SHEN 本神 presented on the TAI JI
symbol as a mushroom in which SHEN 神, HUN 魂 and
PO 魄 are the cap, and YI 意 and ZHI 志 are the stem 35
Figure 19. Five ZANG 臟 presented on the TAI JI symbol....................36
Figure 20. Kidney YIN and Kidney YANG presented on the TAI JI symbol......45
Figure 21. Five emotions (WU ZHI 五志) presented on the TAI JI symbol......48
Figure 22. The character QING 情 'emotion, passion, color of
Consciousness' in ancient seal and classical script......................49
Figure 23. The characters XI 喜 'joy' and LE 樂 'pleasure' in ancient
seal and classical script..51
Figure 24. The characters BEI 悲 'sorrow', YOU 憂 'sadness', AI 哀 'grief',
CHOU 愁 'melancholy' in ancient seal and classical script............52
Figure 25. The character NU 怒 'anger' in ancient seal and
classical script..54
Figure 26. The characters KONG 恐 'fear' and JU 懼 'dread' in ancient
seal and classical script..54
Figure 27. The character SI 思 'thought, worry' in ancient seal
and classical script..56
Figure 28. *Heaven in me is* DE 德, *Earth in me is* QI 氣.
DE *flows downwards,* QI *blooms and this is life*..................95
Figure 29. The character DE 德 'virtue', 'efficiency', 'link from DAO 道'
to Man in ancient seal and classical script...........................96
Figure 30. *Life comes from what is called* JING 精. *Confrontation
between the two* (aspects of) JING 精 *is called* SHEN 神..............100
Figure 31. The character JING 精 'fundamental vitality' in ancient
seal and classical script..101
Figure 32. *Following* SHEN 神, *going away and coming back,
that is called* HUN 魂..105

Figure 33. *Together with* JING 精, *exiting and entering, that is called* PO 魄 107
Figure 34. *When Heart-Consciousness* (XIN 心) *has reminiscences, this is called* YI 意. *When* YI 意 *is established this is called* ZHI 志 114
Figure 35. YI 意 and ZHI 志, *Center-North axis of the* TAI JI *symbol* 117
Figure 36. *When* ZHI 志 *is stabilized and transformed this is called thought* (SI 思) 124
Figure 37. *The thought* (SI 思) *which considers the situation from afar is called contemplation* (LU 慮) 127
Figure 38. The character LU 慮 'contemplation' in classical and ancient seal script 128
Figure 39. *Contemplation* (LU 慮) *which arranges beings and objects is called wisdom* (ZHI 智) 131
Figure 40. Anger (NU 怒), SU WEN, Chapter 39 168
Figure 41. Joy (XI 喜), SU WEN, Chapter 39 178
Figure 42. Sorrow (BEI 悲), SU WEN, Chapter 39 181
Figure 43. Fear (KONG 恐), SU WEN, Chapter 39 187
Figure 44. Cold (HAN 寒), SU WEN, Chapter 39 194
Figure 45. Heat (JIONG 炅), SU WEN, Chapter 39 196
Figure 46. Panic (JING 驚), SU WEN, Chapter 39 197
Figure 47. The character JING 驚 'panic' in ancient seal and classical script 198
Figure 48. Exhaustion (LAO 勞), SU WEN, Chapter 39 205
Figure 49. Obsessive thinking (SI 思), SU WEN, Chapter 39 209
Figure 50. The characters CHU 怵 'apprehension' and TI 惕 'distress' in ancient seal and classical script 217
Figure 51. JUE YIN 厥陰 and SHAO YIN 少陰 layers and their meridians in Six Layers (LIU JING 六經) of QI flow 227
Figure 52. Development of melancholy and sadness (CHOU YOU 愁憂) into depression (DIAN 癲) 209
Figure 53. Injury to Master of Heart, Lung and Liver caused by sorrow and grief (BEI AI 悲哀) 209

Figure 54. Sorrow and grief cause injury to JUE YIN 厥陰, Restless ZANG (ZANG ZAO 臟躁), KUANG 狂 and *Plum pit* QI (MEI HE QI 梅核氣) 304
Figure 55. Factors related to the ability to speak according to Chinese medicine 324
Figure 56. Uncontrollable overflowing anger causes confused speech. *YIN Deficiency and Blood Dryness* 209
Figure 57. Uncontrollable overflowing anger causes confused speech. *Blood Flow Congested and Obstructed* 333
Figure 58. Uncontrollable overflowing anger causes confused speech. *Heart and Spleen Dual Deficiency* 334
Figure 59. Onset of DIAN 癲 disease. *Wind-phlegm* obstructs QI flow in face 364
Figure 60. The flow in Six Layers (LIU JING 六經): when QI descends in the YANG MING 陽明 layer, it helps the ascent of QI in the SHAO YIN 少陰 layer 410

Glossary according to subject

DAO 道 the Way, the Ultimate Direction
DE 德 Virtue, personal link to DAO 道
SAN CAI 三才 Trinity of Powers
TAI JI 太極 the Great Summit
TIAN DI REN 天地人 Heaven-Earth-Man
  1. TIAN 天 Heaven
  2. DI 地 Earth
  3. REN 人 Man

YI 一 Unity/oneness
YIN-YANG 陰陽

SAN BAO 三寶 Three treasures
  1. JING 精 vitality, vital principle (essence)
  2. QI 氣 energy, movement
  3. SHEN 神 Individual Spirit

SHEN 神 Individual Spirit
BEN SHEN 本神 Roots of Spirit
  1. SHEN 神 Individual Spirit, represents the Fire aspect of BEN SHEN related to the Heart
  2. HUN 魂 represents the Wood aspect of BEN SHEN and dwells in the Liver
  3. ZHI 志 represents the Water aspect of BEN SHEN and dwells in the Kidney
  4. PO 魄 represents the Metal aspect of BEN SHEN and dwells in the Lung
  5. YI 意 represents the Soil aspect of BEN SHEN and dwells in the Spleen

CHANG XIN 帝心 authentic (original, true) Heart-Consciousness
GUI 鬼 ghost, daimon, represents the centrifugal influence of Earth

LING 靈 Soul, spirit
SAN CHONG 三蟲 Three Worms
SAN SHI 三尸 Three Corpses

SHEN JI 神機 mechanism of SHEN-Spirit
SHEN JING 神精 Spirit transferring the vital essences, vital spirit
SHEN MING 神明 brightness of SHEN-Spirit
SHEN QI 神氣 Spirit transferring QI
TAN ZHONG 膻中 Center of Chest
TIAN XIN 天心 Heavenly Heart
WEI WU WEI 為無為 action without action, spontaneous action
WU YUN 五蘊 five skandas, the five functions or aspects that constitute sentient beings (Buddhism)
XIN 心 Heart, Heart-Consciousness
XING 性 Virtue, Intimate Nature
ZI RAN 自然 spontaneous natural movement, 'naturally; natural; spontaneously; freely; in the course of events'.
ZI SHI 自失 loss of self

WU XING 五行 Five Modalities (Phases, Elements, Movements)
CHENG 乘 Reverse Generation - Abuse, son abuses his mother
HUO 火 Fire
JIN 金 Metal
JUN HUO 君火 Prince Fire (Ruler)
KE 剋 Control, repression, overcoming, grandfather-grandson relationship
MU 木 Wood
SHENG 生 Generation, nourishment, mother-son relationship
SHUI 水 Water
TU 土 Soil
WU 侮 Reverse Control - Destruction, grandson destroys his grandfather
XIANG HUO 相火 Minister Fire

ZANG 臟 Organs-functions, the builders of body tissues
FEI 肺 Lung
GAN 肝 Liver
MING MEN 命門 Gate of Destiny, Kidney YANG
PI 脾 Spleen
SHEN 腎 Kidney
XIN 心 Heart, Heart-Consciousness

XIN BAO LUO 心包絡 the envelope of Heart communication or communication system of Heart, pericardium; XIN ZHU 心主 The Master of Heart (The Viceroy of Heart)

FU 腑 Organs of transition
DA CHANG 大腸 Large Intestine, column
DAN 膽 Gallbladder
PANG GUANG 膀胱 Urinary Bladder
SAN JIAO 三焦 Triple-Warmer, Triple Heater
   1. SHANG JIAO 上焦 Upper JIAO
   2. ZHONG JIAO 中焦 Middle JIAO
   3. XIA JIAO 下焦 Lower JIAO
WEI 胃 Stomach
XIAO CHANG 小腸 Small Intestine

QI HENG ZHI FU 奇恒之腑 **Organs of Extraordinary Longevity**
(JING 精 storage)
   1. BAO 包 uterus
   2. DAN 膽 Gallbladder
   3. GU 骨 bones, skeleton
   4. GU SUI 骨髓 bone marrow
   5. MAI 脈/脉 blood vessels
   6. NAO 腦 brain

QI 氣 energy, movement and body function
DA QI 大氣 Great, Big QI, QI of the Universe (Heaven and Earth), QI of air
GAO 高 Liquid fats found in the bone marrow and brain
JIN YE 津液 body liquids
JING QI 精氣 QI which transfers vitality, vital energies
JING QI 經氣 QI which flows in meridians
KONG QI 空氣 QI of air
MAI 脈/脉 pulse, blood vessels
NI QI 逆氣 rebel QI or counterflow QI, which flows either in a contrary direction or in an exaggerated fashion in the correct direction, provoking congestion and obstruction.
RONG QI 榮氣 Nourishing QI

TI 體 body substances
WEI QI 衛氣 Defensive QI
XING 形 body, matter, substantial forms
XUE 血 blood, complexion
YING QI 營氣 Nourishing QI
YUAN QI 原氣/元氣 Source, Original, hereditary QI
ZHEN QI 真氣 Authentic QI
ZHENG QI 正氣 Upright, True QI
ZONG JIN 宗筋 Muscle of Ancestors, the center of perineum, place of attachment of abdominal muscles; allows the functioning of penis (erection) or clitoris
ZONG QI 宗氣 Ancestral QI, QI of the rhythm of breath and blood flow

MAI 脈/脉 pulses
CHANG 長 long
CHEN 沉 sinking
CHI 遲 slow
DA 大 big
DUAN 短 short
FU 浮 floating
HONG 洪 flooding
HUA 滑 slippery
HUAN 緩 retarded
JIE 結 knotted
RUO 弱 weak
SAN 散 dispersed
SE 澀 choppy
SHI 實 full
SHU 數 fast
WEI 微 minute
WU LI 無力 without force
XI 細 thin
XU 虛 empty
XUAN 弦 wiry
YOU LI 有力 with force

WU ZHI 五志 The five emotions/passions
KONG 恐 fear
NU 怒 anger
SI 思 thinking, obsessive thinking, worry
XI 喜 joy, elation
YOU 憂 sadness associated with worry

QI QING 七情 The seven emotions (passions) which cause disorders
AI 哀 grief, deep sorrow
BEI 悲 sorrow
CHOU 愁 melancholy, sadness
HAO 好 love
JING 驚 panic, startle, dread
JU 懼 dread, fear which paralyses
KONG 恐 fear
LE 樂 pleasure, joy; character 樂 pronounced as YUE is translated as music
LU 慮 contemplation, worry
NU 怒 anger
SHENG NU 盛怒 rage, overflowing anger
SI 思 thinking, obsessive thinking, worry
WU 惡 hate
XI 喜 joy, elation
YOU 憂 sadness associated with worry

XING 性 Virtue, Intimate Nature
LI 禮 observance of the rituals and traditions, ritual propriety, a proper action at the right time, is an Intimate Nature attributed to Fire-Heart
REN 仁 humanity, kindness, benevolence, is an Intimate Nature attributed to Wood-Liver
XIN 信 loyalty, trust, honesty, confidence, is an Intimate Nature attributed to Soil-Spleen
YI 義 justice is an Intimate Nature attributed to Metal-Lung
ZHI 智 wisdom, intelligence, common sense, discrimination between good and evil, is an Intimate Nature attributed to Water-Kidney

JING LUO MAI 經絡脈 **the network of body animation (meridians and vessels)**

JING MAI 經脈 meridians, vessels

DONG MAI 動脈 artery, the nourishing flow in the body

XUE 穴 acupuncture points in the body usually located on the trajectories of the meridians

LIU JING 六經 **Six Layers of** QI **flow in man**
1. TAI YANG 太陽 Great YANG (Bladder and Small Intestine Meridians)
2. SHAO YANG 少陽 Small YANG (Gallbladder and Triple Warmer Meridians)
3. YANG MING 陽明 Bright YANG (Stomach and Large Intestine Meridians)
4. TAI YIN 太陰 Great YIN (Spleen and Lung Meridians)
5. JUE YIN 厥陰 Exhausted YIN (Liver and Master of Heart/Pericardium Meridians)
6. SHAO YIN 少陰 Small YIN (Kidney and Heart Meridians)

QI JING BA MAI 奇經八脈 **Eight Extraordinary Meridians/Vessels**
1. CHONG MAI 衝脈 Surging Meridian/Vessel
2. DAI MAI 帶脈 Girdle (Belt) Meridian/Vessel
3. DU MAI 督脈 Governing Meridian/Vessel
4. REN MAI 任脈 Conception Meridian/Vessel
5. YANG QIAO MAI 陽蹻脈 YANG Heel Meridian/Vessel
6. YANG WEI MAI 陽維脈 YANG Linking Meridian/Vessel
7. YIN QIAO MAI 陰蹻脈 YIN Heel Meridian/Vessel
8. YIN WEI MAI 陰維脈 YIN Linking Meridian/Vessel

HUANG DI 黃帝 **The Yellow Emperor**
QI BO 岐伯 The teacher of the Yellow Emperor

HE SHANG GONG 河上公 The philosopher, represents the Daoist school of thought

ZHENG 證 **syndrome**
BAI HE BING 百合病 Lily Bulb Disease

ZHONG FENG 中風 *Wind in the Center*

JING SHEN FEN LIU 精神分裂 schizophrenia, separation and rupture between JING and SHEN

ZANG ZAO 臟躁 *Restless ZANG organs*
DIAN 癲 quiet (YIN) body-mind-spirit disorders
TAN HUO 痰火 *Phlegm-fire*
TAN RE 痰熱 Phlegm-heat
TAN YIN 痰飲 *Phlegm-mucus* of cold origin
YU ZHENG 鬱證 depression syndrome caused by constrained QI
MEI HE QI 梅核氣 *Plum pit QI*
XIAN 癇 or DIAN XIAN 癲癇 epilepsy
FENG XIAN 風癇 *Wind epilepsy*
KUANG 狂 agitated (YANG) body-mind-spirit disorders

Treatments
DA 達 vomit
FA 發 perspiration
DUO 奪 purge
XIE 泄 stimulate urination
ZHE 折 regulate water flow

Meridians (abbreviations in the names of acupuncture points)
Bl – Bladder
CV – Conception Vessel
GV – Governing Vessel
H – Heart
Ki – Kidney
LI – Large Intestine
Lu – Lung
PC – Pericardium, Master of Heart
SI – Small Intestine
Sp – Spleen
St – Stomach
GB – Gall Bladder
Liv – Liver

Acupuncture points for treatment of disorders described in SU WEN, Chapter 39, LING SHU, Chapters 8 (3,4) and 22, arranged by meridians. Major treatment points appear in black

	Anger			Joy pleasure			Sorrow grief			Melancholy sadness		Fear dread			Apprehension, distress obsessive thinking worry			Panic	DIAN	KUANG	NI
	SW 39	LS 8-3	LS 8-4	SW 39	LS 8-3	LS 8-4	SW 39	LS 8-3	LS 8-4	LS 8-3	LS 8-4	SW 39	LS 8-3	LS 8-4	SW 39	LS 8-3	LS 8-4	SW 39	LS 22		
BL2																			V		
BL5																			V		
BL8			V																	V	
BL10																			V		
BL11																			V		V
BL13								V		V											V
BL14																			V		
BL15			V		V		V	V	V	V	V	V			V	V	V		V	V	V
BL17	V	V	V	V						V	V	V				V					
BL18	V	V	V		V			V	V			V									V
BL19												V									
BL20		V						V	V	V	V	V					V		V		
BL21																	V				
BL22																			V		V
BL23		V						V		V							V		V	V	V
BL27																					V
BL28																			V		V
BL39																			V		V
BL40					V			V													V
BL42					V			V											V		
BL43			V	V			V	V		V					V				V		V
BL44	V									V	V		V		V			V		V	
BL46																			V		
BL47					V			V		V		V							V		V
BL52	V	V		V							V					V					V
BL58																			V		V
BL60																			V		V
BL61		V																	V	V	V
BL62		V																V	V		
BL63																			V	V	V
BL64											V										V
BL65											V										
BL66											V		V								
BL67																					V

Acupuncture points for treatment of disorders described in SU WEN, Chapter 39, LING SHU, Chapters 8 (3,4) and 22, arranged by meridians. Major treatment points appear in black, continued

	Anger			Joy pleasure			Sorrow grief			Melancholy sadness		Fear dread			Apprehension, distress obsessive thinking worry			Panic	DIAN	KUANG	NI
	SW 39	LS 8-3	LS 8-4	SW 39	LS 8-3	LS 8-4	SW 39	LS 8-3	LS 8-4	LS 8-3	LS 8-4	SW 39	LS 8-3	LS 8-4	SW 39	LS 8-3	LS 8-4	SW 39	LS 22		
CV4	V									V	V					V					
CV6		V					V			V		V	V								
CV7												V									
CV10																V					
CV11							V														
CV12			V		V	V	V			V	V		V		V	V	V				
CV13		V										V			V						V
CV14	V				V		V					V	V					V		V	
CV15		V													V				V		
CV18	V					V	V	V	V												
CV19							V											V			
CV22										V								V			
CV23		V								V		V	V								
CV24																		V			
GB1		V																			
GB8		V																		V	
GB13										V								V			
GB17			V				V														
GB20		V		V														V			
GB24													V					V			
GB29		V																			
GB30		V																			
GB34	V					V		V		V						V					
GB35													V			V					
GB36		V																			
GB37																	V				
GB38	V																				V
GB39																V				V	V
GB40		V				V			V							V		V			
GB41	V											V	V								
GB43	V					V		V		V						V		V		V	
GB44																					V
GV1												V								V	V	V
GV4										V											
GV11							V					V									
GV12	V		V																		
GV14	V		V		V	V				V	V	V								V	V
GV16		V																V			
GV18										V											
GV19		V	V							V	V									V	
GV20										V	V	V			V	V	V	V			
GV22	V	V									V									V	
GV24	V	V		V	V						V			V			V			V	
GV26	V		V	V	V	V		V	V	V			V						V	V	

Acupuncture points for treatment of disorders described in SU WEN, Chapter 39, LING SHU, Chapters 8 (3,4) and 22, arranged by meridians. Major treatment points appear in black, continued

	Anger			Joy pleasure			Sorrow grief			Melancholy sadness		Fear dread			Apprehension, distress obsessive thinking worry			Panic	DIAN	KUANG	NI
	SW 39	LS 8-3	LS 8-4	SW 39	LS 8-3	LS 8-4	SW 39	LS 8-3	LS 8-4	LS 8-3	LS 8-4	SW 39	LS 8-3	LS 8-4	SW 39	LS 8-3	LS 8-4	SW 39	LS 22		
H3				V																	
H5			V	V			V		V		V						V			V	
H6					V	V		V	V		V		V				V	V			
H7	V	V	V	V	V	V			V	V	V	V	V	V		V	V	V	V	V	
H9				V														V			
KI1							V		V						V		V	V			V
KI3		V			V	V		V	V	V			V			V	V	V			
KI4							V					V	V								V
KI5			V									V								V	V
KI6			V						V			V									
KI7	V	V	V	V							V	V								V	V
KI8			V									V									
KI9	V		V																		V
KI10									V							V					V
KI14																					V
KI16			V																		V
KI20												V						V			
KI21	V						V											V			
KI22																					V
KI25													V								
KI26											V										
K27												V									V
LI1																		V			
LI4	V		V			V		V	V	V								V	V	V	V
LI5				V		V												V		V	
LI6																		V		V	
LI7																		V		V	V
LI8																		V			
LI9																		V			V
LI11						V			V			V	V					V			
LI13																		V			
LIV1																					V
LIV2	V	V	V		V	V		V	V		V							V		V	
LIV3	V	V							V	V		V	V	V						V	
LIV5			V				V				V				V					V	
LIV6	V	V	V				V			V	V	V	V		V						
LIV8	V	V										V	V							V	V
LIV13										V	V	V			V	V					V
LIV14		V	V							V	V	V		V	V		V	V		V	V
LU1	V		V																		
LU2							V														
LU3	V																				
LU5	V											V			V						V
LU6												V									
LU7							V	V				V						V	V	V	V
LU9	V																		V	V	
LU10	V																				
LU11			V																V	V	

Acupuncture points for treatment of disorders described in SU WEN, Chapter 39, LING SHU, Chapters 8 (3,4) and 22, arranged by meridians. Major treatment points appear in black, continued

	Anger			Joy pleasure			Sorrow grief			Melancholy sadness		Fear dread			Apprehension, distress obsessive thinking worry			Panic	DIAN	KUANG	NI
	SW 39	LS 8-3	LS 8-4	SW 39	LS 8-3	LS 8-4	SW 39	LS 8-3	LS 8-4	LS 8-3	LS 8-4	SW 39	LS 8-3	LS 8-4	SW 39	LS 8-3	LS 8-4	SW 39	\multicolumn{3}{c}{LS 22}		
PC1	V																				V
PC3				V		V															V
PC4							V	V				V									
PC5		V	V			V	V	V	V		V							V		V	
PC6		V	V			V	V	V	V			V	V		V			V		V	
PC7	V		V	V	V	V	V	V	V	V	V	V	V			V				V	
PC8	V		V	V	V	V			V	V			V							V	
PC9																			V	V	
SI1																				V	
SI3															V					V	
SI4				V																V	
SI5				V																V	
SI7						V							V						V	V	
SI8											V								V	V	
SI19																	V			V	
SP1		V																		V	V
SP2																					V
SP3											V										
SP4	V		V				V					V		V						V	V
SP5																					V
SP6	V	V	V		V	V		V	V	V	V		V			V	V			V	
SP7							V				V						V				V
SP8										V	V				V	V	V				
SP9	V															V	V				V
SP10			V			V			V		V									V	
SP15							V	V													
ST4																			V		
ST5																				V	
ST6																			V		
ST8									V												
ST14							V	V							V						
ST15							V					V			V						
ST18							V	V							V	V					
ST25	V			V		V			V											V	V
ST26																		V			
ST27					V				V			V						V		V	V
ST28																		V			V
ST30												V									
ST34												V									
ST36		V	V							V	V	V			V	V	V			V	V
ST37																			V		V
ST40	V		V	V	V	V			V	V	V		V		V		V		V	V	V
ST41		V					V						V							V	V
ST42																				V	V
ST44	V	V		V		V			V	V		V			V					V	V
ST45																					V

Acupuncture points for treatment of disorders described in SU WEN, Chapter 39, LING SHU, Chapters 8 (3,4) and 22, arranged by meridians. Major treatment points appear in black, continued

	Anger			Joy pleasure			Sorrow grief			Melan-choly sad-ness		Fear dread			Apprehension, distress obsessive thinking worry			Panic	DIAN	KUANG	NI
	SW 39	LS 8-3	LS 8-4	SW 39	LS 8-3	LS 8-4	SW 39	LS 8-3	LS 8-4	LS 8-3	LS 8-4	SW 39	LS 8-3	LS 8-4	SW 39	LS 8-3	LS 8-4	SW 39	LS 22		
TW1																		V			
TW2												V								V	V
TW6	V					V			V											V	
TW8																					V
TW10							V													V	
YIN TANG										V											

Bibliography

A.G.M.A., *Punctologie générale*, Librairie You Feng, 2011

Ameisen, J. C., *La Sculpture du vivant. Le suicide cellulaire ou la mort créatrice*, Seuil, Paris, 1999

Atlan, H., *Entre le cristal et la fumée. Essai sur l'organisation du vivant*, Seuil, Paris, 1979

Barreau, H., *Le Cerveau et l'esprit*, CNRS Editions, Paris, 1992

Beck, S., *Dao de Jing Way Power Book by Lao-zi*, 1996 http://www.daoisopen.com/ddjtranslations.html

Damasio, A., *Descartes' Error: Emotion, Reason, and the Human Brain*, Putnam, 1994; revised Penguin edition, 2005

Damasio, A., *The Feeling of What Happens: Body and Emotion in the Making of Consciousness*, Harcourt, 1999

Damasio, A., *Looking for Spinoza: Joy, Sorrow, and the Feeling Brain*, Harcourt, 2003

Damasio, A., *Self Comes to Mind: Constructing the Conscious Brain*, Pantheon, 2010.

Deadman, P., & Baker, K., *A Manual of Acupuncture* Journal of Chinese Medicine, 2001

Diagnostic and Statistical Manual of Mental Disorders, Fifth Edition, American Psychiatric Association, 2013

Despeux, C., *Prescriptions d'acupuncture valant mille onces d'or : Traité d'acupuncture de Sun Simiao du VIIe siècle*, Paris: Trédaniel, 1987

Eyssalet, J.M., *La Rumeur du Dragon et l'Ordre du Tigre*. Paris: Tredaniel. 1999

Eyssalet, J.M., *Les Cinq Chemins du Clair et de l'Obscure*, Paris: Tredaniel, 1989

Eyssalet, J.M., *Le Secret de la Maison des Ancetres*, Paris: Tredaniel, 1990

Eyssalet, J.M., *Shen-l'instant createur*. Paris: Tredaniel, 1990

Eyssalet, J.M., *Montee des Nuages, Descente des Pluies*. Paris: Tredaniel, 1999

Eyssalet, J.M., *Dans l'Ocean des Saveurs, l'Intention du Corps*. Paris: Tredaniel, 2002

Eyssalet, J.M., *Au Confluent Du Ciel-Terre, Emotions Et Passions*, Tredaniel, 2011

Flaws B. & Lake J. *Chinese Medical Psychiatry*, Blue Poppy Press, 2001

Granet M. *La pensée chinoise,* Albin Michel, 1968

Mussat, M. & Grison, P., *Nan-King: les 81 difficultés de l'acupuncture.* Paris, Masson, 1979

Guillaume, G. & Chieu Mach, *Dictionnaire* des points d'acupuncture Guy Trédaniel, 1995

Husson A., *Huang di nei jing su wen, A.S.M.A.F.* Paris, 1989

Jullien, F., *Detour and Access. Strategies of Meaning in China and Greece,* The MIT Press, 2004

Kalinowski, M., *Cosmologie et divination dans la Chine ancienne: le compendium des cinq agents* (*Wuxing dayi, VIe siècle*) traduit et annoté Paris: Ecole française d'Extrême Orient, 1991

Larre, C., & Rochat de la Vallee, E., *Rooted in Spirit. The Heart of Chinese Medicine.* Barrytown, N.Y.: Station Hill Press, 1995

Legge, James (1872). *The Ch'un Ts'ew, with the Tso Chuen.* The Chinese Classics V. London: Trübner, Part 2 (books 9–12). Revised edition 1893, London: Oxford University Press.

Le Grand Ricci Online - Brill. www.brill.com

Levi J., *Les Oeuvres de Maître Tchouang - Tchouang-tseu*, Paris, ed. de l'Encyclopédie des Nuisances, 2006/2010

Lin Shi Shan, *Traitement des syndromes en acupuncture traditionnelle*, Institut Yin Yang, Forbach, 1994

Lin, Yutang, *The Chinese theory of art, translations from the masters of Chinese art.,* Panther, London, 1969

Milsky, C., & Andres, G., *Ling Shu Pivot Merveilleux,* éd. La Tisserande, 2009

Moashing, N., *The Yellow Emperor's Classic of Medicine*, Boston & London: Shambhalla, 1995

Needham, J. & Lu Gwei-djen, *Science and Civilisation in China* volume 6/06 *Medicine,* Sivin, N., ed., Needham Research Institute, 2000.

Pigeaud, J., *La maladie de l'âme. Étude sur la relation de l'âme et du corps dans la tradition médico-philosophique antique*, Les Belles Lettres, Paris, 1981

Porkert, M., *The Theoretical Foundations of Chinese Medicine: Systems of Correspondence*, Cambridge, Mass. and London: MIT Press, 1974

Rochat de la Vallée, E., & Larre, C., *Su Wen: Les 11 premiers traités*, Moulins-lès-Metz: Maisonneuve, 1993

Ryckmans, P., *Les propos sur la peinture du Moine Citrouille-Amère: Traduction et commentaire de Shitao*, France, Plon, 2007,

Sivin, N., *Huang Ti Nei Ching* 黃帝內經 *In Early Chinese Texts: A Bibliographical Guide*, Michael Loewe (ed.), Berkeley and Los Angeles: University of California Press, 1993.

Soulié de Morant, G., *Chinese Acupuncture*, Paradigm Publications, 1994

Sterckx, P., & Chen Jun, *Diagnostic des syndromes. Comparaisons*, 2002

Unschuld, P. U., Tessenow, H., *Huang Di Nei Jing Su Wen: Nature, Knowledge, Imagery in an Ancient Chinese Medical Text*. Berkeley and Los Angeles: University of California Press, 2003

Van Nghi, N. & Recours-Nguyen, C., *Hoang Ti Nei King So Ouenn*, Marseille: NVN ed., 1973, 1975, 1988, 1991.

Van Nghi, N., Viet Dzung, T., Recours-Nguyen C., *Huangdi Neijing Ling Shu*. Translated from the French by Garbacz, E., S. 2002

Vincent, J., D., *Biologie des passions*, ed. Odile Jacob, 1986

Vincent, J., D., *La Chair et le Diable*, ed. Odile Jacob, 1996

Vincent, J., D., *Le Cœur des autres - Biologie de la compassion*, ed. Plon, 2003

Vincent-Buffault, A., *The History of Tears: Sensibility and Sentimentality in France*. Basingstoke and London: Macmillan, 1991

Watson, B., *The Complete Works of Chuang Tzu*, Columbia University Press, 1968

Wong M., *Ling Shu, traduction* et commentaires, Massons, Paris, 1987

Wieger, L., *Etymological lessons*, NY: Paragon Book Reprint corp., Dover Publications NY, 1965.

Wilhelm, R., Jung C. G., & Hug-yang Liu, *The Secret of the golden flower, a Chinese book of life*, New York: Harcourt, Brace & World, 1962.

http://www.zhongwen.com/ Web version of Chinese characters, Yale press

List of books in Chinese

CHANGYONG BIAOZHUN GUOZI JIEXI 常用标准國字解析, *Analysis of Chinese characters, Chen Shanhu, Taipei, Yuanli chubanshe,* 1983

CHANGYONG GUWENZI ZIDIAN 常用古文字字典, *Dictionary of characters of classical language, Wang Yanlin. Shanghai, Shanghai shuhua chubanshe,* 1987

DAOXUE CIDIAN 道學辭典, *Dictionary of Daoism, Dai Yuanchang, Taipei, Zheng shan mei chu ban she,* 1971

GUJIN YITONG DAQUAN 古今医统大全, *Medical Complete Book, Ancient and Modern, Chun Fu* (Ming dynasty), *Taipei, Xinwenfeng chuban gongsi*

GUWEN ZIXUE XINLUN 古文字学新論, *New treatise on study of the ancient Chinese characters, Kang Yin. Beijing. Rongbaozhai,*1983

HANYU GUWENZI ZIXINGBIAO 漢語古文字字形表, *The Writing System of Scribe Zhou: Evidence from Late Pre-imperial Chinese, Sichuan chubanshe,* 1981

HUANGDI NEIJING LINGSHU YIJIE 黃帝內經靈樞譯解, *Commentary to Nei Jing Ling Shu of the Yellow Emperor, Yang Weijie, Taipei, Mingjian shuju,* 1982

HUANGDI NEIJING SUWEN YIJIE 黃帝內經素問譯解, *Commentary to Nei Jing Su Wen of the Yellow Emperor, Yang Weijie, Taipei, Tailian guofeng chubanshe,* 1984

JINGXUE SHIYI HUIJIE 经穴释义汇解, *A Compilation of Explanations of the Meaning of the Acupuncture Points Names, Shengxing Zhang and Gan Qi, Shanghai, Shanghai fan yi chu ban gong si,* 1984

NANJING BENYI 難經本義, *Original Meaning of Nanjing, Hua Shou* (Yuan dynasty), *Taipei, Jiwen chubanshe,* 1982

SHUOWEN JIEZI 說文解字, *Explaining Graphs and Analyzing Characters, Xu Shen,* (early 2nd-century Chinese dictionary from the Han Dynasty), *Beijing: Zhonghua shuju,* 1963

WENZI YANLIU QIANSHOU 文字源流淺說, *Treatise on the origin of Chinese characters, Kang Yin, Beijing: Rong bao zhai,* 1979

WUXING DAYI 五行大義, *The Great Meaning of the Five Modalities, Xiao Ji* (Sui dynasty), *Taipei, Xinwenfeng chuban gongsi,* 1987

ZHONG YI ZHENG HOU JIAN BIE ZHEN DUAN XUE 中医证候鉴别诊断学, *A Study of Differential Diagnosis and Patterns in Chinese Medicine, Zhao Jin Ze*, Beijing, People's Health Publishing, 1987

ZHONG YI BIAN ZHENG XUE 中医辨证学, *A Study of Differential Diagnosis in Chinese Medicine, Ke Xue Fan, Shanghai, Shanghai zhong yi xue yuan chubanshe*, 1987

ZHONG YI XI TONG BIAN ZHENG XUE 中医系统辨证学, *A Study of Differential Diagnosis and Syndromes in Chinese Medicine, Lei Shunqun zhu, Hebei ke xue ji shu chu ban she*, 1987

ZHONGGUO YIXUE DACIDIAN 中國醫學大辭典, *Guan Xie. Taipei, Taiwan Shangwu Yinshu Guan*, 1958.

XI MING, ZHANG ZAI ZI (Song dynasty, 1020-1077) ZHENG MENG, TAI HE BIEN DI YI, Chapter 1

Contents

Introduction 3

1. Five Modalities (WU XING 五行) **on the Three Levels of the Universe** (Heaven, Earth and Man) 10
   A. Man, through his Heart-Consciousness (XIN 心) and Spirit (SHEN 神), is the witness to all that happens in the Universe 12
   B. Five Modalities (WU XING 五行) as the music of the Universe 16
      Wood Modality (MU 木) 17
      Fire Modality (HUO 火) 18
      Metal Modality (JIN 金) 19
      Water Modality (SHUI 水) 20
      Soil Modality (TU 土) 21
      Laws of change of Five Modalities (WU XING 五行) 22
   C. Man on the Three Levels (Heaven, Earth and Man) expressed by Five Modalities (WU XING 五行) 26
      Three Levels of Man (Heaven, Man, Earth) expressed by Five Modalities
      Upper Level (Heaven): five aspects of SHEN (BEN SHEN 本神) 27
         Fire Modality - South on the TAI JI symbol - SHEN 神 28
         Metal Modality - West on the TAI JI symbol - PO 魄 29
         Wood Modality - East on the TAI JI symbol - HUN 魂 31
         Water Modality - North on the TAI JI symbol - ZHI 志 33
         Soil Modality - Center on the TAI JI symbol - YI 意 34
      Three Levels of Man (Heaven, Man, Earth) expressed by Five Modalities
      Lower Level (Earth): five ZANG 臟 - centers of body formation 35
         Fire Modality - South on the TAI JI symbol – Heart (XIN 心) 38
         Metal Modality - West on the TAI JI symbol – Lung (FEI 肺) 41
         Wood Modality - East on the TAI JI symbol – Liver (GAN 肝) 42
         Water Modality - North on the TAI JI symbol – Kidney (SHEN 腎) . 43
         Soil Modality - Center on the TAI JI symbol – Spleen (PI 脾) 46
      Three Levels of Man (Heaven, Man, Earth) expressed by Five Modalities
      Middle Level (Man): five emotions (WU ZHI 五志) 48
         Fire Modality - South on the TAI JI symbol - joy (XI 喜) and pleasure (LE 樂) 50
         Metal Modality - West on the TAI JI symbol - sorrow (BEI 悲), sadness (YOU 憂), grief (AI 哀), melancholy (CHOU 愁) 52

Wood Modality - East on the TAI JI symbol - anger (NU 怒) 53
Water Modality - North on the TAI JI symbol - fear (KONG 恐)
and dread (JU 懼) 54
Soil Modality - Center on the TAI JI symbol – thought,
worry (SI 思) 55

2. SHEN 神, ethics and emotions 57
A. Emotions according to ZHUANG ZI 莊子, Chapter 15 57
B. Emotions according to HUAI NAN ZI 淮南子, Chapters 7 and 1 59
C. Intimate Natures (XING 性) and emotions (QING 情) according to
Fundamentals of the Five Modalities (WU XING DA YI 五行大義),
Chapter 18 62
    HUN 魂 and Intimate Natures (XING 性); PO 魄 and emotions 70
    HUN 魂 and PO 魄 according to WU XING DA YI and 'fragmentary
    autonomous psychic systems of the unconscious' by C. Jung 72

3. Emotions, QI of the Universe, lifestyle and society 76
A. Heaven and Man - QI and emotions, HUAI NAN ZI, 淮南子, Chapter 7 ... 76
B. Heaven and Man - seasons, QI and emotions, SU WEN, Chapter 5 77
C. Influence of emotions and cold on man, LING SHU, Chapter 4 78
D. Influence of emotions and life events and interaction with society,
SU WEN, Chapter 77 80
E. Influence of emotions and lifestyle on the five ZANG, NAN JING,
Chapter 49 84

4. LING SHU, Chapter 8, Roots of SHEN (BEN SHEN 本神). Life stages and development of Consciousness 89
A. *The first step in the art of acupuncture is rooting in SHEN 神,*
LING SHU, Chapter 8-1 89
B. The Yellow Emperor's questions, LING SHU, Chapter 8-1 92
C. QI BO replies. The first phase. Entities 1,2,3: DE 德, QI 氣,
life (SHENG 生). Spontaneous eruption of individualized life
guided by Heaven and Earth 95
    The first entity, DE 德 - Heaven in Man 96
    The second entity, QI 氣 - Earth in Man 97
    The third entity, life (SHENG 生) 99

D. QI BO replies. The second phase. Entities 4, 5: JING 精 and SHEN 神. Self-identity is based on impersonal support (JING 精) in space and time 100
   The fourth entity, JING 精 - fundamental vitality 101
   The fifth entity, SHEN 神 - Individual Spirit....................................... 103
E. QI BO replies. The third phase. Entities 6,7: HUN 魂, PO 魄. Putting into motion and accompaniment of SHEN 神 104
   The sixth entity, HUN 魂 104
      HUN 魂 and ethics.. 106
      HUN 魂, the first name and transmission between generations 106
      HUN 魂 and adaptation to the changing environment 106
      HUN 魂 and neurology... 107
   The seventh entity, PO 魄 107
      PO 魄, the autonomic nervous system and the hypothalamus 108
      Interactions between HUN 魂 and PO 魄.. 110
F. QI BO replies. The fourth phase. Entities 8, 9, 10: Heart-Consciousness (XIN 心), intent (YI 意), ability to realize life (ZHI 志). Consciousness gathers information to realize life.. 113
   The eighth entity, Heart-Consciousness (XIN 心)............................... 113
   The ninth entity, intent, ideas (YI 意).. 115
   The tenth entity, the ability to realize life, determination (ZHI 志) 116
      Association between YI 意 and ZHI 志 117
      YI 意 - ZHI 志 and modern theories of memory 118
      The relationship between the genome (inborn) and the environment (acquired) in Chinese and in Western philosophy..... 120
G. QI BO replies. The fifth phase. Entity 11: thought (SI 思) 123
H. QI BO replies. The sixth phase. Entities 12 and 13: LU 慮 and ZHI 智. Development of thought: contemplation and wisdom 126
      The twelfth entity, consideration, contemplation (LU 慮) 127
      The thirteenth entity, wisdom, intelligence, use of knowledge (ZHI 智).. 131
      Knowledge and intelligence in the works of Damasio 132
      Speech, storytelling and communication 135
      YI 意, images (XIANG 象) and words (YAN 言) according to WANG BI 王弼 137
I. LING SHU, Chapter 8-1, continues 145

5. Interaction between the Three Levels of Man according to LING SHU, **Chapter 8-2, and** SU WEN, Chapter 62.................. 147

   A. The influence of QI excess and QI deficiency on the functioning of the five ZANG 臟 according to LING SHU, Chapter 8-2........................ 148
      1. Liver, Blood and HUN 魂, LING SHU, Chapter 8-2 148
      2. Spleen, Nourishing QI (YING 營) and YI 意, LING SHU, Chapter 8-2.... 149
      3. Heart, conduits and blood vessels (MAI 脈) and SHEN 神, LING SHU, Chapter 8-2... 152
      4. Lung, breath (QI 氣) and PO 魄, LING SHU, Chapter 8-2................. 155
      5. Kidney, JING 精 and ZHI 志, LING SHU, Chapter 8-2 156
   B. The five vital aspects stored in the five ZANG 臟, and their pathologies expressed in the body and the mind according to SU WEN, Chapter 62 158
      1. The five vital aspects and the five ZANG 臟, SU WEN, Chapter 62..... 158
      2. YI 意 and ZHI 志, and the five ZANG 臟, SU WEN, Chapter 62 160
      3. YI 意 and ZHI 志, and the five ZANG 臟, LING SHU, Chapter 47......... 162
      4. Signs of deficiency and excess of the five vital aspects of man, SU WEN, Chapter 62 163

6. The nine fluctuations of QI flow expressed as emotions, SU WEN, Chapter 39

   1. Anger (NU 怒), SU WEN, Chapter 39 165
      Regulating QI by acupuncture in cases of anger................................ 168
   2. Joy (XI 喜), SU WEN, Chapter 39... 175
      Regulating QI by acupuncture in cases of excessive joy 178
   3. Sorrow (BEI 悲), SU WEN, Chapter 39 181
      Regulating QI by acupuncture in cases of sorrow............................. 184
   4. Fear (KONG 恐), SU WEN, Chapter 39 187
      Regulating QI by acupuncture in cases of fear................................. 189
   5. Cold (HAN 寒), SU WEN, Chapter 39... 194
   6. Heat (JIONG 炅), SU WEN, Chapter 39 196
   7. Panic (JING 驚), SU WEN, Chapter 39 197
      Regulating QI by acupuncture in cases of panic 202
   8. Exhaustion (LAO 勞), SU WEN, Chapter 39 205

9. Obsessive thinking (SI 思), SU WEN, Chapter 39 208
   YU ZHENG 鬱證 constrained (tied) QI syndrome expressed as
   depression 211
   Regulating QI by acupuncture in cases of obsessive thinking 212

7. Damage caused by six combinations of emotions, LING SHU, Chapter 8-3 215

A. Apprehension, distress, obsessive thinking, worry (CHU TI SI LU
   怵惕思慮) damage SHEN, cause fear and dread (KONG JU 懼恐)
   and the anchor of life (JING 精) is lost, LING SHU, Chapter 8-3 216
   Syndromes in Chinese medicine which describe situations similar
   to the damage to SHEN 神 and JING 精 caused by apprehension,
   distress, obsessive thinking, wory 219
   1. *Deficient Kidney JING*, SHEN JING BU ZU 腎精不足 220
   2. *Dual QI and Blood Deficiency*, QI XUE LIANG XU 氣血兩虛 221
   3. *Liver and Gallbladder QI Deficiency*, GAN DAN QI XU 肝膽氣虛 222

B. The *loss of life* in sorrow and grief (BEI AI 悲哀), LING SHU,
   Chapter 8-3 223
   Syndromes in Chinese medicine which describe situations similar
   to the *loss of life* caused by sorrow and grief 229
   1. *Heart and Lung QI Deficiency*, XIN FEI QI XU 心肺氣虛 229
   2. *Liver Fire Assailing the Lung*, GAN HUO FAN FEI 肝火犯肺 230
   3. *Heart Deficiency and Lung Heat*, XIN XU FEI RE 心虛肺熱 231

C. Storage is lost in joy and pleasure (XI LE 喜樂), LING SHU,
   Chapter 8-3 232
   Syndromes in Chinese medicine which describe damage caused
   by joy and pleasure with euphoria and laughter for no reason 234
   1. *Heart Fire Hyperactivity and Exuberance*,
      XIN HUO KANG SHENG 心火亢盛 234
   2. *Heart and Liver Fire Effulgence*, XIN GAN HUO WANG 心肝火旺 ... 235
   3. *No Interaction between Heart and Kidney*, XIN SHEN BU JIAO
      心腎不交 236
   4. *Phlegm Fire Harassing Heart*, TAN HUO RAO XIN 痰火擾心 237

D. Melancholy and sadness (CHOU YOU 愁憂) disrupt QI flow,
   LING SHU, Chapter 8-3 238
   Syndromes in Chinese medicine which describe obstructions caused
   by melancholy and saness 241
   1. *Lung and Spleen QI Deficiency* FEI PI QI XU 肺脾氣虛 242
   2. *Heart and Spleen Dual Deficiency* XIN PI LIANG XU 心脾兩虛 244
   3. *No Interaction between Liver and Spleen* GAN PI BU JIAO 肝脾不交 ... 245
   4. Lily Bulb Disease BAI HE BING 百合病 246
      a. *Lung and Heart* YIN *Deficiency* XIN FEI YIN XU 心肺陰虛 246
      b. *Phlegm-heat or Phlegm-fire* TAN RE/TAN HUO 痰熱/痰火 247
      c. *Liver* YIN *Deficiency* GAN YIN XU 肝陰虛 248
      d. *Heart and Lung QI Deficiency* XIN FEI QI XU 心肺氣虛 249
      e. *Lung and Kidney* YIN *Deficiency* FEI SHEN YIN XU 肺腎陰虛 250
      f. *No Interaction between Heart and Kidney* XIN SHEN BU JIAO
         心腎不交 251
      g. *Loss of Interaction between* YIN *and* YANG, YIN YANG SHI JIAO
         陰陽失交 252

E. Organization and control are lost in overflowing anger
   (SHENG NU 盛怒), LING SHU, Chapter 8-3 253
   Overflowing anger separates QI and Blood 255
   Overflowing anger and wind 257
   Overflowing anger and QI of war 259
   Syndromes in Chinese medicine which describe the loss of
   organization and control caused by overflowing anger 259
   1. *Liver QI Congested and Knotted,* GAN QI YU JIE 肝氣鬱結 261
   2. *Congested QI Transforms into Fire,* QI YU HUA HUO 氣鬱化火 261
   3. *Liver and Gallbladder Fire Flaring Upwards,*
      GAN DAN HUO SHANG YAN 肝膽火上炎 262
   4. *Dual Liver Blood and Kidney* YIN *Deficiency,*
      GAN XUE SHEN YIN LIANG XU 血腎陰兩虛 263
   5. *Loss and Deficiency of Liver* YIN, GAN YIN KUI XU 肝陰虧虛 264
   6. *Confusion of the Heart and* SHEN, XIN SHEN HUO LUAN 心神惑亂 265

F. Ability of being oneself is lost in fear and dread (KONG JU 懼恐),
   LING SHU, Chapter 8-3 266
   Types of fear 268
   Action without action as a treatment for fear according to
   ZHUANG ZI 271
   Art of Nourishing Life (YANG SHENG 養生) as the treatment for fear
   according to LAO ZI 272
   Syndromes in Chinese medicine which describe the loss of ability to
   be oneself caused by fear and dread 274
   1. *Blood YIN Deficiency*, XUE YIN XU 血陰虛 274
   2. *Heart and Gallbladder QI Deficiency*, XIN DAN QI XU 心膽氣虛 275
   3. *Phlegm Fire Harassing the Heart*, TAN HUO RAO XIN 痰火擾心 276
   4. *Heart Fire Hyperactivity and Exuberance*,
      XIN HUO KANG SHENG 心火亢盛 277
   5. *Blood Deficiency and Liver QI Congested and Knotted*
      XUE XU GAN QI YU JIE 血虛肝氣鬱結 278

8. Damage caused by six combinations of persistent emotions, LING SHU, Chapter 8-4 279

A. Damage to Heart, SHEN 神 and flesh caused by apprehension,
   distress, obsessive thinking and worry (CHU TI SI LU 怵惕思慮),
   LING SHU, Chapter 8-4 280
   Syndromes in Chinese medicine which describe the damage to
   Heart, SHEN and flesh caused by apprehension, distress, obsessive
   thinking and worry 282
   1. *Heart and Spleen Dual Deficiency* XIN PI LIANG XU 心脾兩虛 282
   2. *Phlegm-dampness and QI Deficiency* TAN SHI QI XU 痰濕氣虛 283
   3. *No Interaction between Heart and Kidney*
      XIN SHEN BU JIAO 心腎不交 284
B. Damage to Spleen, YI 意 and limbs caused by melancholy and
   sadness (CHOU YOU 愁憂), LING SHU, Chapter 8-4 286
   Syndromes in Chinese medicine which describe the injury to
   Spleen and YI 意 caused by melancholy and sadness 288
   Constrained QI syndrome (YU ZHENG 鬱證) expressed as
   depression, which describes injury to Spleen and YI 意 caused
   by melancholy and sadness 290

a. *Liver* QI *Congested and Knotted,* GAN QI YU JIE 肝氣鬱結 291
   b. *Congested* QI *Transforms into Fire,* QI YU HUA HUO 氣鬱化火 292
   c. *Phlegm and* QI *Congested and Knotted,* TAN QI YU JIE 痰氣鬱結 293
   d. *Loss and Deficiency of Heart* YIN, XIN YIN KUI XU 心陰虧虛 294
   e. *Loss and deficiency of Liver* YIN, GAN YIN KUI XU 肝陰虧虛 294
   f. *Blood Flow Congested and Obstructed,* XUE XING YU ZHI
      血行鬱滯 295
   g. *Heart and Spleen Dual Deficiency,* XIN PI LIANG XU 心脾兩虛 296
   h. *Confusion of the Heart and* SHEN, XIN PI LIANG XU 心脾兩虛 297
C. Damage to Liver, HUN 魂 and JING 精 caused by sorrow and grief
   (BEI AI 悲哀), LING SHU, Chapter 8-4 298
   Syndromes in Chinese medicine which describe the damage to Liver,
   HUN 魂 and JING 精 caused by sorrow and grief 302
   1. *Injury to* JUE YIN 厥陰 305
   2. *Agitated insanity,* KUANG 狂 306
   2a. *Congested* QI *Transforms into Fire,* QI YU HUA HUO 氣鬱化火 306
   2b. *Phlegm-fire Harasses the Upper Body,* TAN HUO SHANG RAO
       痰火上擾 307
   2c. *Excess Fire in* YANG MING, YANG MING HUO SHENG 陽明火盛 308
   2d. *Blood Flow Congested and Obstructed,* XUE XING YU ZHI
       血行鬱滯 309
   2e. YIN *Deficiency and Fire Effulgence* YIN XU HUO WANG 陰虛火旺 ... 310
   3. *Restless* ZANG *organ,* ZANG ZAO 臟躁 311
   3a. *Liver* QI *Congested and Knotted,* GAN QI YU JIE 肝氣鬱結 311
   3b. *Phlegm-fire,* TAN HUO 痰火 312
   3c. *Loss and Deficiency of Heart* YIN, XIN YIN KUI XU 心陰虧虛 313
   3d. *Heart and Spleen Dual Deficiency,* XIN PI LIANG XU 心脾兩虛 314
   4. Plum pit QI syndrome, MEI HE QI 梅核氣 314
   4a. YIN *Deficiency and Liver* QI *Congested and Knotted,*
       YIN XU GAN QI YU JIE 陰虛肝氣鬱結 315
   4b. *Liver* QI *Congested and Knotted,* GAN QI YU JIE 肝氣鬱結 316
   4c. *Lung and Kidney* YIN *Deficiency and Phlegm-Fire Harasses
       the Upper Body,* FEI SHEN YIN XU TAN HUO SHANG RAO
       肺腎陰虛痰火上擾 317

D. Damage to Lung, PO 魄 and sanity caused by excessive joy and pleasure (XI LE 喜樂), LING SHU, Chapter 8-4 318
  Syndromes in Chinese medicine which describe the damage to Lung and PO 魄 caused by excessive joy and pleasure 320
  Treatment of skin diseases (eczema, psoriasis) 321

E. Damage to Kidney, ZHI 志 and back caused by uncontrollable overflowing anger (SHENG NU 盛怒), LING SHU, Chapter 8-4 322
  Syndromes in Chinese medicine which describe the damage to Kidney and ZHI 志 caused by overflowing anger, LING SHU, Chapter 8-4 328
  1. Confused Speech 329
  1a. *YIN Deficiency and Blood Dryness*, YIN XU XUE ZAO 陰虛血燥 330
  1b. *Liver QI Congested and Knotted*, GAN QI YU JIE 肝氣鬱結 331
  1c. *Phlegm-fire*, TAN HUO 痰火 332
  1d. *Blood Flow Congested and Obstructed*, XUE XING YU ZHI 血行鬱滯 332
  1f. *Heart and Spleen Dual Deficiency*, XIN PI LIANG XU 心脾兩虛 334
  2. 'Overflowing anger in Kidney' and modern psychiatry 335
  2a. Personal space invasion 335
  2b. Adolescent identity crisis 336
  2c. Schizophrenia 338
    ▪ Schizophrenia - outbreak YIN 339
    ▪ Schizophrenia - outbreak YANG 340
  2d. Uncontrollable overflowing anger in epilepsy, XIAN 癇 341
    ▪ *Liver Fire and Phlegm-heat*, GAN HUO TAN RE 肝火痰熱 340
    ▪ *YIN Deficiency and YANG Excess*, YIN XU YANG SHENG 陰虛陽盛 342
    ▪ *Blood flow Congested and Obstructed*, XUE XING YU ZHI 血行鬱滯 343

F. Damage to Kidney, JING 精 and bones caused by fear and dread (KONG JU 恐懼), LING SHU, Chapter 8-4 345

9. LING SHU, **Chapter 22,** DIAN KUANG BING 癲狂病, **madness and insanity** 352

  1. Eye examination (SHEN 神 is reflected in the eyes), LING SHU, Chapter 22-1 355

2. Treatment of the DIAN 癲 disease - quiet (YIN) body-mind-spirit disorders 358
   A. First signs of the onset of DIAN 癲 disease, LING SHU, Chapter 22-2 360
   B. Onset of DIAN 癲 disease together with restlessness and face muscle contractions, LING SHU, Chapter 22-3 363
   C. Onset of DIAN 癲 disease together with muscle rigidity and backache, LING SHU, Chapter 22-4 366
   D. Observation of blood coagulation in crisis of DIAN 癲 disease with signs of excess, LING SHU, Chapter 22-5 368
   E. GU DIAN 骨癲, disease in bones together with depression and loss of body liquids, LING SHU, Chapter 22-6 370
   F. JIN DIAN 癲筋, disease in tendons and muscles together with loss of body liquids, LING SHU, Chapter 22-7 373
   G. MAI DIAN 癲脈, disease in MAI - blood vessels, channels (meridians) and nervous system, LING SHU, Chapter 22-8 375
      1. *Wind in the Center* (ZHONG FENG 中風) 376
      2. *Wind Epilepsy* (FENG XIAN 風癇) 377
      3. *'Tightening'* (obstruction) *of Belt Meridian* (DAI MAI 帶脈) 377
   H. DIAN 癲 disease develops into KUANG 狂 disease, LING SHU, Chapter 22-9 378
3. Treatments of KUANG 狂 disease, agitated (YANG) body-mind-spirit disorders 378
   I. Onset of KUANG 狂 disease: sorrow, stress and hunger, memory loss, anger and fear, LING SHU, Chapter 22-10 379
   J. KUANG 狂 disease onset develops into a manic episode accompanied by insomnia, loss of appetite, excessive self-esteem, agitation and cursing, LING SHU, Chapter 22-11 382
      1. *Phlegm-fire Harasses the Upper Body*, TAN HUO SHANG RAO 痰火上擾 384
      2. *Excess Fire in YANG MING*, YANG MING HUO SHENG 陽明火盛 384
   K. KUANG 狂 disease caused by fear, accompanied by agitation and euphoria, LING SHU, Chapter 22-12 385
      No Interaction between Heart and Kidney, XIN SHEN BU JIAO 心腎不交 387

- L. KUANG 狂 disease caused by QI deficiency, accompanied by screaming and visual and auditory hallucinations, LING SHU, Chapter 22-13 388
- M. KUANG 狂 disease, caused by excessive joy, with bulimia and seeing ghosts, LING SHU, Chapter 22-14 390
  1. *Liver and Gallbladder Fire Flaring Upwards*, GAN DAN HUO SHANG YAN 肝膽火上炎 392
  2. *Blood Flow Congested and Obstructed*, XUE XING YU ZHI 血行鬱滯 393
  3. *Confusion of Heart and* SHEN, XIN SHEN HUO LUAN 心神惑紀 393
- N. KUANG 狂 disease - acute psychotic episode, LING SHU, Chapter 22-15 395

4. Treatments of rebel QI (NI 逆) which provokes QI congestion and obstruction 396
   - O. Congestion of cold and edema of limbs caused by invasion of rebel wind (FENG NI 風逆), LING SHU, Chapter 22-16 397
   - P. Sudden internal cold caused by rebel QI (JUE NI 厥逆) in Kidney Meridian, LING SHU, Chapter 22-17 401
   - Q. Congestion in trunk caused by rebel QI (JUE NI 厥逆), LING SHU, Chapter 22-18 405
   - R. Lower JIAO obstruction and urinary retention caused by rebel afflux, LING SHU, Chapter 22-19 407
   - S. Liver rebel QI (QI NI 氣逆) invades Spleen, LING SHU, Chapter 22-20 409
   - T. Obstructions of QI flow in SHAO YIN 少陰 (Source QI) and YANG MING 陽明 (postnatal QI) in severe diseases, LING SHU, Chapter 22-21 411
   - U. Two types of Kidney JING 精 deficiency, LING SHU, Chapter 22-22 413

Conclusion 418
Glossary according to subject 422
Acupuncture points proposed here to treat emotional disorders 433
Bibliography 438

www.ingramcontent.com/pod-product-compliance
Lightning Source LLC
Chambersburg PA
CBHW031603210526
45464CB00004B/1407